£65 -

ANGLO-NORMAN MEDICINE

VOLUME II

SHORTER TREATISES

ANGLO-NORMAN MEDICINE

BY

Tony Hunt

Fellow of St Peter's College, Oxford

VOLUME II
SHORTER TREATISES

D. S. BREWER

First published 1997
D. S. Brewer, Cambridge

ISBN 0 85991 523 9

D. S. Brewer is an imprint of Boydell & Brewer Ltd
PO Box 9, Woodbridge, Suffolk IP12 3DF, UK
and of Boydell & Brewer Inc.
PO Box 41026, Rochester, NY 14604–4126, USA

A catalogue record for this book is available
from the British Library

Library of Congress Cataloging-in-Publication Data
card number 94–14486

This publication is printed on acid-free paper

Printed in Great Britain by
St Edmundsbury Press Ltd, Bury St Edmunds, Suffolk

CONTENTS

PREFACE

A recent volume entitled *Manuscript Sources of Medieval Medicine: A Book of Essays*, ed. Margaret R. Schleissner (New York / London, 1995), contains not a single contribution on Anglo-Norman or continental French. This fortifies my resolve to promote French-language medical texts and to secure for them the sort of long-term familiarity enjoyed by at least some Middle English medical works.

In Volume Two of *Anglo-Norman Medicine* I complete my edition of the vernacular medical texts contained in MS Cambridge, Trinity College 0.1.20 by presenting a treatise on visiting the sick (Chapter One) and a translation of the first part of the celebrated gynaecological compilation known as 'Trotula' (Chapter Two). To these I add the two most extensive medical compendia employing French to have survived in this country, the *Euperiston* (Chapter Three) and the Trinity 'Practica' (Chapter Four). It is unlikely that this exhausts the existing material: indeed, the large collection of medical receipts mixing Latin, French and English found in MS Cambridge, Corpus Christi College 388 is already reserved for a future publication. The insular character of this and the two compendia edited here is not in contention, but, as briefly indicated in the Preface to Volume One of *Anglo-Norman Medicine*, lexical features of the Trinity translations nourish doubts about their origin, however clear it may be that they were copied in England. In my Introduction I have therefore chosen to amplify somewhat discussion of the problems posed by the lexical evidence.

The works edited in *Anglo-Norman Medicine* represent a considerable investment of time and energy by compilers, translators and copyists. It has been a pleasure to build on their efforts at disseminating the experiences and insights of the medical profession, our dependence on whom is equalled only by our scepticism. There is much that has stood the test of time. At the moment of writing much publicity has been given to a report on the anti-depressive properties of St John's Wort (Hypericum perforatum) and considerable attention concentrated on the value of the anti-clotting agent in the saliva of the medicinal leech for the treatment of cardio-vascular cases. The world contains all that is needed to sustain life, yet we continue to destroy it and invent expensive remedies. Those world populations which have not been cured to death still have much to tell us about the skills of our ancestors. We cannot afford to ignore them.

Medieval Studies are already enormously and continuously in debt to Dr Richard Barber. He has also a strong family interest in medicine. It seems right, therefore, that I should repay the faith he has shown in the project by dedicating *Anglo-Norman Medicine* to him.

INTRODUCTION

At the bottom of the page below the chapter 'De fistula et cancro' in a copy of Ricardus Anglicus's *Micrologus*[1] in MS Oxford, Balliol College 231 (late thirteenth century) has been inserted the following in a contemporary hand:

> [f.61v] + In nomine Patris + et Filii + et Spiritus Sancti, Amen + Jeo cray ben en nostre Seynur Jhesu Crit que jeo ceste home .N. puisse ayder de verme e de rauncle e de kaunker e de felun e gutefestre e de tuz maus + In nomine Patris + et Filii + et Spiritus Sancti, Amen + Seinte Susanne fu a tort criminé, [la] dilivera nostre Seynur. Jesu, si verraiment cum vus deliverastes seinte Susanne de perile, issi deliverez cest homme .N. de verme, de rauncle e de kauncre e de felun e de gutefestre e de tuz maus + In nomine Patris + et Filii + et Spiritus Sancti, Amen + Pater Noster et Credo in Deum. Iceste charme deyt trey fez estre dite outre le malade e a checun feyz un Pater Noster e un Cre[do] [f.62r] e trays jours .iii. fez e en num e aprés + Christus vincit, Christus regnat, Christus imperat. Christus te .N. ab isto malo et ab omnibus malis liberet et defendet, Amen + In nomine Patris + et Filii + et Spiritus Sancti, Amen + Devaunt ice ke acune charme seit fete, si deit l'em fere chaunter trays messes de Seinte Esprit.[2]

Three things immediately strike us. A reader of the Latin text has felt moved to supplement it in the vernacular in an operation now referred to as code-switching. The supplement is drawn from the realm of religious faith rather than from that of scientific medicine. The element of faith represented by the charm is expressed through ritual repetition. This juxtaposition of contrasts is entirely characteristic of medieval medicine in the Anglo-Norman period. Indeed, all students of medicine in medieval England are quickly obliged to confront the problem of multilingual documents and, more specifically, the phenomena of code-switching and code-mixing. Even those manuscripts which transmit extensive treatises in Latin, if they are at all used, reveal the influential presence of the vernacular and of popular medical beliefs of a non-scientific nature, some of which go back to very early authorities. Many manuscripts prove to be valuable repositories of rare words and lexical treasures and deserve a study to themselves. Others are significant for revealing patterns of transmission, where certain texts, as we shall see, come to be grouped together forming textual constellations which are readily recognizable. Frequently, too, the manuscripts display another feature of medical texts which should not be overlooked, namely their extraordinary elasticity. Thus copies of ostensibly the same treatise differ considerably in the extent of the material, some versions offering highly condensed texts, others

---

[1] Cf. K. Sudhoff, "Richard der Engländer", *Janus* 28 (1924), 397–403 and *id.*, "Der *Micrologus*-Text der *Anatomia* Richards des Engländers", *Archiv für Geschichte der Medizin* 19 (1927), 209–39 (repr. 1965).

[2] Cf. Hunt, *Pop. Med.*, p.89 no.32.

embodying a striking degree of amplification. The purpose of the present Introduction is to illustrate these observations through the example of a single work, the compendium known as the *Speculum medicorum*.

The manuscript transmission of this work involves the unusual case of an apograph. The medical texts constituting MS Oxford, Bodleian Library, e musaeo 219 (SC 3541) of the late thirteenth century are repeated, with every vernacular item (English and French) and gloss intact, in MS Oxford, Merton College 324, which was copied over 150 years later. A survey of the contents of these two manuscripts will provide an idea of the staple medical works over a number of centuries, furnishing evidence of the inseparability of *materia medica* from vernacular names, and providing a context for the *Speculum medicorum*. Folio references in square brackets indicate the Merton MS, which is more complete.

1. [f.1r–2r] acephalous collection of medical excerpts beginning 'Galienus de sobrie-tate' (inc. 'Sobrietas memoriam servat, sensum acuit') and including [f.1v] 'De ponderibus et mensuris' (inc. 'Siclus et stater et tenarius') (ThK 1479).[3]

2. [ff.2r–94r] *Speculum medicorum*, a medical compendium arranged topically and attributed to Asclepius, 'Incipiunt capitula in librum sequentem qui dicitur Speculum medicorum', a list of chapters up to and including 'Qualiter cauteria debeantur fieri. . .' on f.94r (e mus. 219 f.84r). The rest of the contents of the MS, up to and including 'Liber de practica equorum . . .' on ff.187v–189v, are listed on f.3r 'Preter predictum librum hii libri sequentes in hoc volumine continentur'. The *Speculum* proper begins on f.3r 'Incipit prologus in librum Asclepii qui dicitur Speculum medicorum', inc. 'Ne tibi displiceat quod sic sum corpori parvus . . . Cum animadverterem quamplurimos medicorum non solum minores verum etiam qui doctores videbantur . . .' (ThK 907 & 282) and 'De universalibus et particularibus capitis egritudinibus, complexionibus et curis tam interioribus quam exterioribus' (including [f.14r] 'Experiencia parisii abbatis de dolore capitis').

The *Speculum* is acephalous in MS Bodl. e mus. 219 which begins at f.38r (med.fol.) [f.44r] with a red rubric halfway down the page 'De effectu catapuciorum et modo sumendi . . . 'De vomitu' [f.44v]. The text contains charms against mice, flies etc (f.65v) [f.73v]. There is a variety of vernacular annotation. Sometimes a whole receipt has been added, as at the bottom of f.54v (in hand of the text) [f.60v]:

> Pur ydropesie freide e chaude mellee: Pernez les racines de fenoil e de persil ana e la meité tant de raiz e les debresez en un morter. Puis le quisez en cerveise estale e le bever [M bevez] a mangir e devant e aprés e quel hore ke vus vodriez.

The annotation may be confined to a gloss, as on f.70*r [f.79v] in a receipt 'ad guttam vel pleuresim' where the words 'codenam baconis' are accompanied by an interlinear gloss .i. *coane*. Vernacular words also appear in the text:[4] f.61v 'faverolam .i. *lemeke*';

---

3   References marked 'ThK' are to L. Thorndike and P. Kibre, *A Catalogue of Incipits of Mediaeval Scientific Writings in Latin* 2nd ed. (Cambr., Mass., 1963). In the present case note also MS Dublin, Trinity College 517, ff.22v–23v.

4   I give only the folio references for the Bodleian MS, but the entries all occur in the Merton MS too.

f.63v 'tapsiam barbastam .i. *moleygne*', 'ameroscam .i. *amerose* /.i. *maghere*/', 'ficus qui foris apparet et dicitur *fi od broches* gallice', 'ficus cum aculeis . . . .i. *broches*'; f.65r 'solsequie jus .i. *golde*'; f.67r 'linguam canis quam rustici vocant *bage* et aquileam .i. *pukenedle*', 'cimas ligni qui vocatur *gazre*'; f.70r 'aree (sic) .i. *hove*', 'resta bovis .i. *matefelon*'; f.70v 'brionie .i. *wilde nep*', 'morum .i. *chikenemete*', 'yrisillicum, *flambe* vel *gladene*'; f.71r 'accipe pisces qui vocantur *roches*'; f.74r 'attramentum et scrotulam que vocatur *waghet*'[5]; f.75r 'alleluiam .i. *surele dé boys* .i. *wdesure*'; f.78v 'corticem interiorem de succo .i. anglice *eldre*'; f.79r 'accipe herbam que bugla vocatur et saniculam et similam quod anglice vocant *smerewort*'; f.79v 'accipe radicem cuiusdam herbe que dicitur *medewrt*', '*wdesure*'; f.80v 'rasura alluti .i. *de cordewan*'. In addition we find latinized forms of vernacular terms: f.77v 'coldram teneram tunde'; f.80r '*saieterolam*'.

Apparently incorporated in to the *Speculum* are a number of familiar items:

On f.80v [f.88v] there are 12 verses, inc. 'Hec olus urtica tribulus canabs tanasita' (Walther, *Initia* 7565).

On f.81r/v [f.89r/v] 'De signis mortiferis secundum Galienum', inc. 'Hiis signis moriens certis cognoscitur eger' (Walther 8211, ThK 629)[6] and 'Item de signis mortiferis: frons rubet, supercilia declinantur, oculus sinister minuitur' (and other rubrics).

On ff.81v–83r [ff.89v–91r] *Capsula eburnea*[7] 'Incipiunt secreta Ypocratis in pronosticum vite vel mortis', inc. 'Peritissimus omnium rerum ex domestica sapientia . . .', 'Explicit liber Ypocratis qui inventus fuit in sepulcro eius sub capite illius in pixide eburnea'. The first section consists of signs topically arranged.

On f.83v [f.91r/v] Galen's *De signis mortis et vitae*, 'Pronostica .G. dierum timendorum in inceptione omnium egritudinum', inc. 'Quisquis in die prima uniuscuiusque mensis in infirmitate deciderit' (ThK 1250).

Further miscellaneous excerpts and entries including f.84r [f.91v] *De ranculo*, followed (f.84v) [f.92r] by *Carmen pro rancula* and f.85r [f.92r/v] *De ossibus fractis* (inc. 'Racio medendi ossa fracta hec est').

3. ff.87Av, 88r–105r [ff.94r, 98r–113r] *Trotula*, 'Incipiunt capitula in librum Trotule de egritudinibus mulierum'. A list of 39 chapters interrupts the table of contents of pseudo-Cleopatra, *Gynaecia* which begins on the same folio with the rubric 'Incipit prologus in librum Trotule de infirmitatibus mulierum et earum curis' (the complete text ends on f.87Dr 'Explicit'). The *Trotula* texts represent what Monica Green calls the 'traditional ensemble',[8] rearranged topically with new material added. On f.88r [f.98r] is the red rubric 'Incipit prologus in librum trotule de morbis mulierum et curis'.

---

5 This is an early attestation of a difficult word (see *OED* sub *watchet*) and deserves to be quoted in its full context: 'Ad cancrum et ad fistulam: accipe nigras fabas, farinam siliginis, attramentum et scrotulam de panno qui vocatur *waghet*, ana combure et pulverem cum penna in foramen loci pacientis insuffla et permitte sic per .ii. vel per .iii. dies. Signum curacionis est: si foramen siccum inventum fuerit'.

6 See T. Hunt, *Popular Medicine in Thirteenth-Century England* (Cambridge, 1990), pp.102, 371 (n.96).

7 P. Kibre, *Hippocrates latinus* (New York, 1985), p.114.

8 See below ch.2.

On f.90v we read 'accipe urticam maiorem que dicitur *culrage*' and on f.92v 'succus rapistri' is glossed by English *kedelot* (error for *kerloc*).

4. ff.87Dr–87Ev [ff.96v–98r] a uroscopy under the title 'Magister Walter Agulon de retencione menstruorum', inc. 'Regula urina alba in colore tenuis in substantia' (ThK 1346), which is restarted on f.87Dv [f.97r], with further rubrics f.87Er [f.97v] 'De fluxu nimio menstruorum' (inc. 'Regula urina nigra in colore spissa in substantia'), f.87Ev [f.98r] 'De urina alba livente significante precipitationem matricis' (inc. 'Regula urina alba in colore spissa in substantia').

5. ff.105r–10r [ff.113r–117v] Constantine the African, *De coitu*, 'Incipiunt capitula in librum magistri Alexandri de coitu', f.105v [f.113v] 'Incipit liber Alexandri de coitu et eius effectu', inc. 'Creator volens omne genus firmiter ac stabiliter permanere' (ThK 273).

At the end of *De coitu* there is keyed to the bottom of the page a text which employs cipher[9] (found elsewhere in the MS). 'Experimentum quo scire potes an aliqua debeat esse tibi bmkcb vel non. N. je vus par Deu e par Damnedeu ke fist cel e tere ke si tu deyves .mb.bmkf estre, sur ta teste met ta mbkn destre, si tu ne deives .mb.bmkf estre, sur ta teste met ta mbkn [Merton mkkn] sfnfstrf et post dic tfr Pater Noster et sic reverta [Merton: peverta] tfr vel qubcfr donec videris quod alterum fecerit, sed vide quod videris gestum eius et quod dixeris ea non audiente'. This relates to the last entry of *De coitu*, which is a charm 'Ad habendam .N.', that is for possessing a woman.

6. ff.110r–113v [ff.117v–120v] 'Incipiunt capitula in librum fleubothomie', 'Incipit liber de fleobotomia. Primo de qualitate sanguinis', f.110v inc. 'Sanguis alius est naturalis, alius non naturalis' (ThK 1374).

7. ff.113v–116v [ff.120v–123v] 'Incipiunt capitula magistri Walteri Aguluni de urinis', f.114r [f.121r] 'Incipit liber de coloribus et qualitatibus urinarum et de contentis' (incl. verses, Walther *Initia* 3465), f.115v [f.122v] 'Incipit liber m[agistri] W[alteri] Aguluni de contentis urinarum'.

8. ff.116v–122v [ff.123v–128v] 'Incipiunt capitula in librum m[agistri] R[icardi] Salern[itani] de urinis et febribus', f.117r [f.123v] 'Incipit liber magistri Ricardi Salernie medici de hiis que sunt consideranda in omnibus urinis', inc. 'Qui cupit urinas mea per compendia scire' (ThK 1205).

9. ff.122v–124r [ff.128v–129v] 'Incipit liber de urinis secundum magistrum Alexandrum', inc. 'Igitur a multis philosophorum describitur . . .' (ThK 656).

10. A fragment ff.123Br–v (half leaf) [f.129v], Hippocrates, *Epistola ad Maecenatem* (ThK 817)[10] 'Incipit liber Ypocratis de complexionibus, urinis et morbis et medicinis et de sanitate conservanda regi mecenati missus', inc. 'Libellum quem rogasti mihi tibi promisi'.

---

[9] See for a series of examples MS Oxford, Bodl. Digby 69 f.195v where cipher is used in receipts and experimenta as part of the indication and for names of herbs; similarly on f.201r.
[10] Kibre, *Hipp. lat.*, p.151.

11. ff.124r–127r [ff.129v–132r] *Experimenta Ypocratis* 'Incipit Liber Ypocratis', inc. 'Sicut sunt quatuor tempora anni' (ThK 1498).[11]

12. ff.127r–129r [ff.132r–134r] 'Incipit Liber Ypocratis de urinis', inc. 'Corpus humanum patitur cotidie duo detrimenta' (ThK 269).[12]

13. ff.129v–131v [ff.134r–136r] 'Incipit prologus in librum de pulsibus', inc. 'Qua te devotione teneam mi Johannes qua diligentia complectar' (ThK 1155).

14. ff.132r–133r [136r–137v] 'Incipiunt experimenta Cophonis de febribus', inc. 'Quoniam humanum corpus ex quatuor humoribus constituitur' (ThK 1277).

15. ff.133r–138r [ff.137v–142r] 'Incipiunt experimenta parisii abbatis de febribus', inc. 'Sciendum est quod ex nimia ciborum comestione' (ThK 1393).[13]

16. ff.138v–139r [f.141v–142v] 'Liber de virtute aquile', inc. 'Secretissimum regis cateni persarum de virtute aquile. Est enim aquila rex omnium avium' (ThK 1416/508),[14] f.139r [f.142v] 'Explicit iste tractatus a magistro Willelmo anglico de lingua arabica in latinum translatus'.

17. ff.139r–141r [ff.142v–144r] 'Incipit liber de virtutibus bestiarum', inc. 'Regi egipciorum Octoviano Augusto salutem' (ThK 1343/1360).

18. ff.141r–145r [ff.144r–150v] 'Incipiunt questiones naturales arti phisice competentes', inc. 'De complexionibus: Omnia corpora ex quatuor elementis composita' (ThK 989).

19. ff.145v–149r [ff.150v–154r] 'Incipit liber anathomie', inc. 'Constituencia corporis humani tria sunt .s. humores, spiritus et menbra' (ThK 258/614), f.147r [f.152r] inc. 'Incipit pars quedam libri magistri Ricardi Salernie de anathomia'.

20. ff.149v–176r [ff.154v–180v] Gerard of Cremona's *Summa de modo medendi*, 'Incipiunt capitula in summam magistri Geraldi', f.150r [f.155r] 'Incipit summa magistri Geraldi de modo tractandi', inc. 'Cum omnis scientia ex fine et utilitate sua naturaliter sint appetenda' (ThK 327), f.176r [f.180v] 'Explicit summa magistri Geraldi'.

21. ff.176r–183v [ff.180v–187v] 'Incipit prologus in librum de virtute simplicis', [f.180v] 'Incipiunt capitula libri de virtute simplicis medicine', f.176v [f.181r] 'Incipit liber de virtute simplicis medicine', inc. 'Cogitanti mihi de simplicium medicinarum virtutibus' (ThK 229), f.183v 'Explicit liber de virtute simplicis medicine magistri Geraldi medici'.

22. ff.184r–185v [ff.187v–189v] 'Incipit de practica equorum et aliorum animalium

---

[11] Kibre, *ibid.*, p.165.
[12] Kibre, *ibid.*, p.230.
[13] The details given are inaccurate.
[14] See S.E. Sheldon, "The Eagle: Bird of Magic and Medicine in a Middle English Translation of the *Kyranides*", *Tulane Studies in English* 22 (1977), 1–31. Sheldon refers to the Bodley and Merton copies on pp.18–19, whilst declaring that she has not seen them.

et avium' (ThK 1277), inc. 'Quoniam humana jocunditas in equorum incolumitate plurimum delectetur'. On f.185v [f.189v] we read 'cimas caprifolii .i. *wdebinde*'.

23. ff.186r–188r [ff.189v–191v] various 'experimenta', inc. 'Experimenta pro furtis: si vis scire quis ille sit qui res tuas furatus sit . . .'

The Merton MS continues with

[ff.192r–220v] Macer *de viribus herbarum*[15] [f.192v inc. 'Herbarum quasdam dicturus carmine virtutes'] preceded by a list in two columns of plant names, some with vernacular equivalents, [f.192r] 'Quere has herbas in margine presentis libri'.

[ff.220v–229v] Marbod's Lapidary,[16] ending 'Explicit Liber Marbodi de lapidibus habens versus septingentos .xxx.'

[ff.229v–234r] Miscellaneous 'experimenta', inc. 'Ad dissolvendum fleumaticos humores'.

Although the *Speculum medicorum* has never been studied, a number of other copies are recorded. For example, there is one in the library of St Mark's, Venice[17] and in the Stadsbibliotheek, Brugge.[18] The 'Speculum medicinae' in the Laurenziana, Florence, contains only the opening of the work (incl. *De dolore capitis*),[19] but there is a full text in Prague MS XIV.H.28 [2673] (s.xiii) ff.27r–50r.[20] Particularly notable for its early date is the text in MS Oxford, Bodl. Libr. Rawlinson C 235 ff.9r–31v which was copied shortly before 1200. The opening rubric in green, red and blue reads *Incipit comentum in libro qui vocatur speculus* [sic]. Twelve lines of verse inc. 'Ne tibi displiceat . . .' are concluded with a rubric in red and blue *Explicit comentum*. There follows (f.9v) the prose preface 'Cum animadverterem . . .', which sanctions the title, 'Speculum medicine' and twice refers to 'Paulus' as an authority.[21] It concludes with a red rubric *Explicit prefatio* (f.10r). The text ends incomplete with 'cataplasma ad sciaticos' (f.31v). This is a remarkably early and neat copy of a work which was to go on being copied for at least another two and a half centuries.

For our purposes, though, it is the subsequent insular copies which are of interest, particularly for their inclusion of vernacular material. I noted just two vernacular entries in the fourteenth-century copy in MS London, Wellcome Historical Medical

---

15 *Macer Floridus de viribus herbarum* ed. L. Choulant (Lipsiae, 1832). To the bibliographical information contained in Hunt, *Plant Names of Medieval England* (Cambridge, 1989), p.xl add T.M. Capuano, "Medieval Iberian vernacular versions of the herbal called Macer Floridus", *Manuscripta* 35 (1991), 182–202.

16 See J.M. Riddle (ed.), *Marbode of Rennes (1035–1123) 'De lapidibus'*, Sudhoffs Archiv, Beiheft 20 (Wiesbaden, 1977). There is also a text in Migne, *PL* 171, cols.1737–70.

17 See G. Valentinelli, *Bibliotheca manuscripta ad S. Marci Venetiarum, Codices mss latini* t.5 (Venetiis, 1872), pp.75–6 (L.VII,XVII).

18 A. de Poorter, *Catalogue des manuscrits de la Bibliothèque Publique de la ville de Bruges* t.2 (Paris, 1934), p.533 (MS 471).

19 Plut. LXXIII, cod.xix f.35, see Bandini's *Catalogus codicum latinorum Bibliotecae Mediceae Laurentianae* t.3 (Florentiae, 1776), p.43

20 See J. Truhlár, *Catalogus codicum manu scriptorum latinorum qui in C. R. Bibliotheca publica atque universitatis pragensis asservantur*, pars posterior (Pragae, 1906), p.349.

21 f.9v 'Pauli auctoritatem secutus', f.10r 'non solum prelibati Pauli auctoritatem secutus sum'.

Library 544, pp.154a–184a: p.164b 'succus persicarie gallice *coylrage*' and p.177a 'radices sacre spine que vulgariter dicitur *grouseler*', but it is probably of continental French origin.[22]

The text in MS London, B.L. Sloane 420 (s.xiv) ff.269ra–276rb, an insular copy, has no vernacular entries at all, but perfectly illustrates the elasticity of medical compendia. In this version the *Speculum* is highly abbreviated, little more than a personal anthology, containing very short receipts.[23] It bears the title 'Speculum medicine' and contains both prefaces ('Ne tibi displiceat . . .' and 'Cum animaverterem . . .'). The main text then begins 'Oportet ergo diutius permanente [f.269rb] capitis dolore materiam detrahere per os et nares . . .' and ends on f.276rb with a receipt *Ad dolorem pedum*.

In complete contrast, at the beginning of the fifteenth century a copy was made, now MS London, B.L. Royal 12 E xxii, ff.18r–105v, which is highly amplified. Despite its relatively late date, it contains more French material than English. An initial red rubric reads *Incipit liber de cura pauperum id est speculum medicorum a curiosis medicis appellatus* followed by 'Cum animaverterem . . .' New material is inserted immediately after the prologue: *Incipit de capillis. Ad delongandos capillos et procreandos ubicumque volueris.* The names of plants receive explanations in both Latin and the vernacular:

f.35r   accipe herbam que vulgo vocatur ablata – quoddam genus titimalli est[24]
f.62r   ypia minor .i. chykenmete
f.62v   fragrarie a[nglice] strebery
f.76r   primula veris a[nglice] dayesegh
f.100r   cimas sarmenti a[nglice] cuttynges of the vyne crop

There are other words glossed in either French or English:

f.41r   verucas 'wartes' (interlinear)
f.50r   lupas id est truytes
f.53r   scabronem .i. escarbot
f.63r   epatis a[nglice] lyver

The receipts themselves mix Latin, French and English forms in the way which characterizes most insular medical receipts. Take for example, *Emplastrum ad pedes inflatos et tibias* (f.68r):

> Accipe sepum ovinum et pinguednem porcinam nova[m] et liquefiant ana succum de tansay, de plauntayne a[nglice] rybwort, mellis despumati, dregges de cervisia veteri, de jubarbe, de lempe, de grundeswall, de omnibus supradictis ana et

---

22 The title is given as *Speculum medicinarum* and after 8 lines of verse ('Ne tibi displiceat . . .') there is an introduction beginning 'Opusculi huius series cuncta quedam morborum remedia tam consimilium quam officialium quibus magister .G. probatissima experimenta hucusque fidem asserit adhibendam . . .'

23 The same is true of the fifteenth-century copy in MS B.L. Harley 2390 ff.25r–57v which begins (f.25v) 'In hoc parvissimo libello quem speculum medicine appellare volo, ordinaliter colligere volere . . .'

24 See T. Hunt, *Plant Names of Medieval England* (Cambridge, 1989), p.1 (*ablacta*).

bulliendo bene move cum spatula semper imponendo novum bran quousque sit ita spissum sicut unum tansay (?) et tunc appone circa pedes et tibias inflatos.

Following receipts which contain 'celydoyne, bugle, marygold, centori, ambrose', we have (f.68r–v),

> ... walwort et wormode, smalache et pety morell, radices feniculi, radices petrocilli a[nglice] percell ana manipulum unum, lava bene herbas et radices et extrahe les pethhes de radicibus in medio et cut al thys small et cape unam novam ollam terream et pone intus illas herbas cum una lagena boni vini rubii vel cervisie defecate et una quarta mellis bene clarificati.

A number of French receipts are imported in to the text of the *Speculum*:

> Item pur ptisi que ad longement tenu: donez a boyver jubarbe et peluet et toust garra od l'ayde Dieu. Item ptisyke, etyke, palsy et dropsy garrer: quisez en vyn ment, aloyne, rewe et puleol reale et veez que la poote seit bien covert et qaunt il sera quise .iii. ou .iiii. jours aprés, bevez de ceo nut teve et matyn chaude et garra netment. (f.62v)

> Item pocioun pur ptisyke garryre: pernez la racyne de elena campana que l'en appele horselme une poigné e la mountaunce de la tierce partie de lycoris e fetez le lycoris parer e bien debrisere ov un martell e pus les boilliez ensembell en un galoun de eawe tanque il ne eit forsque une potell e beyve le malade au matyn de ce chaude e au vesper freide. (f.63r)

> Item pur chaude ydropesy homme doit prendre .ix. groses vermes de la terre e couper toutz les chiefs e enjettez e puis moldrere les vermes e distemperez eux od ewe benet e ceo donez al ydropyke a boiver e ensi le fetz par .ix. jours en amenusaunt / le coun[t]e des vermes e mettez y de suger ou de mele pur le boiver endoucer e bien se garde la malade de aukes aucis e de oynouns e de nusauntz viaundes, si garra certeinement saunz defaut. (f.64r/67r)

> Item pur ydropesy. Cest bure ouste ydropesy e autres enflures del corps e fest grele e salve le corps: quisés orge en ewe jeskes il soit depescé,[e] quater herbes ou tut – avance, plauntayne, matfeloun, alehost (sic).[25] Triblez bien e beyve de cely ly malade au matyn freyde e au seire chaude, si garra bien toust. E lavés trois seirs les jaumbes e les plauntz des piés de ewe froyde e reez bien e frotés les bien de aille triblé par dymenge einz le solaile levant. Quisez alehost e les autres trois herbes qaunt voldrez en une altre eawe deskes la tierce part remaint e les tiercez partiez soient quisez einz. (f.67v)

Folio 65 is a single leaf insertion in the hand of the principal scribe which contains a receipt in Latin, one in English, and on the verso, written upside down, the following receipt in French:

> Item pur ydropysy, bone medecyne esprové: de ache le jus pernez atant que aver purrez, jus de solsequy deus ataunt e de percell, altretaunt de centorye, e de scaryele ne soit oblié, e toutz ceus juses ensemble builliez e a boiver le malade donez. Item

---

[25] Apparently for *alekost* = 'alecost'. If this is so, it is the earliest recorded example.

pro eodem: pernez sauge demy livre e atant de warance .i. madyr e ataunt de
polipody e ataunt de mistell, derechief .i. iterum pernez de geneste .i. brome le pois
de .ii. unces e mesmes le peis de eglentere e ataunt de la racine de fenoile e donqes
pernez cervoise estale ou vine blanc a la mesure d'une galun e quisez toutz ces
herbes en cele cervoise ou en vine jesques a la tierce partie seit quit id est si seit
.iii. quarte licoris, bulliatur ad unam quartam, et donqes le pacient beivera une
poicyoun le vesper teve e le matyn par .iii. jours continueles e puis beivera en ewe
chaude bien medlé ov feivefauche [sic] devaunt le fest seint Johan le Baptist.[26] E
si il ne soit my del tut saine, derechief beive jesqes il soit entierement garri. Bien
est prové par experiment etc.

One of the French receipts is attributed to John of Scarborough, about whom we
otherwise know nothing:[27]

Item: une femme avoit un male entour le cuer e en la coste destre e ele prist rowges
urtices, marigold, percel e saffron e les quist en bone cervoise e les buist e garrist
bien e nettement. Expertum est per Johannem de Scardeburgh. (f.70v)

More receipts in French follow on ff.76v–77r and 104v–105r. The point of these
examples is to illustrate how supplementary material in French was still being
imported in to such a compendium as late as the early fifteenth century, whilst the
incidence of material in English is almost negligible:

Unguentum vade mecum: tak the jus of celydoine, funter, borache, scabiouse and
the red dok, of ilkene a quarteroun, and tak lytarge, ceruse, es ustum ana demi
uncie and meng tham wyth feus of vine eger and gres of a wolde bore / [or] swyne,
of ayther ana, and temp al togyder and than set tham over the fyre and sethe tham
over the fyre and when thay sethe, cast in the pulder and styr tham fast togyder
wyth a sklyte and thys unement is gude for scabbes and for oucornes and many
other thynges. Of the lytarge, ceruse, es ustum make thy pulder. (f.100v/101r)

On f.105v a receipt begins 'Item for swelyng heved and soore woundes so at the
bone be noght broken', but is then continued in Latin. Formal recognition of the
vernacular in a Latin context is given in a receipt for leprosy in which the patient,
unbeknown to himself, is given to eat 'cor catuli' and then asked ' "Petre, quomodo
est tibi?", ita dicendo "Petre, Deus fecit tibi bonum quia tu commedisti cor canis". Et
ita dices ter et hoc materna lingua' (f.102v).

The compendium in the version of MS Royal 12 E xxii contains a number of charms
(ff.30v–31r, 36r/v; 58v–60v against fevers; 80r incl. the celebrated 'sator arepo'
charm[28]). Whilst the contents are largely receipts of a popular kind, many of which
find their way into the 'Trinity Practica' edited below, there are references to 'mag.

---

[26] Note that such directions are already found in the Flos medicinae in Renzi, Collectio Salernitana 5,
   p.91 'Has herbas circa Baptistae collige festum' (3109) and p.92 'Succus betonicae Baptistae nocte
   legatur' (3130).
[27] See C.H. Talbot and E.A. Hammond, The Medical Practitioners in Medieval England: A Biographical
   Register (London, 1965), p.181.
[28] See T. Hunt, Popular Medicine in Thirteenth-Century England (Cambridge, 1990), p.358 n.100.

G. de Monte Pessulano' (ff.25r,42r), 'mag. Bartholomaeus' (f.25v), 'Salernitane mulieres' (f.28v), 'secundum magistrum Johannes Cometam' (ff.36r,82r/v).

The next significant stage in the fortunes of the *Speculum medicorum*, after abbreviation and expansion, is translation. A full and careful Middle English version is found in MS London, B.L. Add. 34111 ff.40r–190r of the second quarter of the fifteenth century, a large compilation which includes references to 'experimenta' of William Somers (f.174r).[29] Eleven introductory Latin verses beginning 'Ne tibi displiceat . . .' are followed by an English translation, also in eleven lines. Then comes the following preface:

> Her begynneth a boke þat is clepid þe Spectacle of Medicines, þe wyche wyse men
> ad seen for help of mannes body. And þis boke was made and icompild of divers
> auctors and be ordre han gadred fro þe heved þat is begynnyng of þe body and be
> oþer divers [f.40v] membres suyng to be soles of þe fete, þat curiouse leches may
> fynd wiþoute travail and noye liȝtliche what shalle falle to every membre and þe
> iuseers of þis litel bok shalle have knowleche and of oþer doctours assayed for soþe
> þynges þat bien seen profitable. And for to worche liȝt þingges han þes doctours
> put to þis litel boke þat seke men shal noȝt long perish and þat leches unconyng
> may be holpyn of many þenges.

To begin with each receipt is separated by double spacing but this ceases on f.57r. On two occasions it seems that the translator explains that he has been unable to execute his original plan because of illness. Thus, on f.51v he declares:

> I be hight in þe begynning of þis litel boke for to agone doune to þe sole of þe fote
> from þe coppe of þe heved, ȝif þat it hadde lykyd unto me, bote for I am broght in
> sekenesse and may noȝt geder alle þinges, and alle medicines endyd þat bien from
> þe heved þat is þe begynning of all þe body unto þe chekes of þe throte, bote nevere
> þe lesse all þo thinges þat bien most profitable unto þe forsaid I have done my
> diligence to save and helpen þat bien in sekenesse broȝt.

This, however, illustrates a common pitfall in the study of texts which are compilations or translations, namely the temptation to attribute to the compiler or translator *in propria persona* observations which are already part of the source. Thus de Poorter, in his description of MS Brugge, Stadsbibliotheek 471, cites the following passage which occurs at the end of the first chapter devoted to the head and which marks a rearrangement of material in the Brugge MS:

> Reminiscor me, in proemio libelli huius, promisisse usque ad plantam pedis
> descendere, et fecissem si licuisset, sed fractus infirmitate, nequeo cuncta examu-
> sim colligere. Finitis omnibus medicamentis que ad caput, quod est principium

---

[29] See *Catalogue of Additions to the Manuscripts in the British Museum in the years MDCCCLXXXVIII–MDCCCXCIII* (London, 1894 repr. 1969), pp.198–200 and Talbot and Hammond, *op. cit.*, p.416 (William of Sumery). 'Experimenta' attributed to 'Willelmus de Sumereye' are found in MS Cambridge, Corpus Christi College 297 f.127. The 'Virtutes Aquile' (ff.195r–196v) is edited by Sheldon, *art. cit.*, 21–8. The 'Liber Cophonis' on ff.218r–230v is edited together with a facsimile in P. Fordyn, *The 'Experimentes of Cophon, the Leche of Salerne'* (Brussels, 1983).

corporis, pertinent, et ubicumque sensus hominis sedem haberet usque ad gutturis fauces descendens, curiosos moneo medicos ut studiose suos revolvant libros, et quecumque vitia que a faucibus nasci solent curanda susceperint, ne pigeat illos diversarum specierum medicamenta componere, et tantum ego quecumque potui invenire que aptiora mihi videntur, predictis medicamentis que ad caput pertinent prudenter subjunxi.[30]

Yet this passage is actually found in the earliest witness, MS Rawlinson C 235, where it occurs on f.30v after a receipt 'Ad raucedinem vocis', with only the variant 'subiungam' at the end. In both MSS the compiler proceeds 'ad neufreticos et qui lapides habent in renibus aut in vesica'.

Nevertheless, the translation in MS Add.34111 seems full and deserves a detailed study.[31] The receipt against flies in the house (MS e mus. 219 f.65v), for example, is reproduced (f.70v) along with material which is lacking in some of the MSS.

The other real interest of MS Add.34111 is that the Middle English translation of the Speculum medicorum is followed by translations of texts which are transmitted with it in MS e mus. 219. Thus on ff.190v–194v there is a translation of the 'Experimenta parisii abbatis de febribus' (cf. ThK 1393), on ff.195r–196v that of the 'Liber de virtute aquile',[32] on ff.197r–217v a version of the Trotula, what Green calls "a hugely condensed and rearranged translation of selections from the intermediate Trotula ensemble . . . the only one of the five English translations to include many of the cosmetic as well as the obstetrical and gynecological remedies",[33] and on ff.231r–233v a translation of the 'Capsula eburnea'.

This brief survey of the fortunes of one medical compendium thus illustrates the twin processes of continuity and adaptability, whilst showing that even in the fifteenth century the process of translation into English had not excluded the retention of material in French.

But what of beginnings? What do we know of the provenance of such medical works? The answer is often all too little. In one case there is a particularly difficult problem and it unfortunately concerns the most precious of all the insular collections, Cambridge, Trinity College 0.1.20, which is the source of four of the texts printed in Anglo-Norman Medicine. As was pointed out in the introduction to volume 1, three points can be made about the contents of this manuscript.

First, the Latin originals are mostly Salernitan, and certainly not insular. Secondly, the language of the translations is not unambiguously Anglo-Norman and, in some cases, certainly not Anglo-Norman. Thirdly, the scribes, on the other hand, are definitely insular and leave clear linguistic traces, predominantly in the matter of spelling, but not exclusively so.

---

30 A. de Poorter, "Catalogue des manuscrits de médecine médiévale de la biblothèque de Bruges", Revue des Bibliothèques 34 (1924) [271–306] 295–6.

31 On the background of Middle English medical translations see F.M. Getz, "Charity, Translation and the Language of Medical Learning in Medieval England", Bulletin of the History of Medicine 64 (1990), 1–17.

32 See Sheldon, art. cit.

33 Green, "Handlist of Trotula MSS", see below p.70 n.11.

If we turn back to the versified *receptarium* called the *Physique rimee*,[34] since this is the first vernacular treatise in the Trinity MS, we read in a cure for gout:

717–18   O jus de evele bien seit pestri / et de *bibuef* autresi.

The word *bibuef* signifies Artemisia vulgaris, what we call mugwort, but it is not a word of Latin origin, rather of Germanic ('biboz'), whence it enters the language of N.E. France.[35] It certainly is not standard French or any type of Anglo-Norman. When we check the reading in MS D 4 of St John's College, Cambridge and also the text of this receipt as it has been excerpted in MS Sloane 146,[36] we find an entirely different line: 'Pus freez ceo ke jeo vus di'. In the Trinity text *bibuef* appears once more:

1605   E le bibues tot bien triblez

but when we look at two other witnesses, the St John's copy and Trinity 0.8.27,[37] we find that instead of *bibues* they have *artemese* and *artimese* respectively. What hypothesis does this support? That insular copyists replaced a word they judged unfamiliar, yet nevertheless understood the meaning of? Or is the simpler hypothesis that a N.E. French copyist substituted a local form, *bibues*, for the transparent *artemese* and that the Trinity text is alone in being copied from an exemplar which contained this substitution? But these are not the only examples in the Trinity MS, so that the question is wider than the problems of the *Physique rimee*. After this text in the Trinity MS there are a number of prose receipts, one of which (f.24rb) contains as an ingredient *blaunc bibuef*: an Anglo-Norman graphy followed by a lexeme of N.E. French origin! A little later the fragment of a French translation of Roger Frugard's *Chirurgia* contains (f.27rb) 'Pernez aloine, bibuef . . .' (I,13; the full translation has 'armaise'). This is not all. The second example in the *Physique rimee* occurred in a section on childbirth. Later in the Trinity MS there is a vernacular verse translation entitled 'Les secrés des femmes', which consists of certain passages on fertility and conception drawn from the first redaction of the *Liber de sinthomatibus mulierum*, generally known as 'Trotula maior'. Here we read:

[f.23ra] *Por mort enfaunt*
Pernez moi avrone et muschet (?) / et *bibuef* autretaunt i met

The Latin source has 'Accipiatur ruta et arthimesia'. On the same folio we find the word again, where the Latin has no reference to mugwort:

Autre: Ou *bibuef* le jus pernez / Od peivre beivre li donez

---

[34] See Hunt, *Pop. Med.*, pp. 142 ff.
[35] See J. Haust, *Médicinaire liégois du XIIIe siècle et médicinaire namurois du XVe (manuscrits 815 et 2769 de Darmstadt)* (Bruxelles / Liège, 1941) p.63 which records the forms *bivut, biveut, bivueut, bivueul*. See FEW 1,352.
[36] See *Pop. Med.*, p.270 no.18.
[37] See Hunt, "Recettes médicales en vers français", *Romania* 106 (1985), [57–83] 76, l.455.

Still on f.23ra is a third example in another section on childbirth, where the Latin has 'arthimisia':

Pernez mai rue et *bibuef*

So there are four works in the Trinity MS, three of which have Latin originals, containing the word *bibuef* as a lexical innovation or substitution.

The importance of lexical traces is illustrated elewhere in the same MS. For example, an 852-line verse translation of the *Liber de sinthomatibus mulierum*, which begins in decasyllables and graduates to alexandrines, includes the following lines which are not in the Latin:

233 O le fon de la terre en fais cist bevement,
    'Gris con' et 'con canu' l'apelent laie gent.

The reference is to fumitory, 'earthsmoke' (Fumaria officinalis L.). The word 'canu' (= 'chanu') means hoary, resembling the other epithet 'gris'. These names are nowhere in the dictionaries. But in MS BL Sloane 3126, a continental MS which contains a much amplified version of the 'Lettre d'Hippocrate', we find in the supplementary material a number of distinctively N.E. French forms, including (f.59v) 'fine terne [error for fume terre] c'est une herbe que l'en apelle con chanu [MS conchani]'. Also in the *Chirurgie de l'abbé Poutrel* (ed. Södergård p.46 f.44,17) we have 'fumeterre, c'est concennu'.[38] In Daems's dictionary of *synonyma*[39] we find under 'Fumus terre' the synonyms *grisecom, gryston, grisecont(e)* and *grisetum*. Finally, MS Wellcome Historical Medical Library 546 (s.xiv), of continental French provenance, has (f.30b) 'por desechier les malvés humeurs batez le con chanu'. Interestingly, the Trinity verse translation of the *De sinthomatibus mulierum* renders 'artemisia' in the source with *armoyce, ermo(i)se, hernise, hermoise* and *mere herbe*, but never 'bibuef'!

A third lexical trace is *anblete*, a plant name of uncertain meaning (spurge, euphorbia?) and origin (only continental examples have been registered, and just a very few of those). It occurs at line 628 in the *Physique rimee*, where the St John's MS has *amplette*. Conversely at line 369 the St John's MS has *amblette* where the Trinity text has 'bete'. *Amblette* appears in a twelfth-century collection of receipts in MS BL Royal 12 C XIX and in the Trinity 'Practica' (to be discussed later) [83] (f.15v) 'jus de amblette' and [145] (f.28r) 'folia de amblette'. Is it Anglo-Norman?[40]

In fact, there is only one translation in the Trinity MS which has any distinctively insular *lexical* traits and that is the complete translation of Roger Frugard's *Chirurgia*. The relevant items are English words and the manner of their incorporation in the

38 See also Cl. de Tovar in *Romania* 103 (1982), 359–60 who quotes TCC O.1.20 and remarks (presumably apropos the *Chirurgie*) 'gricon n'apparaît que dans des copies très picardisantes'.
39 W.F. Daems, *Nomina simplicium medicinarum ex synonymariis medii aevi collecta: semantische Untersuchungen zum Fachwortschatz hoch- und spätmittelalterlicher Drogenkunde*, Studies in Ancient Medicine 6 (Leiden etc., 1993), p.172 no.309.
40 There is an example on f.169r of MS Exeter Cathedral Chapter Library 3519 (s.xv) which is certainly insular, but the receipts may be of diverse origins.

text leaves room for the possibility that they began life as glosses before being attracted into the main text:

I,xlvi Pernez de la semence jusquiami, que en engleis est apelé *hannebane*
I,liv   la semence de chenillé, qui est apelee *hannebanne*
II,iii les verms qui issent hors del ventre de l'home e que li Anglés apelent *maddokes*
II,iv   gipsus, qui est en englés apelé *cockel*
III,x   foilles papaveris [nigri], qui est apelé en engleis *popi neir*

The last entry suggests some linguistic confusion concerning 'engleis' and one wonders also about the significance of 'franceais' in I,liii 'une maladie que est apelé serpigo e en franceais *derte*', since *derte* is common in Anglo-Norman and fairly transparent in ME *tetter*.

The other translation in Trinity O.1.20 is of the Salernitan *De instructione medici* attributed to Archimatthaeus and abbreviated in a treatise known as *De adventu medici aegrotum*. The copy is clearly insular, but there is no lexical trace which points unambiguously in an insular or continental direction, and we do not have the evidence of rhyme.

The single most important anthology of Anglo-Norman vernacular medicine turns out, therefore, to be entirely ambiguous so far as the provenance of its contents is concerned. Certainly the teaching that it embodies is continental, but it has been copied in England, and so the question becomes 'Is that fact sufficient to justify speaking of Anglo-Norman medicine?', especially given that we do not yet know of continental French translations of some of the works in question.

There is, on the other hand, no reason to doubt the insular production of *Euperiston* and the Trinity 'Practica', printed in the present volume, for they mingle Anglo-Norman and English in an apparently spontaneous way.

All these texts, of course, simply demonstrate what medical knowledge was available to practitioners in medieval England.[41] They do not give us any idea of how these practitioners were regarded or how effective they were.[42] This is a subject for another study! As an indication of the sort of material which survives one might cite the testimony of Guiot de Provins. Guiot was a court poet, probably originating, despite his name, from the Ile-de-France, studying at St Trophime, Arles, and the author of a number of lyrics, who became a Cistercian, first at Clairvaux, and soon after at Cluny. In 1206 he completed his satirical *Bible*, the second part of which concentrates on the clergy, especially the various orders. It concludes with an account of doctors:[43]

How I marvel at physicians and the treatments and advice they dispense! There's no other life like theirs for sheer diversity and perversity. 'Doctor' is what they are generally called, but in my opinion there is not one who is not to be feared. It

41 The identities of the practitioners are the subject of C.H. Talbot and E.A. Hammond, *The Medical Practitioners in Medieval England: A Biographical register* (London, 1965).
42 See for some suggestions E.J. Kealey, *Medieval Medicus: A Social History of Anglo-Norman Medicine* (Baltimore, 1981).
43 See J. Orr (ed.), *Les Oeuvres de Guiot de Provins* (Manchester, 1915), ll.2523–2686.

pleases them to find absolutely noone free from some disability. They're always concocting an ointment or a bath without rhyme or reason. If you escape their treatment, it's like being released from a loathsome prison. If you know how to swindle and cheat whilst giving the impression of conducting yourself honourably, you can't go wrong; what really does them good is the faith people place in them. There's a thousand who become doctors who know no more than I do. The truly skilled are mortified, for there's no profession in which there are so many charlatans. They see off scores of folk. There are no friends or relatives whom they would be happy to pronounce healthy. They really are rascals. To entrust yourself to the hands of doctors is to enter loathsome bonds. Why? Well, they had me in their clutches – and never was there a more disgusting experience. I'm not partial to their company, so help me God, as sure as I'm in good health – to fall in to their hands is to endure such disgusting treatment! To think of it! When I'm ill, I have to suffer their interference. You should just hear them inspecting urines, nothing but lies and guesswork, or pronouncing on some condition using the foulest words. They find a malady in everyone. If the patient has a fever or a dry cough, then they say he's phthisical, or dropsical, melancholical, or tumerous, asthmatic or palsied. You should hear them going on about the choleric or the phlegmatic! One person has an inflamed liver, the next wind. Their practises are most devious, their language disgusting, nothing but filth . . . Any old rascal with the gift of the gab, so long as he's capable of reading, can take in dim-witted folk. They're all physicians and masters! And when they're in a good town they deceive each other, the best physicians praising someone who knows nothing. The master accommodates quacks. Why? To hoodwink people. And so that he may be left in peace, the scabby accommodates the foul-smelling and the foul-smelling the scabby. Neither is the slightest put out. Why? Because they both stink! I'd be better off a prisoner in Beirut than undergoing treatment from doctors for a whole year. They're mighty expensive, too, charging far too much, and they forbid the most delectable foods. But they can keep their pills, which are not very nice! If they come from Montpellier, their electuaries are very expensive, and then they claim that they contain ginger and pliris, tragacanth and rose-sugar, barley-sugar and sugar with violets – with their 'diarhodon' and 'julii' they've taken in many people. They're much esteemed and praised. They declare there's ginger and aloes in their 'diamargariton', but I'd prefer a fat capon any day to their pill-boxes, foul and moist. And someone who comes from Salerno pulls the wool over our eyes by pretending that sloes and quince are Babylonian spices, and if someone were to swallow them, he'd have such loose bowels as to be disgraced at once. I'd rather stick with good foods, good clear wines and strong sauces. Their own practises are false.

Fortunately, Guiot, despite the élan of his diatribe, is willing to recognize exceptions.[44]

They're not all the same. The good, reliable physicians, good men and well-read, have often given sound advice. Many people who were in a bad way have gained

---

44 Cf. the defence of medicine at the end of the *Flos medicinae* and the criticisms under the heading 'medicaster', Renzi, *Collectio Salernitana* 5 (Naples, 1859), pp.102–3 ('Fingit se medicum quivis idiota, prophanus, / Iudaeus, monachus, histrio, rasor, anus, / sicuti alchemista medicus fit aut saponista, / aut balneator, falsarius aut oculista. / Hic dum lucra quaerit, virtus in arte perit').

from this advice. When a man fears death, he really needs to be comforted and sound advice has brought comfort to many a worthy man who was in distress. And when sound practice is well known it is right that it should be properly appreciated. Yet the good towns have been so inundated by the tricks of the charlatans and quacks that the good men are not so esteemed as they should be. They often see each other and meet together, but their works are not sufficiently known, though quite distinct. Yet beside thorns roses do not lose their beauty or their scent or their goodness. I've seen the rose bush grow and bloom beside the nettle patch. If nettles sting, cause pain and smell, roses are beautiful and precious. Good works, complete, true and reliable are like precious metal which is separated from clinker. Everyone knows that there is a worm that makes silk. In other words, bad works do not shut out good ones. Reliable and learned physicians ought to be properly respected, esteemed and cherished. I certainly hold dear the good, reliable doctor when I need him – I'm only too glad to see him brought before me. When sickness assails me, he is a great comfort. But, when my sickness leaves me and I no longer suffer, then I'm happy for a boat to transport him promptly to far-away Salonika, him and his medicine, and for him to stick strictly to his journey, so that I never see him again!

Few physicians seem to have achieved high social status or unqualified approval in medieval England, as Kealey shows.[45] Yet he is able to identify ninety physicians in the first half of the twelfth century alone.[46] It is to be hoped that future research will help us to get to know those who may have used some of the materials printed in *Anglo-Norman Medicine*.

---

[45] E.J. Kealey, *op. cit.* For the later period, however, see C. Rawcliffe, "The Profits of Practice: The Wealth and Status of Medical Men in Later Medieval England", *Social History of Medicine* 1 (1988), 61–78. For an overview of the variety of practitioners see K. Park, "Medicine and Society in Medieval Europe, 500–1500" in A. Wear (ed.), *Medicine in Society: Historical Essays* (Cambridge, 1992), pp.59–90.

[46] On pp.31–3 he lists 8 physicians for the Anglo-Saxon period, 11 for 1066–1100, and 90 for 1100–54. The latter are identified in greater detail on pp.121–51.

CHAPTER ONE

Visiting the Sick

A vernacular treatise on visiting and treating the sick in MS Cambridge, Trinity College 0.1.20 ff.196r–213v, which begins with considerations concerning what would today be called the physician's bedside manner, was first identified by the indefatigable Paul Meyer,[1] who appreciated that it was based on an anonymous work of Salernitan origin, edited by Henschel and published by Renzi.[2] He recognized, nevertheless, that this view needed qualification:

> Seulement notre traducteur a dû avoir sous les yeux un texte pourvu d'un prologue qui manque dans le ms. de Breslau et dont il s'est borné à donner un résumé en forme indirecte. La traduction est du reste fort libre et renferme bien des passages que je n'ai pas trouvés dans le latin.[3]

Meyer's impression of the qualities and scope of the translation derived from the mistaken notion that the source was the anonymous De adventu medici ad aegrotum. In fact this text is an abbreviated version of a longer treatise, attributed to the Salernitan Archimatthaeus, known as De instructione medici which was printed from a fourteenth-century copy (Paris, Bibl. Imp. f.lat. 7091) by Renzi.[4] This text provides a model for all the variant readings and interpolations which had struck Meyer when comparing the vernacular treatise with the De adventu. There is, unhappily, no modern edition of the De instructione and the text printed by Renzi is unsatisfactory at many points. A Latin text much closer to the vernacular treatise is found in MS Oxford, Bodleian Library, Digby 79 (s.xiii[2]) ff.119v–129v which I print in the following pages. In addition, a very similar text of the opening is found in MS Oxford, Pembroke College 21 (s.xiii ex) ff.189r–192r and a reliable text of the complete treatise is also found in MS Winchester College 26 (s.xiii) ff.36ra–42vb. There is no list of surviving manuscripts of the De instructione and little is known about Archimatthaeus.[5] Henschel's annotations to the De adventu show that the main sources are passages drawn from Galen (especially concerning the taking of the patient's pulse and the choice of site for bleeding) and Hippocrates, with no trace of Arabic influence.

1 P. Meyer, "Les Manuscrits français de Cambridge", Romania 32 (1903) [18–120] 86–7.
2 Collectio Salernitana 2 (Napoli, 1853), pp.74–80 (introduction pp.72–3). The vernacular treatise corresponds in scope to p.74, l.1 – p.79, l.25.
3 art. cit., 86.
4 Coll. Sal. 5 (Naples, 1859), pp.333–49. The vernacular translation corresponds to pp.333, l.1 – 342, l.26.
5 See F. Hartmann, 'Die Literatur von Früh- und Hochsalerno und der Inhalt des Breslauer Codex Salernitanus . . .' diss. Borna-Leipzig, 1919, pp.20–23.

It was, of course, principally Hippocrates who transmitted to the Middle Ages an informed discussion of medical ethics.[6] There is some relevant material in Galen's fourth commentary on the sixth of Hippocrates' *Epidemia* and in a very short treatise 'Quomodo visitare debes infirmum'.[7] After the two Salernitan treatises which are the subject of the present chapter there is the important work *De cautelis medicorum* attributed to Arnald of Villanova.[8] In the fourteenth century an interesting picture of medical deontology can be gained from individual chapters in medical works by Jan Yperman, John of Arderne, Guy de Chauliac, and Henri de Mondeville who all display increased knowledge obtained from translations of Greek and Arabic works.[9] The *De cautelis* bears some resemblance in intention to the similarly titled work by the fourteenth-century Bolognese physician Albertus de Zancariis.[10] It is in fact a composite work which includes a treatise on uroscopy and a reworking of the first third of the *De adventu*.

The *De adventu* is also reworked in verse in a vast compendium of seven books printed by Renzi.[11] This compendium, found in MS Paris, Bibl. Imp.8161 A (s.xiii[2]), begins with two books dealing with cosmetics and the diseases of women based on texts circulating under the attribution *Trotula*. Books 3–6 constitute a surgery derived almost wholly from the *Chirurgia* of Roger and Roland (of Parma), and Book 7 is based on the *De adventu* (versified in 27 chapters), on Copho's *De modo medendi* and on Arnald of Villanova. The prologue to the compendium runs as follows:

> In sublime volet fixus stilus hactenus imis,
> Et prerupta maris sicco pede transeat, absque
> Remigis auxilio vel classis; transeat Alpes
> Incedens pedibus metricis; doceatque mederi
> Ex antiquorum scriptis archana revelans

---

6   Cf. W.H.S. Jones, *The Doctor's Oath* (Cambridge, 1924) and G. Weiss, "Die ethischen Anschauungen im Corpus Hippocraticum", *Archiv für Geschichte der Medizin* 4 (1911), 235–62. See especially *Precepta* 3–13 in W.H.S. Jones (ed. and transl.), *Hippocrates* 1 (New York, 1923), pp.317–29. Also L.C. MacKinney, "Medical Ethics and Etiquette in the Early Middle Ages: The Persistence of Hippocratic Ideals", *Bulletin of the History of Medicine* 26 (1952), 1–31 and V. Nutton, "Beyond the Hippocratic Oath" in A. Wear *et al.* (eds.), *Doctors and Ethics: The Earlier Historical Setting of Professional Ethics* (Amsterdam / Atlanta, GA, 1993), pp.10–37 (with full bibliographical references).

7   Printed in Renzi, *Coll. Sal.* 2, p.73 and H.E. Sigerist, "Early Mediaeval Medical Texts in Manuscripts of Montpellier", *Bulletin of the History of Medicine* 10 (1941) [27–40], 31. For early MSS see Beccaria, *I Codici di Medicina*, Index of Incipits (p.424) and see also Index sub *deontologia*.

8   See H.E. Sigerist, "Bedside Manners in the Middle Ages: The Treatise *De cautelis medicorum* attributed to Arnald of Villanova" in F. Marti-Ibañez (ed.), *Henry E. Sigerist on the History of Medicine* (New York, 1960), pp.131–40. Sigerist prints an English translation. The Latin translation I have consulted in *Arnaldi Villanovani philosophi et medici summi, Opera omnia* (Basilieae, 1585), cols. 1453–1458.

9   See M.C. Welborn, "The Long Tradition: A Study in Fourteenth-Century Medical Deontology", in J.L. Cate and E.N. Anderson (eds.), *Medieval and Historiographical Essays in Honor of James Westfall Thompson* (Chicago, 1938), pp.344–57.

10 M. Morris, 'Die Schrift des Albertus de Zancariis aus Bologna, De cautelis medicorum habendis', diss. Leipzig, 1914.

11 *Coll. Sal.* 4, pp.1–176 ('De secretis mulierum, de chirurgia, et de modo medendi libri septem') and pp.177–84. The reworking of the *De adventu* is found on pp.145–55.

Nexibus artatum metrice compaginis istum
Rhetorico ritu florescere nemo libellum
Autumet. At veniam, si quid peccaverit auctor,
Largius expectat dum res gravis ipsa recusat
Esse resolvenda metrico vel carmine stringi.
Qui licet incomptus incedens gnaviter artes
Per calles, doceat que sit cautela medendi
Quotque modis variare decet medicaminis usum,
Que sit et utilitas, quibus actis musa laborem
Compleat; at metuat primo livoris ocellum,
Dente venenoso ne conterat hoc opus omne,
Ne nimis exposita vilescat pagina presens,
Incultam faciem lenonibus abdita velet,
At lector licitus omnino revolvat eandem,
Cuius ad obsequium nuper processit ad ortum.

The contents of the *De instructione medici* may now be summarized. The chapter headings of the versified Latin *De adventu* are provided for the purpose of comparison. The basic structure corresponds to three stages of treatment: before the crisis, during the crisis, and after the crisis.

After a prologue which is not included in the *De adventu*, the introduction [2] deals with the physician's preliminary gathering of information concerning the patient, so that if the latter's urine and pulse are not sufficiently instructive, the physician will be able to convince the patient that he understands his condition and thus command confidence [c.1 *Qualiter se habeat medicus invitatus ad egrum*].[3] The physician is advised to secure the patient's agreement to confession, if this has not already taken place, for to request it after the commencement of treatment might suggest lack of confidence on the part of the physician and cause despair in the patient. Everything is to be done to express approval of the patient's surroundings and to put him at his ease [c.2 *Qualiter se habeat ingrediens domum egri*; c.3 *Qualiter se habeat ad egrum ingressus*].[4] The patient's pulse is to be taken in the left arm, allowing time for both physician and patient to calm down after the initial excitement of their meeting, taking into account the exertion of the physician in making his journey and the hopes and fears of the patient [c.4 *De iudicio pulsus*].[5] There follows inspection of the patient's urine, which will provide firmer evidence than the pulse alone [c.5 *De iudicio urine*].[6] The patient should be given a favourable prognosis, but the physician should cover himself against possible disaster by informing members of the household that the patient's chances are only moderate, thereby enhancing his own standing if things go well and minimising the damage to his reputation if things go badly. It is important to keep up the patient's spirits and achieve a good relationship with him – he must not be upset by ill-judged behaviour on the part of the physician such as unseemly staring at examples of female beauty in the house. If invited to stay for a meal, the physician should conduct himself with humility and sensitivity, avoiding placing himself at the head of the table and at all times affecting appreciation of the food and service.[c.6 *De confortatione egri et pronunciatione iudicii*; c.7 *Qualiter se habeat medicus ad prandium invitatus*; c.8 *Qualiter sollicitus sit de egro in prandio*; c.9 *De visitatione mulierum in domo*; c.10 *Qualis debeat medicus eligi*].[7] It is important to show at all times a real concern for the patient, so that he never feels forgotten and is pleased that his hospitality is appreciated.[8] A section follows on the administration of food, which must take place at the right times, according to the patient's condition [c.11 *De modo et diversitate cibandi infirmum*].[9] Dietary procedure must be based on the patient's habit, illness, age, the time of the year and the region [c.11, ll.95f 'morbi genus, etas, / Mos, regio, victus et constipatio, fluxus']. [10–11] There follows a digestive receipt [c.12 *De quatuor modis medendi et primo de digestivis*; ll.97ff 'Cumque modos medici dent quatuor esse medendi, / Digerat et primus, alter dissolvat, et alter / Constringat vel mortificat, restauret et alter']. [12] We are reminded that the physician's task is to work with nature in combatting the malady.[13] Digestives, working on the humours, must be applied according to the cause of the malady. A number of oxymels are recommended [c.15 *De variatione digestivorum secundum locum et materiam*].[14] The inspection of urines for signs of digestion [c.14 *De signis manifeste digestionis*].[15] Observations that digestives are employed in the case of impending maladies and not maladies that have already taken hold [c.14, ll.173ff].[16] Instructions on how we assist nature, depending on whether hot or cold matter is the source of the malady [c.14, ll.178ff. c.15 *De alterantibus materiam*; c.16 *De evacuantibus materiam sive purgantibus*].[17] A section on phlebotomy, its times and conditions [c.18 *De evacuatione sanguinis et quot sint attendendo circa flebotomiam*; c.19 *Que complexio magis aut minus sit flebotomanda*; c.20 *Quod secundum vires magis aut minus sit flebotomandum*; c.21 *Quo tempore magis sit flebotomandum*].[18] Discussion of the times of bleeding from the left arm and the right arm, of specific precautions for bleeding from the cephalic, median and hepatic veins, and instructions for lowering the ambient temperature when bleeding [c.22 *Qua parte corporis minuendum sit secundum diversa tempora anni*; c.23 *Quibus locis magis sit flebotomandum*; c.24 *Qua etate magis aut minus sit flebotomandum*; c.25 *Qualiter secundum consuetudinem sit flebotomandum*; c.26 *Quod secundum qualitatem regionis sit flebotomandum*; c.27 *Qualiter secundum qualitatem sexus sit flebotomandum*].[19] Bleeding has two purposes – to draw off the noxious matter of a malady or to preserve the patient from a greater malady.[20] Consideration of the symptoms of impending crisis according to the location of noxious matter, as issuing in vomiting, diarrhoea, urine, haemorrhoids, menstrual discharge, nosebleed and sweating.[21] Remedies for the different cases when recognized before the critical day.[22] Occurrence of the crises according to the time of year, and the recommended remedies.[23] The conditions determining tertian and quartan crises.[24] The use of decoctions, syrups, pills and electuaries to draw out noxious matter, and receipts for them.[25] Receipts and treatments.[26] Receipt for a laxative syrup and other remedies.[27] The critical hours when medication should be withheld.[28] A list of principal symptoms.[29] Instructions for making suppositories.[30] Instructions for making clysters (enemas).[31] Receipt for a caustic clyster.[32] The treatment of constipation by constrictive medicines.[33] The preparation and administration of a cleansing clyster.[34] The preparation of constrictive medicines.

[f.196r] *Issi comence le sotil enseignement Ypocras a ces disciples, que mult li aveient requis coment il deusent visiter li malades.*

[1] Li auctor dist au comencement de cest livre et parole a ses disciples, qui l'avoient requis de cest livre faire, et dist qu'il a grant joie et grant leesse totes les foiz que il pense a lor peticion pur le preu que lor est a venir de sa doctrine, s'il volent retenir, et dist qu'il ne lor dira se choses espruvees non et coneues. Et si lor dist qu'il n'eient[12] pas sa doctrine pur vil por ce qu'il ont assés livres de fisique, que om estanche bien sovent sa soif d'un roissel com l'en ne poet venir a la funtaine. Ore nos dirons dunques un poi de bons comandemens que serront autresi com introductions de practique. Car a la fiez si vaut mut l'art ové la main, c'est a dire que le practique vaut mut ové la theorique. Ore vus doig donques un novel comandement que vus façés trestoz autresi come jo faz et que vo[s] overés sicom jo vus enseigneray. [f.196v]

[2] O tu mires, com hom te requera que tu viengies veoir aucun malade, le nun Nostre Segnur te puisse aider, et li angeles Deu, ke fist compaignie a Thobie cum il ala en Ninive et le guiout[13] et menout, puisse guier et conduire vostre cors et vostre alme en totes vos ovres. Ore vus amoneste donques que vus enquerez et encerchez par chemin, tot com vos irrés pur veoir le malade, dou messager com longement li malades avera geu et en quele manere la maladie li avint, que vus puissez estre certefiez de la maladie par les signes que li messager vus dirra, si que vus ne seez pas esbais cum vus vendrez devant le malade, et, ja soit ice que vus ne parcevez riens de sa maladie par l'orine ne par son pous, cum vus le averez veu et tastez, que vus puissiez conustre et deviser lui et sa maladie par les signes et par les accidens que vus averez[14] enquis dou messager, et que il puisse aver fiance en vus autresi cum en ce[f.197r]lui qui li devra doner sauneté.

[3] Et cum vus vendrois devant lui, si enquerés si il avra esté confés. Si nun, si li devez amonester qu'il se face confés ou qu'il promette qu'il se fra confés. Car come vus l'averez regardé et pris en cure et vos après l'amonestez de fere sei confés, il sei des[es]pera par aventure de aver santé, kar il quidera par aventure que vus li diez ice por ce que vus quidez que il murge. Et ceste chose ne fait pas a lasser, kar plusors maladies avienent et sordent par pecchiez, des queles, come hom ad lavés ses pecchiez des lermes de bone conscience, hoem garist soventesfoiz par la misericord dou soverain mire. Dont Nostre Sire dist en le ewangeile: 'Alez et ne pecchiez plus, ke vus ne aviengne pis que devant'.[15] Et come vus entrez au malade, n'aez pas le chere orgoilluse ne fere ne chiere de coveitise ne de malice. Et si tost cum il leveront encontre vos et vus salueront, si les resaluez et come se aseent, se vus aseez ovec eus. Et cum vus averez repris [f.197v] vostre parole, se vos fablés ovesques eux et loez la region et la disposition de la mesun.

---

12 MS *naveient.*
13 MS *gruout.*
14 MS *averas.*
15 John 5, 14.

[4] Et a la fin seez vus vers le malade et li demandez coment il sei sent et li maundez que il vus tende son bras. Et ces choses que jo vos ai dit si sont necessaires pur aquere l'amur et la bone volenté dou malade et des gens que sont entor. Et si poet on estre tost deceu en pous garder por[16] ce que les esperiz se sun[t] esmeu en vos par chemin, por[17] ce que les [esperiz] dou malade sunt esmeus pur la joie de vostre venue ou pur ce qu'il pense come hoem avra de son avoir et pur autres diverses causes, que de vus que de lui, en poez estre tost deceu a conustre le pous. Donques come vus serrez bien reposes et vus avrez le malade bien asseuré, si devez taster son pous el senestre braz, kar ja soit ice que li quers souffle en la destre partie, si conust on neporquant plus legerement les motions dou quer el senestre braz, pur ce que [f.198r] il est plus pres dou quer que la destre. Et pernez garde que li malade ne gise pas sor la senestre coste, kar ce desturbereit les esperiz a mover. Et gardez que li malades n'ait pas les dois trop estendus en la paume ne trop fermement clos. Et vus devez bien sagemen[t] mettre les somerounez des dois de la destre main sor le pous et sustenir le braz de la senestre, kar par la sensibilité de la destre partie aparceverez plus legerement les variances dou pous. Et li malades, come cil qui est febles, a bien mestier que vus li sustenez sun braz dou vostre main senestre. Et s'il ad le bras pleins et carnels, si li serrez bien vos dois sor le pous por aprocher as arteres bien qui sunt repostes. Mes si il ad les braz gresles et megres, si devés taster le pous en la superficé dou bras trestot suavet. Et devés bien regarder le pous jusc'a .c. coups pur conustre et aparceivre la diverseté dou pous et por ce que icil qui i sont oient plus volentiers et plus diligen[f.198v]tement vostre jugement et vostre respuns pur la longe atente.

[5] Et aprés comandés que l'en vus mostre sa urine, kar ja soit ice que la variance dou pous vus signefie sa maladie, l'urine vus certefiera miels et plus apertement. Et li malades encore quidera que vus ne conusseez mie sa maladie par le pous tant solement, ainz le conoissiés par l'un et par l'autre, ce est asaver par le pous et par l'urine. De garder l'urine: come vus regarderez l'urine, si devez mettre grant cure et grant entente a regarder la color,[18] la substance, la qualité, la quantité et ce que est contenu dedens, de la diverseté des queles choses conoist l'en la diversité[19] des maladies, sicome nos avon enseigné en nostre tratié des urines.

[6] Et aprés si devez promettre saunté au malade, que mult desire a oir vostre respons. Mes come vus departirez de la meisun, si dirrez a ceus que le gardent que mult est malades. Et ce dirrez pur ce que si il eschape, que vus en [f.199r] soiez le plus loez, et s'il mourt, que il tesmognent que del comencement desesperiez vus de sa sancté. Estre ice jo vus amonest[e] une chose, que vus ne covoitiez ne sa femme ne sa fille ne sa chambrere, ne que nule beauté vus deceoive que vus veez en eaus. Kar icés choses en asotent soventefeiez le mire et li fait encore la male volenté de Nostre Seignur et perdre la grace de lui en son overaigne et fait le mire desplaire au malades et [le] malade desespeir de avoir aide del mire. Et pur ce vus amoneste jo que vus soi[e]z de beles

---

16 MS *que por.*
17 MS *quei por.*
18 MS *colere.*
19 MS *diversites.*

paroles et que vus attendez l'aide Nostre Seignur et appellés en totes vos ovres. Et come il avient et sout avenir que li sires ou cil qui sont maistre gardein de la meisun[20] vus retenent a manger oveques eus, gardez vus de trop fierment contenir, ne elisez pas le premer leu en la table, kar au mire et au prestre sout on appareiller le premer leu en la table. Ne despisez nul boivre [f.199v] ne nul manger que l'en vus tende ne ne blamez riens que viengne sor la table, kar par aventure vus n'avez pas apris de sauler vostre ventre de mil ne de viandes de vile.[21] Et si vus ensi le faites, si aquerrez la bone volenté de tuz et trestuz se peneront de vus loer et de honorer.

[7] Pur faire li malade enfier en vus:[22] Por faire que li malades ait grant fiaunce en vos, come vus averez plus diversitez des mes devant vus, si faites enquere par aucon des sergans coment li malades le fait et ce sovent. Et ce sachez que se vus si faites, que li malades avra grant fiance en vus com il verra que vus ne l'obliez pas entre vostre solaz. Et come vus leverez de la table et vus vendrés devant lui, si vus demandera coment vus avez esté servi, si li direz que richement et bien, de la quele chose il en avera mult tresgrant joie pur ce ke il n'avra pas esté [poi] ententif a ce.

[8] Et come il eirt tens que l'en lui doinst a manger, [f.200r] paissez lui vos meimes et lui donez a manger. Et eliseez une hore covenable a lui doner a manger come quant l'accés l'avera laissee[23] et serra plus en repos, en [fevre] continuel ou tens de faus repos, kar hom ne les[24] trovera ja san[s] fevre dusc'a la declination cretique. Et notez que es fevres entrepolates qu'on [ne] lor doit tant[25] doner a manger devaunt l'accession,[26] kar autrement sera la nature en double bataille come ele ne porra defire la viande que est a deffire[27] ne sormonter son enemi. Mes si l'accession s'avance[28] tant, si que vus ne porrez trover covenable hore de doner li a manger, si attendez tant que l'accession soit alee. Mes neporquant ne li donez pas a manger maintenant après l'accession, kar les membres que sont lassez et travaillez de la bataille devant et de l'assaut de lor enemi si n'ont cure de nule charge de viande, ains vourunt un poi reposer come [f.200v] cil qui sunt las après la victoire de lor enemi. Et por ce si devés attendre a doner li a manger après l'accession une hore ou dous au meins.

[9] Diete: Si le devés dieter solonc la manere de la maladie et le tens de l'an et solonc l'age, et li variés la qualité et la quantité de la viaunde, kar vus devés dieter de greinor viande celui que travaille de maladie interpollate que celui que travaille de maladie continue, et plus sotille diete en la continue que en le interpollate, et de plus grant

---

20 MS *moisun*.
21 The translator has not correctly rendered the Latin 'de iure et genere rusticano miliaceo pane'.
22 Rubric in MS.
23 Renders the Latin 'in interpolatis'.
24 The Latin similarly changes to the plural when dealing with general observations: 'quando sunt in vera quiete . . . sine febre non inveniuntur'.
25 The Latin has 'tanto tempore ante accessionem'.
26 There follows in the Latin 'ut cum ventum fuerit ad tempus accessionis, cibus ex toto sit digestus. Aliter . . .'
27 The Latin has 'escam importune ingestam'.
28 MS *sa avance*.

diete en yver et en veir que en esté. Mes en aust si suffrent eus malement grant diete. Et si devez regarder l'age dou malade, kar as enfanz doit l'en doner plus sovent a manger que a juvenciax, kar la consumption est plus grant en eux por la liquidité de lor moisteté et por ce qu'il[29] ont mester de viandes pur norir lur membres et por croistre les et por restorer lor ce qu'eles perdent chescun jor en la maladie. Mes les viels homes deit l'en dieter de poi de viande et [f.201r] por la feblesce de lor natu[r]el chalor[30] et por la petite force qui il en ont. De l'acoustomance dou malade devés vos prendre garde, kar cil ke un[t] apris grosse diete et grant doit l'en dieter autrement que ceus qui ne l'ont mie apris. Et si devez prendre garde si il ad le ventre serré ou mol ou moine entre ces dous. Kar si il ad le ventrail laissiés, si le devez dieter de grosse diete, come des poires et de[s] coins, kar il estouperont le fons de l'estomac de lor groscesse et serront[31] le ventrail de lor qualité. Mes si il ad le ventrail dur et serré, si li donés avant choses moles et bones a deffire et l'eue de la decoction de prunes, et, aprés, grosses choses qui facent la viande plus tost descendre par lor pesantime. Mes si li ventrail n'est ne trop dur ne trop mol, meis moiene entre dous, si li donez avant mole diete, kar plus est profitable au malade et preservatif de greignor nuisanse[32] come li ventres fait bien son office. Kar ce que l'en vait bien a chambre ne conforte pas solement les membres nutritives, ens [f.201v] conforte[33] totes les membres.

[10] Donés li donques premerement prunes quites en ewe ou greins ou la[i]t d'alamandes, que vos aparellerés en teu manere: pregne l'en les almaundes et les mete l'en en ewe chaude tant que les puisse l'en[34] peler. Et après les triblez fortment et metés un poi de ewe froide et movez bien trestot ensemble et le colés parmi une touaillie et ce qu'en istra doigne l'en au malade. Mes si il est quit un poy en un pot, si est plus legere a deffire que si il le beust cru. Et notez que come la alemandes serra appareillez, si le deit on mettre un poi reposer. Et aprés doit on suffler hors la cresse que est en la superficé qui serroit noreture et viande al chalor de la fevre.

[11] Et autresi doit on fere quant on done l'eue ou la geli[ne] a esté[35] quite ou l'eue ou l'en a [mis] mie pain dedens. Et aprés li donez orgee a manger, que vus devez apareiller en tele manere: vus prendrez l'orge et la elirez mult bien. Et après le moilliez fortment et le frotez bien sor une aspere piere tant que il soit bien [f.202r] eschorchés. Et après le batez bien en un morter ou vus l'esquartelés entre dous moles. Et après le mettez quire mult tresbien. Et en la fin de la decoction si metés ens le lait d'alemandes. Et après le donez au malade. Et si vos volés faire ptisane, si en colez l'eue et donez li a boivre ou ewe ou avra esté esmie dou pain. Et notez que, come l'amande est en l'estomac, que vus ne devés doner ne ewe[36] ne syrop, car ce fait issir la viande defite ou ce retarde[37] la digestion.

---

29 MS *qui il.*
30 MS *cholor.*
31 MS *seerront.*
32 MS *que g. quisance.*
33 MS *conforter.*

34 MS *puissent p.*
35 MS *estre.*
36 The Latin specifies 'aqua diuretica'.
37 MS *detarde.*

[12] Et notez que li mires au comencement de la maladie doit overer contre la maladie de choses digestives, kar li mires est le sergant nature come sen maistre en totes ses ovres et ele si doit aler devant come mestresse et dame. Kar sicome nature travaille a afebler la force de la maladie et a avoir la victoire de lui et a fere crisim et a varier[38] la mateire de sa mauveise qualité et a departir la matere par les membres por mels boter le hors, a la queu chose fere ele tent plus, autresi deit li mi[f.202v]res appareillier ce que mestiers est a lui et a nature a boter fors la maladie et la mateire de lui. Dont Ypocras dist: 'Il covient mediciner les choses deffites et movir les choses qui sun[t] pas crues'.[39]

[13] Come l'en a donc regardé la cause de la maladie, si doit l'en varier les choses digestives des humors. Car si colere ou autre humor chaut et sech est cause de la maladie, si li donez sirop aceptous por deffire la, mes si fleume naturele ou si fleume acetouse ou fleume verrigne ou melancolie naturele ou colere vitelline, et meimement en yver, si li donés oximel, si il ne chiet en continue ou si li tens de l'an ne seit trop chaut.

Syrop acetous fait on en tele manere: pregnez les dou[s] pars de vin eagre et la terce de zucre et les metez boilir desque la maité soit degasté. Et si vos le volez plus espés, lassiés le plus boilir et metez un poi plus de zucre. Mes sacez qui il ert meins divisif[40] et ara mendre efficace, ja soit ce qu'il soit plus [f.203r] dous et plus soef a guster. Et autresi fait on oximel zaqueran dou jus de poumes grenates acetouses et de zucre. Oximel simple fait on en tele manere: escumez vostre mel premerement mult bien sur le fu en un vaissel d'estaim et come vus avrez geté hors le escume, si metez ens les dous pars de vin egre et faites tot boilir desc'a la moité. Oximel composte fait on en tele manere: hom met temprer les rascines d'ache, de fenoil, de perresil, sparge, brusci, rafani, siuere, squilla en vin egre et si le lassce on dous jors au meins. Et gete on hors le fust, ce ke l'en trovera dedens[41] les racines, et aprés les colés. Et come vus les averez colez, si mete om mel en coleure. Ou si vus volez plus tost aver fait, si triblez les racines et le faites boilir en vin egre et donés au malade.

[14] Dongne on oximel ovesques ew chaude au matin come il [n']i a viandes en menbres nutritives qui lor nurisent et empeechent [f.203v] por afieblier la vertu des viandes, ovesques ewe chaude por afieblier la substance et por aoster l'abhominable savor et por desoudre la fente. Si dogne on icés choses tant que les signes de la digestion apergent, la queu chose vos regarderez en l'ur[i]ne et en la matere de l'affliction. Par l'urine en dou maneres, kar l'urine si est a la fiez coloree et a la fiez descoloree et a la fiez tenve et a la fiez espesse. Se ele est donques des le comencement descoloree et tenve et ele devigne[42] aprés coloree et espesse, si signefie que la matere que fu devant

38 MS *verier*.
39 *Aphor*. I,22. Cf. G. Lafeuille (ed.), *Les Amphorismes Ypocras de Martin de Saint-Gille 1362–1365* 1 (Genève, 1954), p.57, 'Il esconvient evacuer par medecine laxative la matiere digeree, et non mouvoir la matiere crue . . .'
40 MS *mels divisiet*, cf. *De instructione* 'minus erit efficax ad dividendum'.
41 MS *dui dedens*.
42 MS *dovigne*.

est desteinte. Kar primes come la matere que fu compacte et que recevoit feble action de chalor en soi, si ne peut pas l'urine prendre color et por ce que poi [remaint] ovesques l'urine de la matere que fu serré et dure si fu ele tenve et cliere. Mes aprés par le ovres des choses digestives et par la vertu que vus li averez doné, si en ist une greignor flambe et une greignor chalor de la matere que est [f.204r] ja quite. Et come la conpaction de la matere et des humors est ja amoli et relasscé, si s'en ist et se melle plus essemblement ovesque l'urine, dont ele est plus espesse et plus coloree. Mes come l'urine est descoloree au comencement et espesse, icele espesseté disons nos qui vient de la multitude des superfluitez, kar ele ne vient pas de[43] la force ne de l'ovre de nature, ains vient de la malice de la maladie come ele est espessie au matin et ele remaint espesse. Mes come ele rasiet et atenvist, signefie la digestion des humors et que l'astat de la maladie est prochein. Mes come ele devient tenve aprés que ele avra esté espesse, si covient a force que ce aviegne de l'un de ces dous choses, de ce que la matere est ravie et montee amont el chief ou par ce que la matere est degastee. Et por ce se ne devez pas estre hastif de juger l'urine, einz devez encercher et enquere diligentement la cause de la tenveté de l'urine, come se li malades avra [f.204v] dormi la nuit devant ou veillié, kar s'il a veillié la nuit devant et s'[a]esté [. . .], si saciés que la tenveté de l'urine est de ce que la matere est montee amont; [e] n'est pas de la consumption de lui. Mes si li malades ait esté en sa bone memorie la nuit devant et reposee natureument, se poez dire que la fevre le lasse del tot ou que il a terminé apertement.

[15] Et notés que nos donons choses digestives encontre cause de maladie que est a venir et n'est pas contre cause que est ja ensemble ovesques la maladie. Kar la cause joincte ja ovesque la maladie n'est pas appareillié a faire maladie, ainz la fait ja et est impossible que ele soit changé de sa qualité ne nos traveillons pas a voider le ovesque nos medicines, kar ele se degastera bien de sa propre chalor endementiers que ele fait s'action et dessout en fumez. Mes la matere et la cause de la ma[la]die qui est a venir defisons nos et la purgons come ele est deffite. Et chescun jor indicatif[44] devés vos regarder les signes de la digestion et les [f.205r] ovres de nature. Kar si l'urine ist en ces jors en grant quantité, donques devés ovrer des choses diuretiques. Et si vos volez lascher le ventrail plus qu'il n'est, si li donés choses moles et sorbibles sicome l'eue de la decoction de violettes, de prunes ou de mauves.

[16] Et si deit on aider nature par totes les parties ou ele tendra plus. Ewe diuretique contre chaude matere en caut tens come en esté chaut deit on faire des semences melonis, citrulis, cucumeris, cucurbite triblez et bolliez en ewe. Ou en verse ewe boillans sor eles come eles sunt bien tribleez et en colés l'ewe. Et come ele est fait en teu manere, si ad l'eue plus grant efficace. Mes en froit tens et a home de grant age deit on doner l'eue de la decoction de semence de ache, de fenoil, de peresil, de brusco, de sperago ou des racines de aux. Mes en esté tans come l'en travaille de froide matere ou en yver de caude, si doit on doner ewe diuretique faite de froides herbes et de chaudes. Et notés que on dora les cho[f.205v]ses evacuatives et digestatives contre cause de maladie que est a venir. Kar la cause que est conjoincte ovec la maladie

---

43 MS *del.*
44 MS *medicatif.* See below n.57 and 59.

degaste bien de sa propre chalor come ele font en fumee que fait la fevre, la quele come ele est degasté, si est li malades delivre par la maladie. Et come la matere est deffite, ce poés vos conustre par l'accession que vendra plus tost qu'il ne seut et li lerra plus tard et le tormentera plus. Et notés que autretele comparisun come il i a entre la chalor de nostre complexion[45] et le feu, autretel comparison i a il entre le matere de nostre complexion et la matere del feu. Kar nos veons bien ke si la busche est vert, que li feus se prent a tart et gete fors de lui un(e) poi de [flamme por la] verdeur [et] por la cruesce de lui, mes par longe action de la chalor et come totes les actions sont dessouses en fumee si devient une grant flaume par la secchesce que est la lime de chalor. Tot autresi come la matere de nostre chalor que est le feu de nostre cors est crue [f.206r] et defite, totes les autres choses en sont plus febles. Mes aprés la longe action de la chalor si devient la matere plus avanables a ardoir et aparçoit en soi la destemprance fevreuse et art plus aguement et dure l'accession plus por ce qu'il i a plus appareillé de la matere a ardoir et por ce qu'il remaint mains de la matere par l'ardor, si aproche l'estat de la maladie. Mes come l'accession vient plus tart et come l'affliction est lente et remisse et dure meins et meins et ne veés nul signe de digestion, icés choses sont signes que l'estat de la maladie est loi[n]g. Et come li mires verra ice, si ne doit li mires en nule manere purger le malade, la queu chose, s'il le fait, si fra la maladie estre plus long(n)e. Kar come il avera menees fors les plus soutilles parties de la matere que n'est pas defite, si remaindront les plus grosses et les plus terreuses et en ert li malades plus febles et en sont menees fors les bones humors en leu des mauvesses.

[17] Et notés que por ce que seignee est contenue souz [f.206v] purgation, la quele on deit faire au comence[me]nt dedens le tiers jor ou le quart. Dont Ypocras dist: 'Au comencement deit on movoir ce que on veit que fait a movir'[46] et ce entendon nus que on doit faire par seigné. Mes dou quint en avant n'avons pas apris que on doit seigner le malade, kar come l'en seut traire le sanc et oster qui est le norreture dou cors et le meillor ami que nature ait, s'en est li malades plus febles qui est cuit de la chalor de la fevre. Mes a seignés faire doit on regarder la force du malade et sun age deit l'en regarder, kar enfans et veille gens sont meins covenables a seigner, mes autrement les uns et autrement les autres. Kar les enfans ont les esperiz petiz et soutiz et deliez et s'en issent legerement come il trovent la veine[47] overte et come il ont mester de restauration des choses et de croistre la substance de lor membres, si est certaine chose qu'il perdent et l'un et l'autre come l'en les seig[f.207r]ne. Veille gens ne sont pas a seigner, que par le subtraction de sanc que norrist la chalor naturele ne soit estaint le chalor et que li malades ne muerge par defaute d'esperiz. La force dou malade doit l'en regarder, kar l'en doit bien criembre de seigner home feble devant la maladie et home afebli par maladie, ke il ne moire entre les mains au mire par la subtraction dou sanc, la queu chose, se on le fait, l'en verra bien qu'il en ert. Le tens de l'an doit l'en regarder, kar come li tens et li aier sont chaut mult, si doit on traire poi dou sanc, kar come l'en contrait mult la matere venimeuse et ague, si monte sovent

---

45   On the notion of 'complexion' see L. Thorndike, "*De complexionibus*", *Isis* 49 (1958), 398–408.
46   *Aphor.* II,29. Cf. Martin de Saint-Gille, *ed. cit.*, p.61, "En celles maladies au commencement, s'il est mestier de faire evacuacion, si la fay'.
47   MS *ucine*.

au cervel et met le malade en frenesie ou por la inanition[48] des veines come les ners sont secchiez et retraiz si chiet hom en espasme ou la fevre devient plus ardaunte por la secchesce et les autres accidens en devienent peiors. La converse avient come l'en seigne par trop froidure, kar par froidure doit l'en traire peu ou noient du [f.207v] sanc, kar les froides inspiracions de l'air amortifient les membres si il ne sont noris du sanc et por ce si deit hom regarder la region.

[18] Et notez que des le comencement de veir doit on seigner del senestre bras por les froides humors qui sorhabundent en cele partie. De icel tens en avant et de icele hore ariere doit on seigner du destre por les chaudes humors qui sorhabundent en cele partie. Et por les maladies du chief deit hom seigner du veine capitale, por les maladies des membres esperitez de la moiene veine du braz, et por les maladies des membres nutritives de la veine du foie. Donques come vus voudrés seigner le malade, cachiez tote la maisnie hors et aseurez le malade et enchisés[49] la veine du chief. Et si ce poet estre, si en traie on taunt de sanc ke la male[50] color change en bone et si frotés le chief, le col et la chere. Et premez aval le sanc jusc'a la espaule. Et se vus le seignez de la moine veine, [f.208r] se le premez le piz et les espaules et li commandés a toussir. Et se vos le seignez de la veine dou foie, se le frotez les membres nutritives et meimement de cele part ou vus le seignez. Et li levez un poi les quisses et li traiés le sanc devers la plaie et estopés la plaie a la fiez de vostre doi. Et après l'ostez por fere venir le sanc plus reddement et porter fors les choses noisantes qu'il encontrera.[51] Et ja soit ice que ceste manere de seigné enfeblist le malade par la perdition des esperiz qui en issent ovesques le sanc, si li metez es narines ewe rose ou violettes ou mirre solonc la matere de la seigné por restorer les esperiz qui sont perduz. Ou vus li arosés la chere de ewe froide por les esperiz fere entrer ens et conforter le quoer et les autres membres esperiteus. Et come vus l'averez seignié du sanc tant come mesters est et vus li averez lié bien et bel le bras, moillez vostre main en ewe froide et li aplaniez le bras contremont ou la liure nen est [f.208v] point por retorner le sanc qui fu ameu de venir a la plaie. Et ce deffendera icele partie a enfler. Et come vus avrez ce fait, si dorrez au malade sirop violat ou rosat ovecques ewe froide, si la maladie n'est par aventure reumatiques. Et si la maladie est reumatiques, si li donés penidias destemperees ovesque ewe d'orge. Mes s'il n'est pas reumatiques, si li donez lait d'alemandes ou mie de pain dessouse en ewe, kar icés beverages confortent le seigné et ne soevrent[52] pas en anguiser la colere. Et le couchiez en un leu oscur, que li esperit de la veine n'en evanice par la clarté de l'air. Et si devez un poi refroider la maison par art et meimement s'il fait chaut. Junche on donques la maison des foilles froides come de mirte, de sauz, de roseax et de foilles de vingne et de glaiox. Et face on l'ewe corre d'un vassel en autre et la meson ou il est si ait overt, si il fait chaut, les huis et les fenestres devers bise. Et gardez que li air ne soit corrumpus entor lui de nule male fumosité.

[19] [f.209r] Et notés que on seigne le malade por dous choses: por traire fors la matere de la maladie par conduit fait par art, sicome on fait en sinoque et es autres maladies

---

48 MS *matution*.
49 MS *enchoises*.
50 MS *meillor*.

51 MS *encontrerera*.
52 Apparently for *sueffrent* "allow, permit'.

engendrés du sanc, et por contregarder le malade de greignor maladie. Que quant on voit qu'il est plectoriques et que il ad les veines enflés et les membres pesans et tardifs a movoir et par large diete qu'il avra usé devant, les queles choses totes si sont signe de grant peril a venir,[53] et meimement come le[s] humors et les esperiz sont appareillez a destemprance de la destemprance de l'air, donques com vos averez doné choses digestives, si devés prendre garde es jors indicatifs queu chose et dont nature overe. Kar lors doit on veoir ce que doit avenir el jor cretique. Et si vos ne veez devant le jor cretique nul signe de digestion, si saciés que an jor de cretique que crisis serra nule ou, si il i a point, que ce sera par force de maladie et nient par la force de nature. Et si li malades se sent aleggés aprés, n'est [f.209v] pas a croire, kar ce ne vient pas de force de nature. Dont Ypocras dist: 'A ceus qui se sentent [aleggés] et n'est pas par force de nature ne doit on mie croire'.[54] Dont jo vus comant, si ce poet estre, que vus ne li donez pas medicine laxative si nature n'ait ovré avant, kar si nature a boté fors sicum Ypocras dist, ne covient pas novele chose faire mes fin. Come la matere sera botté tote fors par le ovre de nature, ce puet l'en conoistre par la tenvesce de l'urine et par le inanition dou pous et par ce que come crisis est parfite et bone, si perdera li malades le abhomination de manger, si lur vendra l'apetite de manger. Et li pous se carra en une rarté et l'urine se descolora et reposera li malades de nuit. Mes por ce qu'il i a nus malades qui sont plein de venim d'avarice, que come il veient nature veintre la maladie sanz l'aide dou mire, si detenent la deserte au mire et dient que n'i a fait li mires, donques poez muer et changer lor male opinion se faites qu'il semble que vus li avez [f.210r] aidé mult de saunté aver par doner li sirops et autre onctions fere, si qu'il quide que vus avés fait ce que nature li avra fait. Et li dites que li maladie li revendra plus cruelment aprés que ele n'a fait avant s'il n'a mult bone garde et bone aide des medicines et de autres choses. En tele manere si quidera li malades que vus li avez fait ce que la for[c]e de nature avra fait. Mes se nature ne poet parfitement faire crisim ou jor cretique et ele meine neporquant aucone chose fors du cors, si la devés aider et ce que ele ne porra fere que tu le parfacez par ton art et par ton enging. Et ce que en remandra si la metez fors par la ou nature ranpeira.

[20] Signes diverses:[55] Diverse signes sont de terminement a avenir solonc la sege de la matere, kar si la matere est en la boche de l'estomach, si sentira li maledes une morsure en l'estomac, abhomination, pruritus, li mangeront le levre et tremblera la levre desouz et li corneront les oreilles et [avra] dolor dou front. Totes icés choses sont signe que li [f.210v] malades terminera par voncher. Mes si la dolor est [es] boax et on a le ventre enflé et les costes pesans et meimement des le numbril en aval, icés choses sont signe de terminer par meneison. Mes si la dolor des reins est grans et les egestions petites, si poez savoir qu'il terminera par urine, [meimement] se on a le penil enflé et pesant. Mes mordications et pointures en fondement si son[t] signe que on terminera par flux des emorides et meimement come il ont esté coustomers d'aver les. Es femmes une pesanture es reins et es quisses si est signe de terminer par flux menstruel. Dolor

---

53 MS *tenir*.
54 *Aphor.* II,27. Cf. Martin de Saint-Gille, *ed. cit.*, p.61, "Es corps allegiez non selon raison, il n'esconvient pas croire . . .'
55 Rubric in MS.

ou front et es temples, les veines enflés et tendans, la veue[56] troublé et mangisons es narines si signefie terminement a bien par flux de sanc par les narines. Mes mordications du superficé del cors, tressailer et degeter sei et une chalor en la superficé du cors si sont signe de terminer par suor.

[21] Et de totes iceles choses serez vus plus certain ou jor cretique indicatif[57] et si vus veés iteus signes le[58] jor indicatif[59] devant. Et ce ert mult necessaire a nature qui travaille, kar se vus veés sig[f.211r]ne de voncher, si devez aider a nature par doner li sirop acetous ou ewe chaude solement. Et si vos veé[s] de terminement par egestions, si fetes emplastre sor le ventrail de oile violat ou des mauves, de bran[ca] ursina,[60] de la semence de lin, de fenugrec. Et notez que jo en ovre ensi por deffire la matere. Ou on les boille en ewe et li mete on ens par desouz. Ou on les mette sor le membre, la ou la matere siet pur deffire le, kar icés choses laschent les humors et alargissen[t] les condusz. Mes si vus veez signe de terminer par urine,[61] si li donez ewe chaude ou on avra tempré eins semences diuretiques; si par emorides, et eles soient enflees et eles ne corgent pas, ou vos ovrés d'une seigné[62] ou vos metés sancsues; si par flux menstruel, si mettés sor la matrix mauves quites en ewe. Si vu[s] veés signes de terminer par flux de seigner par les narines, et li sanc ne ne porra issir, si mettés soies de porc en un baston et li botés es narines et le movez en tornaunt tant que vos en rompez les veines et laissez hors le sanc; si par [f.211v] suor, si covrez bien le malade et li mette on une pot pleine de ewe boillante et li boute on desouz sa robe asperement, que ele ne puisse espandir. Et covre on bien le malade, que la chalor ne ne puisse issir, que la calor de l'ewe face ovrir les porres et laisse issir la suor. Et notés que si li malades a pris a suer de legier come il est seins, que l'en nel doit pas trop covrir. Car come les porres sont trop overt, si en issent les humors trestotes en fumee et remaint la suor. Dont vus verrés plusors gens que plus sueront com il sont covert d'un linceol e ouelement que si il fuissent mult tres bien covert.

[22] Et notés que en ver termine on plus sovent par flux de sanc dou nes que par aillors, car li sanc habonde lors del properté dou tens et por ce si seignons nos le malade meismement en icel tens. En esté tens entendon nos tant qu'il termine par voncher ou par suor por ce que les porres se overent par la chalor de l'air que les avirone et laissent fors la suor. Par voncher termine l'en sovent por ce que de la qualité du tens si habondent les humors legeres [f.212r] et chaudes en la boche de l'estomac. Dont nos solion doner vomitum en esté tens. Dont Ypocras dit qu'il covient purger par amont en esté et en yver par aval[63] et meimement come les conduiz esperitex sont plus larges par le inspiration de l'air chaut. Mes en aust et en yver sout on terminer

---

56 MS *veine*.
57 MS *medicatif*.
58 MS *et le*.
59 MS *medicatif*.
60 MS *de bran. de ursina*.
61 MS *brine*.
62 MS *flenie* (?).
63 *Aphor.* IV, 4. Cf. Martin de Saint-Gille, *ed. cit.*, p.71, 'En esté l'en doit purgier par en haut, et en yver par embas'.

par l'urine et par cesession, kar les porres environez de l'air froit si cloent et serent ensemble, si qui[64] suor n'i porra issir. Et por ce en yver si doit on aider le malade des choses laxatives par aval et des choses diuretiques.

[23] Issi parole de une maladie ke l'en apele crisis.[65] Et sachiés que crisis est faite a la fiez par ternaire et a la fiez par quaternaire. Si li malades est fors et movans, et ce poet on conoistre come il se torne et se moet, et si la matere est petite, et ce puet on conoistre par les parfites operations des vertuz et par les veines pleines et par la petitesce des superfluitez, et si la matere est appareillé a digestion, et ce conoistrés vus par l'urine que en espess. . . sera et par l'accession qui s'en avanchera et par l'aguesce de l'affliction come vus [f.212v] [. . .] totes icés choses coure[nt] ensemble, si sachiés que la maladie terminera par ternaire et tost. Et si une partie de ces choses courent ensemble, ja soit que li terminement tarde, si terminera la maladie totes voies par ternaire. Mes si vos veez[66] la converse avenir, si sachiés que la maladie terminera par quaternaire, ja soit que ele tarde come totes ces accidens courent ensemble, c'est a savoir feblesce de vertuz, multitude de matere et de duresce de lui ou tost come aucoune de ces defaillent. Mes la feblesce de nature demaunde que on termine plus sovent par ternaire en esté tens por la chalor de l'air qui ovre les porres. Mes en yver termine on plus par quaternaire, por la froidure que clot et sere les porres. Donques come li jor cretique vendra et vos aiez eu[67] les signes de la digestion de la matere, ne seez en esmai si li malade rebe et veillie et travaille la nuit devant le jor cretique, kar se vus en partés, un autre vendra en vostre leu et queudra le fruit que vus deussiés coillir. Mes crie[m]bre porrés vos, mes ne desesperez pas, kar [f.213r] ce avient sovent de la division de la matere par les membres, come nature se apparaille de terminement faire de la maladie. Mes come ce avient sanz nule signe de digestion que l'en ait eu avant, se poez avoir suspescion que ce est de la force de maladie et n'est pas de force de nature.

[24] Mes come aucoune chose revient de la matere de la maladie que soit a mener fors, si le devez mener fors de pilles et de electuaires. Mes en esté et meimement en tens chaut defendon nos a doner medicines aguisiés d'escamonie et a ceus qui sont purgiés [de] legier et qui ont les egestions coleriques ne a caus qui ont la foie eschaufé par coustume. Mes vus lor poez doner decoctions que vus freez en teu manere: vus boillerés prunes et viollettes en ewe et en cele ewe come vus l'averez colé si i metez une once [ou une] once et demie[68] de cassiavistula et ce est asavoir une once de thamarindes et les colés derechief et après metés i une once ou dous de mirabolans citrins en cele coleure et les laisse on temprer tote nuit la fors a l'air [f.213v] en cele coleure. Et au matin le colés bien et donés au malade. Et le doit on mels[69] [doner] au matin que de nuit, kar la calor qui est grant de nuit par dedens dessoudroit de legier la maladie. Le matin le donons nus plus que a miedi por ce que les membres nutritives sont plus fors de la froydure de l'air dou jor. Et de autre part si om donat itele decoction

---

64 *qui* for 'que'.
65 Rubric in MS.
66 MS *volez*.

67 MS *veue*.
68 MS *o. et demie once et $*.
69 MS *melsa*.

a miedi, le malades n'oseroit[70] manger trestot le jor. Et si doit om mettre en la decoction mirabolans qui sont pesanz et viscos et qui devienont a peine poudre par lor viscosité. Et si tost come vus l'avrés doné la decoction, se li fa[i]tes laver mai[n]tenant sa bouche de ewe froide et li donés un poi de sirop et de zucre a boivre por oster la savor de sa buche.

<hr />

[70] MS *noiseroit*.

GLOSSARY

Abhomination s. 19,20   distaste, disgust, nausea
Accés s. 8   bout, attack, onset [accesio]
Accession s. 8,16,23   bout, attack, onset [accessio]
Accident s. 2,17,23   symptom, sign [sinthoma]
Ache s. 13,16   smallage, wild celery (Apium graveolens L.) [apium]
Acoustumance s. 9   habit, custom [consuetudo]
Action s. 15,16   attack, onset [accessio]
Aguesce s. 23   acuteness [acumen]
Aguisié p.p. 24   sharpened, rendered more acute and pungent
Ai(e)r s. 17,22   air [aer]
Alamande, almaunde, amande s. 11,18   almond [amigdala]
Aleggé p.p. 19   relieved [alleviatus]
Ameu 18 p.p. of **amovoir**   to agitate, move, arouse
Amortifier v.a. 17   to deaden [mortificare]
Anguiser v.n. 18   to sharpen, become more acute [acuere]
Aoster v.a. 14   to remove
Aplanier v.a. 18   to touch, feel
Art s. 19   skill **par art** 18,19   artificially [artificialiter]
Asoter v.a. 6   to bemuse [obcaecare]
Aspere a. 11   rough
Astat s. 14   paroxysm [status]
Atente s. **la longe atente** 4   the long term
Atenvir v.n. 14   to thin [attenuare]
Avanable a. 16   prompt (to), ready (for), suitable (for) [habilis]
Avarice s. 19   avarice [avaritia]
Aventure s. **par aventure** 3,6,18   by chance, perhaps
Bise s. 18   north [septentrio]
Boax s.pl. 20   intestines [intestina]
Branca ursina s. 21   bear's breech (Acanthus mollis L.) [branca ursina]
Brusci, brusco s. 13,16   butcher's broom (Ruscus aculeatus L.) [bruscus]
Busche s. 16   wood, log [ligna]
Carnel a. 4   fleshy [carnosus]
Cassiavistula s. 24   a laxative pulp, purging cassia (Cassia fistula L.) [cassiafistula]
Cesession s. 22   defecation, evacuatiom of bowels [secessus]
Citrulis s. 16   water melon (Citrullus lanatus (Thunb.) Matsum and Nakai) and also
confused with white-flowered gourd (Lagenaria siceraria (Mol.) Standley) [citrulus]
Coin s. 9   quince (Cydonia oblonga Miller) [coctanus]
Colerique a. 24   made up of choler
Coleure s. 13,24   strained material [colatura]
Colere s. 13,18   choler, bile [colera] **colere vitelline** 13 bile the colour of egg yolk (deep
yellow tinged with red) [colera vitellina]
Compact a. 14   compacted [compactus]
Comparisun, comparison s. 16   comparison, resemblance
Complexion s. 16   complexion [corpus]
Conduit, condusz s. 19,21,22   channel, passage [meatus]
Conpaction s. 14   density, compression
Confés a. 3   confessed, shriven [confessus]
Conjoinct a. 16   joined (to), connected (with) [coniunctus]

Contraire v.a. 17   to draw off (blood)
Contregarder v.a. 19   to protect, preserve [preservare]
Converse s. 17,23   converse
Corgent pr.ind.6 of **cure**   to run
Corner v.n. 20   to buzz (of ears) [tinnitus]
Coustomer a. 20   accustomed
Covenable a. 17   suitable [idoneus]
Cresse s. 10   fat, fattiness [unctuositas]
Cretique a. 19,21   critical **jor cretique** 19,23   astrologically significant day of symptom's
first appearance [creticus]
Crisim, crisis s. 12,19,23   crisis [crisis]
Croistre v.a. 9,17   to increase
Cruesce s. 16   immaturity, fact of being unseasoned (of wood) [cruditas]
Cucumeris s. 16   cucumber (Cucumis sativus L.) [cucumis]
Cucurbite s. 16   various cucurbitaceae [cucurbita]
Declination s. **declination cretique** 8   subsiding of the crisis [declinatio cretica]
Decoction s. 9,11,15,24   decoction, liquid [decoctio]
Defaute s. 17   lack, deficiency
Def(f)ire v.a. 8,9,10,11,12,13,15,21   to dissolve, digest, consume [digerere]
Degaster v.a. 13,14   to consume [consumere]   v.refl. 15   v.n. 16 to be consumed
Degeter v.refl. 20   to gesticulate [iactatio]
Delié a. 17   fine, subtle
Delivre a. 16   free, freed (from)
Deserte s. 19   reward, remuneration [meritum]
Dessoudre v.n. 15   to be dissolved v.a. 24 to dissolve   **dessous** p.p. 16,18
Desteint p.p. 14   digested, absorbed [ad digestionem transivisse]
Destemprance s. 16,19   morbid condition [distemperantia]
Detenir v.a. 19   to withold [retrahere]
Digestif, digestatif a. 12,13,16,19   digestive [digestivus]
Diuretique a. 15,16,21,22   diuretic [diureticus]
Efficace s. 13,16   effect, influence
Egestion s. 20,21,24   excretion [egestio]
Electuaire s. 24   electuary [electuarium]
Elire v.a. 11   to select
Eliseez 8 imp.5 of **eslire**   to choose [eligere]
Emorides s.pl. 20,21   haemorrhoids, the five haemorrhoidal veins [emorroidae]
Emplastre s. 21   plaster [cathaplasma]
Enchiser v.a. 18   to cut [incidere]
Enfier v.n. 7   to trust, have confidence (in)
Enging s. 19   skill
Entrepolat a. 8   intermittent [interpolatus]
Escamonie s. 24   scammony (Convolvulus scammonia L.)
Escumer v.a. 13   to skim [dispumo]
Esmie de pain s. 11   crumb, soft part of bread [mica panis]
Espandir v.n. 21   to spill
Espasme s. 17   spasm [spasmus]
Espriz s.pl. 18   spirits, humours [spiritus]
Esquarteler v.a. 11   to grind to pieces [contero]
Essemblement adv. 14   thoroughly [essentialiter]
Estaim s. 13   tin [stagnatus]
Estaint 17 p.p. of **estaindre**   to extinguish
Estat s. 16   paroxysm [status]
Estouper v.a. 9,18   to stop up, block [opilare]
Estre prep. 6   besides, in addition to
Evacuatif a. 16   laxative, emetic [evacuans]

Evanice pr.sbj.3 of **evanir**   to vanish [evanescere]
Ewangeile s. 2   gospel [evangelium]
Ewe rose s. 18   attar of roses [aqua rosacea]
Fabler v.n. 3   to talk, converse (with)
Fenoil s. 13,16   fennel (Foeniculum vulgare Miller) error for fenugreek [fenugrecum]
Fente s. 14   dung, faeces [feces]
Fenugrec s. 21   fenugreek (Foeniculum vulgare Miller) [fenugrecum]
Fevre s. fevre continuel 8   continual fever
Fleume s. fleume naturele 13   uncorrupted phlegm [flegma naturale] **fleume verrigne** 13
congealed, glassy phlegm [flegma vitreum]
Flux s. 20   flow [fluxus]   **flux menstruel** 20,21   menstrual flow   **flux de sang** 20,21,22
flow of blood
Fondement s. 20   anus [anus]
Force s. 17,19   strength [vires]   **a force** 14   necessarily
Frenesie s. 17   madness, delirium [alienatio]
Fume s. 15   vapour [fumus]
Fumee s. 16,21   vapour (fumus)
Fumosité s. 18   vapour, fume [fumositas]
Fust s. 13   woody parts of plant [stipites interiores/exteriores]
Geline s. 11   hen [gallina]
Geu 2 p.p. of **gesir** v.n. to lie
Gise 4 pr.sbj. 3 of **gesir** v.n. to lie
Glajol s. 18   yellow flag (Iris pseudacorus L.), sweet sedge (Acorus calamus L.) [gladiolus]
Huis s. 18   door [porta]
Inanition s. 17   morbid depletion of bodily humours, 19   depletiom of pulse [pulsuum
inanitio]
Indicatif a. 15,19,21   indicative [indicativus]
Inspiracion s. 17,22   movement, current (of air) [inspiratio]
Interpollat a. 9   intermittent [interpolatus]
Juvencial s. 9   youth, young male [juvenis]
Laissié p.p. 9   loose, loosened [fluxus]
Lascher v.a. 15,21   to loosen [laxare]
Laxatif a. 19,22   laxative [laxativus]
Lin s. semence de lin 21   linseed [semen lini]
Liquidité s. 9   liquidity [liquiditas]
Liure s. 18   bandage [ligatura]
Maintenant adv. 8   at once [statim]
Maité, moité s. 13   half [mediocritas]
Malice s. 14   force, virulence [vis]
Mangisons s.pl. 20 itching, irritation [pruritus]
Matrix s. 21   womb [matrix]
Mauve s. 15,21   marshmallow (Althaea officinalis L.), mallow (Malva L. spp.) [malva]
Mediciner v.a. 12   to treat medically [medicare]
Meimement adv. 13,18,19,20,22,24 especially [maxime]
Mel s. 13   honey
Melancolie s. melancholy   **melancolie naturele** 13 black bile unmixed
Melonis s. 16   melon (Cucumis melo L.) [melo]
Memorie s. **en sa bone memorie** 14   in full possession of his wits [compos]
Meneison s. 20   diarrhoea, discharge from bowels containing blood [secessus]
Mes s. 7   dish (ferculum)
Mie de pain s. 18   crumb, soft part of bread [mica panis]
Mirabolan citrin s. 24   citrine myrobalan (Terminalia citrina Roxb.) [mirobolanus citrinus]
Mirre s. 18   myrrh [mirra]
Mirte s. 18   sweet gale (Myrica gale L.) [mirta]
Moiene a. 9   middle, intermediate [medius]

Moire 17 pr.sbj.3 of **murir**   to die
Moisteté s. 9   moistness [humiditas]
Mole s. 11   grindstone [mola]
Mordicacion s. 20   stinging irritation [mordicatio]
Morsure s. 20   biting sensation
Muerge 17 pr.sbj.3 of **murir**   to die
Multitude s. 23   great quantity [multitudo]
Noisant a. 18   noxious [nocivus]
Nuisance s. 9   harm [nocumentum]
Nutritif a. 9,14,18,24   nutritive [nutritivus]
Oile s.   **oile violat** 21   oil of violets [oleum violaceum]
Onction s. 19   ointment [unctio]
Orge s. barley   **ewe d'orge** 18   barley-water
Orgee s. 11   barley flour [far ordei]
Oximel s. 13,14   **oximel simple** 13   mixture of vinegar, herbs and honey [oximel simplex]
oximel composte 13   oximel compounded with other substances [compositum oximel]
oximel zaqueran 13   oximel with sugar substituted for honey and the addition of tart juice
of pomegranates [oxizaccaria]
Paissez 5 imp.5 of **paistre** v.a. to feed [pascere]
Peler v.a. 10   to peal, shell
Penidias s.pl. 18   barley-sugar [penidias]
Penil s. 20   pubes, groin [pecten]
Perdition s. 18   loss [perditio]
Per(r)esil s. 13,16   parsley (Petroselinum crispum (Miller) A.W. Hill) [petroselinum]
Pesantime s. 9   weight [gravitas]
Pesanture s. 20   heaviness [gravitas]
Pille s. 24   pill [pillula]
Plectorique a. 19   plethoric, characterizes by excess of blood or other humours [plectoricus]
Porre s. 21,22,2   pore [porus]
Poume grenate s. 13   pomegranate (Punica granatum L.) [granatum]
Pous s. 2,4,5,19   pulse [pulsus]
Practique s. 1   practice
Premer v.a. 17   to press
Preservatif a. 9   preventative
Preu s. 1   advantage, benefit, profit
Properté s. 22   property, distinctive quality
Prune s. 9,10,15,24   plum [prunus / pruna]
Pruritus s. 20   itching
Ptisane s. 11   infusion, tisane [ptisana]
Pointure s. 20   pricking, stinging sensation [punctura]
Quaternaire s. 23   count of four [quaternarium]
Que de . . . que de 4   partly . . . partly, both . . . and [tum . . . tum]
Queudra 23 fut.3 of **coillir**   to gather, collect
Rafanus s. 13   radish (Raphanus raphanistrum / sativus L.) (wild) radish [raphanus]
Ranper v.n. 19   to creep [repere]
Rarté s. 19   spareness [raritas]
Raseoir v.n. 14   to settle [resideo]
Ravir v.a. 14   to transport, bear away, transmit
Reber v.n. 23   to rave, be mad [alienus essere]
Reddement adv. 18   vigorously [impetuosius]
Refroider v.a. 18   to cool [infrigdare]
Remis p.p. 16   reduced, abated, in remission
Repost 4 p.p. of **repondre**   to hide [occultus]
Restauration s. 17   restoration [reparatio]
Retraiz 17 p.p.   shrunken, contracted [contractus]

Reumatique a. 18   rheumatic [reumaticus]
Rosel s. 18   reed [calamus]
Sancsue s. 21   leech [sanguissuga]
Sauler v.a. 6   to satisfy, satiate [saciare]
Sauz s. 18   willow [salix]
Sege s. 20   position [positio]
Seigné(e) s. 17,18,21   bleeding, phlebotomy [flebotomia]
Seign(i)er v.a. 17,18,19,22   to bleed [flebotomare]
Serer v.n. 22   v.a. 23   to close (become constricted)
Serré p.p. 9,14   constipated; dense, compact [constipatio]
Seut 16,17 pr.ind.3 of **soloir**   to be accustomed (to)
Sinoque s. 19   prolonged, continuous fever [sinochus]
Sirop s. 19,24   **sirop aceptous, syrop acetous** 13,21   decoction of honey and vinegar
[siropus acetosus]   **sirop violat** 18 syrup of violets **sirop rosat** 18   syrup of roses
Siuere s. 13   ?   [–]
Soie de porc s. 21   hog's bristle [seta porcina]
Solion 22 impf.ind.4 of **soloir**   to be accustomed
Someroun s. 4   tip (of the finger)
Sorbible a. 15   digestible [sorbilis]
Sout 6,22 pr.ind.3 of **soloir** v.n.   to be accustomed (to)
Sparge s. 13   asparagus (Asparagus officinalis L.) [sparagus]
Sperago s. 16   asparagus (Asparagus officinalis L.) [sparagus]
Squilla s. 13   squill (Scilla L. esp. Squila maritima Baker) [squilla]
Suavet adv. 4   gently [satis]
Subtraction s. 17   removal, drawing off [of blood]
Suor s. 20,21,22   sweat [sudor]
Superficé s. 10,20   surface [superficies]
Tenve a. 14   thin (tenuis)
Tenvesce s. 19   thinness [tenuitas]
Tenveté s. 14   thinness [tenuitas]
Terminement s. 20   critical culmination [crisis]
Ternaire s. 23   count of three [ternarium]
Terreux s. 16   lumpy, thick? [terrestris]
Thamarinde s. 24   tamarind (Tamarindus indica L.) [tamarindus]
Theorique s. 1   theory
Touaillie s. 10   napkin [gausape]
Tressailer v.n. 20   to leap, bound
Variance s. 4,5   variation [variae motus / mutatio]
Veine s.   **veine capitale** 18   cephalic vein   **veine moiene, moine veine** 18 median vein
[vena mediana]   **veine du foie** 18   hepatic vein   **veine du chief** 18 cephalic vein
Veillier v.n. 23   to lie awake, to be unable to sleep
Veir, ver s. 9,18,22   spring [ver]
Ventrail s. 9,15   stomach, intestines [venter]
Vers prep. 4   together with, in the company of
Vin e(a)gre s.13   vinegar [acetum]
Vingne s. 18   vine [pampinus]
Viol(l)ette s. 15,18,24   violet (Viola L.spp.) [viola]
Viscos a. 24   viscous [viscosus]
Viscosité s. 24   viscosity [viscositas]
Voider v.a. 15   to empty, evacuate   [evacuare]
Vomitum s. 22   vomitory [vomitum]
Voncher v.n. 20,21,22   to vomit
Vourunt 8 fut.6 of **voler**   to wish, desire
Zucre s. 13,24   sugar [zuccarum]

Proper Names

Ninive 2   Niniveh
Thobie 2   Tobias
Ypocras 12,17,19,22   Hippocrates

De instructione medici secundum Archimatthaeum
(MS Oxford, Bodleian Library, Digby 79)[1]

[Prologue]

[f.119v][1]   Cogitanti mihi votum vestrum votum bonum suborta est de affectu vestro leticia et gaudium de commodo futuro. Desideriis igitur vestris satisfaciens nota loquar frequenti [et] usu conprobata, et licet sicienti de fonte satius sit bibere quam de rivo, tamen ardor sitis ab eo extinguitur. Et quia noveram vobis esse paganis variis exeratas,[2] quibus ad conservanda sana et curanda egra vel neutra phisicalia tradebantur precepta, nolui ingratus vestri[3] et invidus antiquorum subiunctura nova condere vetera quod mihi quidem laboriosum vobis foret dispendium. Introductoria ergo quedam ad practicam sub quibusdam preceptis catholicum vobis disponere censui et [quia] quandoque plus [valet] arte per manus, mandatum novum do[4] vobis ut sicut ego facio, ita et vos faciatis.

[Advisable precautions]

[2]   Cum ergo, o medice, ad egrotum vocaberis, adiutorium tuum sit in nomine Domini. Angelus qui comitatus est Tobiam[5] affectum mentis et gressum corporis tui comitetur. In itinere tuo a nuncio sciscitare quantum [est] quod infirmus ad quem vocaberis laboraverit, qualiter ipsum egritudo invaserit, ut sinthomata inquirendo, si fieri potest, de egritudine certificeris. Hec autem sunt necessaria, ut quando ad ipsum accesseris, egritudinis eius non omnino inscius vel videaris esse ignarus, ut postmodum visa urina, considerato pulsu, licet per ea egritudinem non cognoveris, tamen sinthomata que presciveras dixeris, confidet in te, tanquam in auctorem sue salutis, ad quod summopere laborandum est.

[3]   Cum igitur ad eius domum accesseris, antequam ipsum adeas quere si conscientiam suam sacerdoti manifestaverit, quod si non fecerit aut faciat aut se facturum promittat; quia si inspecto infirmo et consideratis egritudinis signis super hiis sermo fuerit, de sua incipit desperare salute, quia et te desperare putabit, et hoc omittendum non est, quia multe egritudines propter peccata emergunt que lacrimis conscientie

1   Corrections have been made from three other witnesses: B = Oxford, Bodleian Library, Bodley 361 (S.C. 2462) pp.432–44 (a truncated and sometimes garbled text); W = Winchester College MS 26 ff.35ra–42vb; P = Oxford, Pembroke College 21 ff.189v–192r.
2   *per paginas variis litteris excecratas* (W).
3   *videri* (B).
4   MS *de*.
5   See Tob. 5, 6 *et seq.*

sorde mundata a summo cura[n]tur medico secundum illud evangelii 'Vade et amplius noli peccare ne tibi deterius contingat.'[6] Ingrediens ad infirmum nec superbientis vultum nec cupidi pretendas affectum, assurgentes tibi pariter et salutantes humili gestu resalutatis, eis sedentibus sedeas. Cum vero pectus resumpseris, quibusdam verbis interpositis quibus debes illius regionis situm commendare, dispositionem domus in qua es,[7] si expetierit, laudare vel curialitatem gentis extollere.

[4] Tandem ad infirmum conversus, qualiter se habeat queras, et brachium tibi exhiberi precipias, et hec que diximus sunt admodum necessaria, ut in omnibus tuis moribus astantium compares favores. Et quia spiritus in te ex itinere moti sunt[8] et infirmus qui in adventu tuo multum delectatur, [f.120r] vel quia iam tamquam avarus de precio cogitat[9] [vel] propter diversas animi passiones, tum de culpa tui tum de infirmi vicio, [in pulsuum cognitione deciperis]. [Data ergo securitate infirmo] in te impetuosior spiritus motu cessante pulsum in brachio sinistro consideres, quia licet cor in dextra parte sufflet, tamen quilibet motus cordis ex propinquitate in sinistro facillime cognoscitur in brachio. Et attende ne super illud latus infirmus iaceat, quia per conpressionem impeditur motus spiritus et neque digitos habeat extensos in palmam neque reductos in pugnum, et tue dextre manus apponens digitos cum sinistra sustentans brachium, quia ex maiori sensibilitate dextre partis tue facilius varios motus discernes et egri brachium tamquam debile tuo indiget adminiculo. Et si brachium plenum est et carnosum, digiti imprimantur, ut occultis aproximent arteriis; si vero gracile et extenuatum, sit tibi satis in superficie pulsus percipere et usque ad centesimam percussionem ad minus pulsum consideres, et ut diversa pulsuum investiges genera et adstantes [ex longa] exspectatione verba tua gratiora[10] suscipiant.

[5] Deinde precipias tibi urinam afferri qua etsi pulsus immutatio ipsum egrotare significet, genus tamen egritudinis melius urina designat et eger egritudinem non solum per urinam sed etiam per pulsum te cognovisse putabit. Cum autem urinam inspexeris, diu intendas colorem, substantiam, qualitatem, quantitatem atque contentum, ex quorum diversitate diversa egritudinum cognosces genera, sicut in tractatu nostro[11] de urinis docetur.

[6] Deinde egro ab ore tuo pendenti salutem promittas. Cum autem ab eo recesseris, domesticis eius dicas ipsum multum laborare quia propter hoc, si liberatus fuerit, meriti maioris eris et laudis, si vero mortuus fuerit, testabuntur te de eius[12] desperasse salute.[13] Unum preterea moneo, nec eius uxorem, filiam vel ancillam respicias [oculo] cupido nec species te decipiat muliebris. Hec enim operantis medici obcecant animum et

6   John 5, 14 'iam noli peccare, ne deterius aliquid contingat'. Cf. P. Diepgen, *Die Theologie und der arztliche Stand* (Berlin, 1922), pp.49ff.
7   MS *inquires*.
8   B adds 'vel propter varios astantes tibi vel ignotos vel quia infirmus . . .'
9   B adds 'vel quia tui nobilitatem et sui parvitatem vel e converso considerat'.
10 MS ?*grandia*.
11 MS *nr̄e*. The reference is omitted in B.
12 MS *eo*.
13 MS *salutem*.

cooperantis dei inmutant sententiam et medicum infirmo efficiunt honerosum et de se minus sperantem. Sis ergo sermone blandus, vite spectabilis, divino expetens auxilio iuvari. Cum autem te ad prandium, ut solet fieri, qui domui presunt invitaverint, nec te importunum ingeras nec in mensa primum eligas locum, licet sacerdoti et medico, ut solet fieri, primus accubitus preparetur. Potum tibi propinatum nullum contempnas, cibos nec vituperes nec fastidias qui forte de iure et genere rusticano miliaceo pane ventris esuriem vix consueveras saciare. Quod si feceris, omnium in te animus conquiescet et notus in tuas laudes inde prorumpet.

[7] Cum autem ferculorum varietate tua fuerit intentio occupata, per aliquem circumstantium sepe infirmi statum requiras. Quod si feceris, de te plurimum confidet [f.120v] infirmus quem videt inter delicias sui oblivisci non posse. Cum autem a cena surgens ad egrum etiam intraveris, dicas tibi fuisse oppi[pa]re ministratum, de quo infirmus valde delectabitur, quia ad hoc non modice sollicitus fuerat.

[8] Si vero tempus cibandi infirmum fuerit, ipsum cibabis. Tempus autem cibandi optimum elige: in interpolatis, quando sunt in vera quiete; in continuis, quando [est] tempus false quietis, quia usque ad creticam declinationem sine febre non inveniuntur. Et notandum quia in interpolatis tanto tempore ante accessionem infirmi sunt cibandi, ut cum ventum fuerit ad tempus accessionis cibus ex toto sit digestus, aliter natura duplici erit in bello dum escam importune ingestam non valebit digerere nec hostem poterit superare. Si vero accessio febrilis anti[ci]pet nec cibandi ante accessionem oportunam horam invenias, exspecta donec accessio cessaverit et non [statim] infirmum cibabis, quia membra ex precedenti bello et hostis insultu defatigata nullum honus ex cibo sibi volunt imponi, sed tamquam post triumphum de hoste quietem desiderant. Exspecta ergo ad cibandum spatium duarum horarum post accessionem vel ad minus unius hore.

[9] Cibabis ergo infirmum secundum genus egritudinis et secundum tempora anni et secundum etatem,[14] variata qualitate et quantitate cibi. Nam ampliori cibo cibabis pacientem in interpolata quam continua et superiori in continua quam in interpolata;[15] ampliori in hieme et vere, minori estate et autumpno gravissime ferunt cibos. Considerabis etatem quia pueros sepius reficies quam iuvenes, quia in eis maior est consu[m]ptio propter liquiditatem humiditatis et quia [cibo] indigent ad augmentum naturale, ut[16] cotidie perdita reparentur.[17] Senes pauciori cibo reficies et propter caloris debilitatem et virium[18] imbecillitatem, tandem secundum eius etiam consuetudinem, quia si ampliori et grossiori ut[ent]i consueverat cibo, non debet sibi esse equalis exhibitio ipsi et sorbili sive modica dieta uti. Tandem te oportet [attendere] constipationem[19] vel fluxum [sive medium] inter hec, quia si fluxus fuerit, a grossiori

---

14 MS *varietates*. The A–N translation 'solonc l'age' presupposes the reading 'etatem', cf. Renzi's reading 'etates'.
15 B has 'fortiori', W 'et frigidiora in interpolata quam continua'.
16 MS *et*.
17 MS *reparantur*.
18 MS *vicium et*.
19 MS *consuptionem*.

incipies[20] cibo [ut] a piris, coctanis, et sorbis, quia hec grossicie sua opilabunt et qualitatibus constipabunt. Si vero constipatio fuerit, incipiens a sorbilibus et lenientibus, dabis pruna et aquam decoctionis prunorum, deinde grossa, que gravitate sua ea cicius exire compellant. Si vero inter hec medium fuerit, a suptilioribus et liquidioribus tamen incipies,[21] quia satis est utile egro et [ad] preservationem maioris nocumenti si ventris procuretur officium, quia superfluitatum emissio non solum nutritiva verum etiam universa membra alleviat.

[10]   Dabis ergo pruna cocta in aqua vel granata vel lac amigdalarum, quod sic[22] preparabitur: amigdale enucleate ponantur in aqua calida ut rigore corticis lentescente possi[n]t mundari. Deinde conterantur fortiter et aliquantulum aque frigide addatur et omnia simul moveantur et per gausape nitidum coletur et quod inde exierit propinetur. Si vero in olla aliquantulum decoquatur cum mica panis, perfectius digeritur quam si crudum bibatur. Et notandum quia postquam amigdalum erit paratum, debet aliquantulum dimitti et postea cum exsufflatione eiciatur unctuositas que est in superficie que esset fomentum caloris.

[11]   Hoc idem facio: propino ius ubi gallina est decocta vel aqua ubi resolvitur mica panis. Deinde dabis far ordei quod sic facies: ordeum bene mundabis et frigida aqua effusa sparsum super lapidem fortiter fricabis ut excorietur. Deinde pistetur in mortario vel inter molas conteratur in grossiores partes et hoc far optime decoquatur et iam circa finem decoctionis adde aliquantulum lactis amigdalarum et postea offeras egrotanti. Si vero ptisanam facere volueris, far odei et quod inde egreditur erit ptisana quam ei propinabis in potu, sive aquam ubi positus sit panis sive aquam bullitam infrigdatam. Et nota quia cibo existente in stomaco neque aquam diureticam ne surupum exhibebis quia ista cogunt cibum indigestum exire vel digestionem retardant.

[Digestives]

[12]   Notandum preterea est quia medicum a principio morbi cum digestivis expedit obviare. Ipse enim minister nature ipsius opera desiderat immutari que semper nobis debet esse preambula et magistra. Sicut ergo natura ad faciendam crisim, ad triumphandum de morbo vires morbi enervare laborat, materiam a sui prava qualitate alterando, ipsam per membra partiendo, ut partibus alterutrum separatis toto effectu debili e[x]pulsioni a[d] quam facilius intendat, celebret. Sed medicus ad expellenda nociva sibi debet preparare viam nature secundum istud: *Medicari oportet digesta et movere non cruda.*[23]

[13] Considerata egritudinis causa variantur digestiva humorum, nam colera si fuerit egritudinis causa[24] vel alius humor calidus et siccus, siropum acetosum dabis ad digerendum. Si vero flegma naturale, acetosum vel vitreum sive melancolia naturalis

[20] MS *incipiens*.
[21] MS *incipiens*.
[22] MS *sic sic*.

[23] Hippocrates, *Aphor.*I,22.
[24] MS *causa e variantur*.

sive colera vitellina, maxime in hieme dabis oximel nisi forte inde fiat febris continua et tempus anni sit calidum.[25] Fiat autem sirupus acetosus sic: in duabus partibus aceti bulliat tercia pars zuccari usque ad mediocritatem et si vultis spissum facere, plus bulliat et aliquantulum zuccari addas. Sed sciatis quia minus erit efficax ad dividendum licet gustui sit suavior. Eodem modo fiet oxizaccaria de succo granatorum acetosorum et zuccero. Oximel simplex sic fit: mel primo dispumetur in stagnato. Eiecta spuma addantur duas partes aceti et bulliat totum usque ad medietatem. Compositum oximel sic facias: radices apii, petrosilini, fenugreci, sparagi [f.121v] et brusci et raphani[26] sive squille[27] dimittantur in aceto ad minus per tres dies et a radicibus eiciantur stipites interiores.[28] Postmodum colato aceto mel addatur vel si cicius volueris facere, bullire in aceto facias radices contritas et adito mele fiat oximel.

[14]   Huiusmodi digestiva dabis cum aqua calida, mane autem dantur quia in nutritivis non inveniunt cibaria a quibus impediantur et virtus eorum debilitetur et sapor abhominabilis reprimatur et feces dissolvantur. Dentur autem ista donec signa digestionis emergantur que in urina et in modo afflictionis discernetis. Per urinam ergo dupliciter quia urina aliquando est discolorata, aliquando est colorata, aliquando tenuis, interdum vero spissa. Si ergo urina a principio est discolorata et tenuis et postmodum fiat colorata et spissa, materiam significat de quadam cruditate ad digestionem transivisse. Primo enim cum materia compacta et cruda debilem in se caloris actionem susciperet, urinam colorare non poterat et quia a se tamquam compacta parum aut nihil emittebat quod sui admixtione inspissaret urinam. Urina autem erat tenuis. Nunc autem cooperantibus digestivis ab excocta materia flamma maior emittitur et relaxata terrestritate humoris materia egritudinis essentialiter admisceatur urine. Unde urina coloracior erit, pariter conspissior. Si vero urina a principio discolorata exit et spissa, hanc substancie turbationem de multitudine superfluitatum dicimus provenire, que non opere nature sed vi sinthomatis admisceatur urine. Et cum urina mane mincta manet spissa, si vero residens attenuatur, digestionem humoris significat et statum propinquum. Si vero post spissam exit tenuis, horum duorum unum non effugiet quin hoc, aut sit ascensu materiei aut de eius consumptione. Et ideo medicus in iudicio preceps esse non debet, sed tenuitatis causa cum diligentia investigetur. Si nocte precedente eger vigiliarum instancia laboraverit et extitit alienus, de ascensu materiei noveris provenisse. Si vero eger sui compos fuerit vel steterit et nocturna quies naturalis precesserit, dicas febrem aut omnino cessasse aut manifestam declinationem habere.

[15]   Et notate quia nos damus digestiva ad antecedentem causam digerendam et non coniunctam, quia coniuncta non paratur ad egritudinem faciendam, immo eam facit. Et impossibile est admodum a sua qualitate alterari nec ad eam evacuandam cum nostra laboramus medicina, quia ipsa proprio calore consumitur dum accessionem facit et in fumum resolvitur. Antecedentem ergo causam digerimus et digestam postmodum evacuamus et nos in singulis diebus indicativis signa digestionis attendamus et opera nature consideramus, quia si in eis maior urine exierit copia,

---

25 P ends here (f.192r).
26 MS *raphanus*.

27 MS *squilla*.
28 MS *exteriores*.

diureticis insistemus,[29] ut aqua decoctionis violarum vel prunorum vel malvarum. [f.122r]

[16] Inde enim natura iuvanda est unde repit. Aquam diureticam contra calida[m] materiam in tempore calida et etate calida facietis de semine citruli, melonis et cucu[meris], et semina contrita bulliant in aqua vel super ea contrita effundatur aqua fervens et semina dilaterentur et aqua coletur et si sic fiat, efficacior erit aqua. In tempore vero frigido et etate superiori[30] contra materiam frigidam detur aqua decoctionis seminum apii, petroselini, fenugreci, sparagi et brusci vel radicum eorum. Si vero in estate de frigida materia laboraverit vel in hieme de calida tam ex calidis quam ex frigidis, aqua diuretica preparetur. Et notate quia tam digestiva quam evacuantia dantur contra causam antecedentem. Coniuncta enim causa proprio calore consumitur dum in fumum facientem febrem exsolvitur, qua consumpta si antecedens est digesta vel evacuata, liberatur infirmus. Per egritudinem digestionem materiei cognoscimus .s. per anticipationem accessionis, per acumen afflictionis, per diuturnitatem affligendi. Sic notandum est quia ignis corporis nostri igni comparatur exteriori, sicut ignis nostri materia exterioris ignis materie est comparanda. Videmus enim quia si ligna viridia sunt, ignis in eis tarde accenditur et propter eorum cruditatem et vi[ri]ditatem modica flamma emittitur, sed diuturna caloris accessione aquosioribus partibus resolutis in fumum siccitate inducta que est luna caloris rogus maior efficitur, sic materia ignis nostri cruda existente et indigera omnia sunt imbecilliora. De vero actione caloris diuturna materia successioni fit habilior et febrilem in se distemperantiam citius suscipit et acutius ardet et succensio diutius perseverat, quia plus de materia ad succensionem paratur et quia minus parandum remanet, status egritudinis apropinquat. Postposita vero remissio vel tarditas affligendi nullo digestionis signo precedente statum narrat esse remotum, quod cum medicus viderit, nullo modo purgare presumat. Quod si fecerit et morbus fiet prolixior, dum indigestione materiei suptilioribus eductis partibus reliquum fiet terrestre et erit debilior cum vice malorum boni educerentur humores.

[Phlebotomy]

[17] Sciendum est quia sub purgatione flebotomia continetur, quam a principio facimus usque ad quartum diem vel ad plus usque ad .v. diem secundum illud Ypocratis: *Inchoantibus morbis si quid videtur movere move.*[31] Hanc motionem maxime per flebotomiam intelligimus. A quinto die in antea facere non consuevimus, quia subtracto sanguine fomento caloris amico nature debilitatur infirmus febrili calore excoctus. Sed ad flebotomiam faciendam considerare oportet vires egri, etatem infirmi, [f.122v] temporis qualitatem et situm regionis. Etatem attendimus, [quia] pueros enim et senes ad fleobotomiam non invenimus idoneos, aliter tamen et aliter, nam in pueris spiritus modicus est et suptilis quia aperta vena facile evaporat et quia ad reparationem

---

29 W adds 'si vis venter plus soluto procuretur, lenientibus et sorbilibus insiste ut aqua . . .'
30 MS *frigidiori.*
31 *Aphor.* II, 29.

perditorum indigent et augmento. Subtracto sanguine certum est utrumque cessare sufficienter. Senes vero flebotomare timemus, ne subtracto sanguine fomento caloris extinguatur calor et propter defectum spirituum mortificetur infirmus. Vires consideramus infirmi quia debilem ante egritudinem et ex egritudine nimis debilitatur fleobotomare timemus ne subtracto sanguine inter manus medici cito exsolvatur, quod si fiat quid inde sequatur tu videris. Tempus anni considerabis quia in vehementer calido aere parum aut nichil sanguinis detrahatur. Nam si multum detrahitur aut furiosa effecta materia superiora petens alienationem inducit aut propter venarum et arteriarum inanitionem desiccatis et contractis nervis sequitur spasmus, aut ex siccitate efficitur febris ardentior et sinthomata ultimantur. E contrario in nimis frigido tempore parum aut nichil sanguinis detrahatur, quia frigidi aeris inspiratione nisi a sanguine foveantur membra mortificantur. Et secundum hoc etiam regionem attendimus.

[18] Et notandum quia a principio autumpni usque ad principium veris de sinistro brachio sanguinem detrahes, quia in hiis temporibus in sinistra parte frigidi humores habundant. A principio veris in antea de dextro brachio, quia in ea parte calidi augmentantur humores. Et propter passiones cerebri venam incidetis cephalicam, propter spiritualium morbos medianam, propter egritudinem nutritivorum epaticam.

Cum ergo egrotantem flebotomare volueris, presentes abice, securitatem indicis, fluentis sanguinis colorem attendas, ut si fieri potest, tamdiu trahatur sanguis donec color malus mutetur in bonum. Et dum cephalica vena inciditur, caput, facies, collum fricetur et prematur usque ad humerum. Si vero mediana, fricentur atque premantur pectus et scapule et ut tussiat precipe. Si vero epatica, nutritiva manibus fricentur et illius partis in qua fit flebotomia crus aliquantulum sublevetur ut illius partis fiat compressio et interdum digito apposito fluentem repellas sanguinem ut iterum impetuosius currens nociva que invenerat impellat facilius, licet hic modus flebotomandi egrum debilitet quia spirituum fit multa perditio. Dum vero sanguis exit, naribus apponas aquam ro[saceam] vel vio[laceam] vel mirtum secundum quod tempus anni exigerit ut fiat spirituum reparatio. Vel aqua frigida rorabis faciem, ut spiritus ad interiora revocati confortent principia. Iam sanguine sufficienter detracto et ligato brachio manum tuam aqua frigida infusam superpones ubi non est liga[f.123r]tura usque ad humerum. Hec enim venientem repellit sanguinem et illius partis tumorem prohibet sive gravedinem. Hoc facto mulsam, siropum ro[saceum] vel viol[aceum] cum aqua frigida propinabis infirmo, nisi forte sit egritudo reumatica, que si fiat, dabis penidias distemperatas in aqua ordei; si vero non fuerit, dabis etiam lac amigdalarum vel micam panis resolutam [in aqua]. Hii enim potus et flebotomatum confortant et subtracto sanguine non permittunt acui coleram. Aer etiam debet obscurus fieri, ne per disgregationem claritate aeris spiritus evanescat. Debet etiam aliquantulum artificialiter infrigdari maxime si aer naturaliter sit calidus. Spargatur ergo pavimentum frigidis frondibus mirte, salicis, calami, pampini, gladioli, junci vel querci; aqua etiam de vase[32] in vase currat ut aer infrigdetur. Domus in qua moratur fenestras et portas habeat versus septentrionem ne aliqua fumositate putredinis quem inspirat aer inficiatur.

---

[32] MS *valle*.

[19]   Notandum vero quia flebotomia propter duo fit .s. ut aliqua egritudinis materia per artificialem detrahamus meatum ut fit in sinochis et in aliis continuis, vel ut egrum a maiori egritudine preservemus. Cum videmus ipsum esse plectoricum, venas turgidas et inflatas habentem, membra gravia et ponderosa ad motum, que omnia dieta larga precedente maiora pericula futura minantur et maxime cum ex resolutionibus et aeris distemperantia distemperatis spiritibus humores venarum parati sunt distemperari, datis ergo digestivis, in diebus indicativis attendas quid et unde natura operatur. Quia tunc indicatur quid sit futurum et si ante diem creticum nulla signa digestionis videris, scias in die cretico aut non futuram crisim aut si fiat non erit vi nature sed vi sinthomatis secundum illud: *Alleviatis et non secundum rationem non oportet credere.*[33] Unde precipio ut, si fieri potest, nisi precedente opere nature medicinam laxativam non detis. Si natura totam nocivam expellit, ut dicit Ypocras, non oportet novum facere, sed finem. Materiam vero totam opere nature expulsam fore cognoscimus per urine tenuitatem, per pulsuum[34] inanitionem, et quia perfecta crisi fastidium cessat quo infestabatur infirmus, pulsus in quadam cadent raritate et urina discolorata cum quiete naturali nocturna. Sed quia quidam infirmi avaricie inebriati veneno dum vident sine medici auxilio naturam triumphare de morbo, meritum medici retrahunt, pariter et retardant dicentes 'quid fecit medicus?', ut autem ab iniqua opinione mutentur, siropis, unctionibus, fomentis videamur adducere salutem quam adduxit natura et in alterius intremus laborem dicentes morbum postmodum futurum graviorem insultum nisi ei medicine auxilio et succursu subveniatur et sic quod nature fuerat imputabitur medico.[f.123v] Si vero die cretico adveniente natura crisim perfectam operari non poterit, tamen aliquid eduxit a corpore, tunc, o medice, iuva naturam et quod natura non fecit artificium tuum perficiat et que remanserint educas unde natura repit.

[Crisis]

[20]   Sunt autem diversa signa crisis future secundum positionem materiei, nam si materia fuerit in ore stomachi, abhominatio, pruritus labiorum, citatio inferioris labii, tinnitus aurium, dolor augmentatus in fronte futuram crisim per vomitum significabunt. Si vero dolor[35] intestinorum, inflatio ventris et laterum gravitas maxime ab umbilico inferius, per secessum crisim exspectabis. Si vero dolor lumborum augmentatur egestione modica exeunte, per urinam fiet crisis, maxime si est gravitas pectinis et tumor. Si vero in ano mordicatio nimia est et punctura, crisis fit per emorroidas, maxime si eas consuevit habere; in mulieribus, per menstrua, si vero gravitas est lumborum, femoris et coxarum et si tempus menstruorum advenit. Dolor frontis, temporum, extensio venarum, perturbatio visus, pruritus aurium, sanguinem a naribus fluere denunciant. Superficiei corporis mordicatio, saltus et quedam iactatio et in superficie maior calor sudorem promittunt.

[33] Hippocrates, *Aphor.* II, 27.
[34] MS *p. et.*
[35] MS *dolorem.*

[21] Et de hiis certiores erimus adveniente die cretico indicativo, si in precedente talia emersere. Et hoc valde necessarium ad cognitionem ut et opem feras laboranti nature. Nam si vomitus est futurus, dato siropo acetoso vel sola aqua frigida seu calida digitis seu penna ori immisa juvetur natura. Si vero per secessum moveatur venter, cum oleo violaceo inungatur, cathaplasmetur cum malvis, branca ursina, semine lini et fenugreci. Et notate quod ego istis utor ad digestionem materiei superponendo ea bullita in aqua membro in quo continetur materia digerenda, quia hec laxant humorem et alargant meatus. Si vero per urinam, dabitur aqua calida in qua dilacerentur semina diuretica. Si vero per emorroidas et ipse fuerint turgide nec tamen sanguinem emiserint, vel flebotomum appones vel sanguissugas. Si vero per menstrua, malvas bullitas in aqua mulier matrici supponat. Si vero sanguinis fluxus[36] ex naribus signa apparent nec tamen sanguis fluit, cum setis porcinis in modum crucis in aliquo ligno impositis frequenter movendo lignum inter nares venas narium rumpens sanguinem[37] provocabis. Si vero per sudorem, egrum cooperietis, urceolum in se habentem aquam ferventem[38] undique obvolutum panno teneat iuxta se sub pannis ut eius vapore apertis poris sudor provocetur. Et notate quod si eger consuevit in sanitate citissime sudare, non debet multis pannis operiri, quia poris immoderate apertis humores in fumositates evaporabunt et sudor nullus emerget. Unde vos videbitis multos magis sudantes cum solo lintheamine quam cum pluribus operimentis.

[22] Sciendum vero est quod in vere[39] [f.124r] crisi[m] per fluxum sanguinis maxime exspectabis, quia de proprietate temporis sanguis habundat et tunc in vere flebotomiam morbo imputamus. In estate[40] sudorem vel vomitum exspectabis; sudorem quia calore aeris circumdante[41] pori sunt aperti, vomitum quia de qualitatibus temporis calidi et leves in ore stomachi habundant humores. Et inde nos in estate exspectare consuevimus secundum illud:[42] Estate purgare oportet per superiora et maxime cum calidi aeris inspiratione spirituales meatus sunt largiores. Autumpno et hieme crisim per urinam vel per secessum exspectabis, quia frigido aere circumdante constrictis poris et eiusdem visitatione[43] spiritibus infrigdatis in hiis temporibus frigidi generati hu[mores] nec educi in vomitum nec parati sunt erumpere in sudorem. Et ideo in hieme cum diureticis et per inferiora laxantibus subveniendum est.

[23] Sciendum vero est quod crisis aliquando fit per ternarium, aliquando per quaternarium. Si eger fortis est, quod per facilem eius motum cognosces, et si materia est pauca, quod ex hoc perpendes quia operationes virtutum perfecte sunt et venarum non est plenitudo nec superfluitatum multitudo, et si materia [apta] ad digestionem, quod in urine inspissatione, [in] veloci anticipatione[44] accessionis [et] acumine afflictionis cognosces, hiis omnibus concurrentibus, per ternarium et cito scias egritudinem terminari. Si vero quedam adsunt, per ternarium sed tarde determinabuntur. Tamen semper et principaliter ad hoc fortitudo virtutis egritudinis exigit. Si vero e

---

36 MS *fluxerit.*
37 MS *et sanguinem.*
38 MS *fluentem.*
39 MS *vera.*
40 MS *estatem.*

41 MS *circumdantes.*
42 Hippocrates, *Aphor.* IV, 4.
43 MS *visitationem.*
44 MS *anticipationem.*

contrario[45] accidit, per quaternarium determinabitur egritudo sive tarde omnibus
convenientibus .s. debilitate virtutis, multitudine materiei et compactione ipsius sive
quibusdam cito deficientibus. Si tamen debilitas nature exigit, et in estate sepius per
ternarium et cito calore aeris apertis meatibus determinacionem egritudinis exspectabis, hieme vero per quaternarium et tardius poris aeris frigiditate constrictis.
Adveniente vero die cretico signis digestionis precendentibus, si in nocte precedente
diem creticum eger alienus sit, vigiliarum instantia laboret, nulla te desperatio
perturbet, quia si recesseris, alius in labore tuo intrabit et laboris tui fructus percipiet.
Timens ergo sed noli desperare quia hec fiunt de divisione materiei per membra, cum
se natura preparat ad faciendam crisim. Si vero hoc fierent nullo signo digestionis
precedente, suspecta essent quod vi sinth[o]matis et non nature acciderent.

[Decoctions, syrups, pills and electuaries]

[24] Si ergo facta crisi aliquid remanserit quod sit educendum, educetis cum decoctionibus, siropis, pillulis vel electuariis. In estate ergo et maxime in regione calida
scamoneatas medicinas dare prohibemus et hiis qui facile purgantur et quorum
egestiones sunt colerice et quibus epar de consuetudine est calefactum. Dabis ergo
decoctiones [f.124v] quas sic facies. Pruna [et] viole bulliant in aqua et in ea aqua
colata resolvatur uncia una vel uncia una et semis cassiafistule et semis tamarindi et
iterum colabis et apponatur uncia una et semis vel duos mirobolanum citrinum et tota
nocte dimittas sub divo si fieri potest. Et mane colatum dabitis. In mane debet dari et
magis quam in nocte, quia in nocte calor in interioribus multiplicatus liquidam
materiam facile exsolveret. Mane magis damus quam in meridie, quia in mane ex
frigiditate nocturni aeris nutritiva sunt fortiora. Est et aliud quia si in meridie daretur
decoctio, eger tota die non auderet commedere et vos in decoctione debetis ponere
mirobolanos qui sunt graviores, viscosiores et qui viscositate sua vix possunt pul-
verizari. Data decoctione statim lavetur cum aqua frigida. Detur aliquantulum siropi
vel zuccari ad potandum ut tollatur malus sapor.

[The Anglo-Norman translation ends here]

Commasticentur aliqua poma vel menta vel fenum grecum. Ligentur brachia fortiter,
ut per talem stricturam constringatur[46] os stomachi ut spiritus et fumositates currant
ad locum constrictum et minor motus circa medicinam sit et sic facilius retineatur.
Iaceat eger supinus, capite aliquantulum elevato et cum eructuaverit, apprehendat
nares et os aperiat ut omnis abhominabilis fumositas evaporet. Cum autem ceperit
assellare, suaviter ducatur ad sellam vel usque ad .iiii. vel .v. assellationes conetur.
Postea vero de aqua frigida bibat et cum iam medicina cessaverit ducere, bibita aqua
frigida vel calida et digitis ori inmissis provocetur vomitus, quia accidit quod per
medicinam est attractum et non evacuatum quod si retineatur digestionem cibi et alias
impedit operationes. Quo facto cibum parabis, sed si febris non fuerit, dabis
pullos elixos, aves minores et vinum album valde limphatum. Si vero adhuc febris

---

[45] MS *v. egro.*   [46] MS *confringatur.*

remanserit, consuetam dabis escam. Si vero fuerit valde debilis, dabis extremitates alarum pulli elixi vel facies gallinam decoqui in aqua diutissime et postea eam positam in mortario simul cum mica panis conteres omnino et proicies aliquantulum iuris[47] desuper ubi cocta fuerit. Et colabis fortiter torquendo et quod exierit dimittatur ut resideat. Unctuosumque quod supernataverit proicies, reliquum propinabis. Et quia vinum adeo desiderat, quod nisi vinum biberet nihil commederet, sic eum decipies. Accipe forte acetum et inde lava linguam, quasi sordes lingue deberes extergere, ut lingua saporem amittat. Deinde digitos tuos infusos in vino forti ad nares egri ducas, quasi aliquid inde tolleres et postea in cipho madidato a vino ponas succum granatorum, acetum vel aquam et micam panis combustam primo infusam in modico aceto vel vino. Et cum biberit auferas ei ciphum ab ore ne totum bibat. Et propter hoc existimet se vinum bibere quod ei cum timore propines. Sic me[f.125r]mini me decepisse quendam comitem. Septem diebus non solum cum decoctionibus, verum etiam cum sirupis laxativis remanentem purgabis humorem.

[25] Sirupus laxativus sic fit. Semina melonis, citruli, cucurbitie, aliquantulum polipodii si vis purgare flegma, sandalos albos et rubeos facies in aqua bullire et colate aque addas zuccarum sic preparatum: zuccarum pulverizabis et pulverem conficies cum albuginibus ovorum et pones in supradicta aqua et cum bene fuerit coctum, appones mediam unciam reubarbari et postmodum siropus colatus erit clarissimus, quod propinabis cum aqua frigida. Et cave ne cum dederis cibus sit adhuc in stomacho.

[26] Hyeme vero dabis pilulas vel electuaria. Pillulas dabis sero, ut in sompno calore revocato ad interiora, ut solida substancia pillularum dissolvatur.

[27] Aut media nocte in antea dabis electuaria ut oxi, psilliticum, electuarium de succo rosarum, diaprunis, chatarticum et si forte hic simplicia vultis scamoneate, in pondere trium terrenorum vel .ii. de scammonea non trita cum aliquot granis masticis in pomo concavo obvoluto pasta facies bullire et postea cum electuario conficies vel, quod melius est, scammoneam et masticem, hec non pulverizata, ligabis in panno lineo suptili et pones in aqua tepida et in mane proiecto panno quod in vase remanebit in modum lactis conficies cum electuario.

[Times when medication is withheld]

[28] Considerare vos oportet horas in quibus natura operatur crisim, ut in illis horis nullam detis medicinam. Verbi gratia: Prima septimana secundum Ypocratem habet sex dies integros et .xvi. horas. Finitis illis sex diebus in .xvi. horis sequentibus nullo modo infirmum [urgabis]. Secunda septimana habet sex dies integros et .xvi. horas, octo de .xiiii. et octo de .xiii. que remanent preter octo qui remanserint de septimo in quibus horis exspectabis crisim et non dabis medicinam. Similiter tertia septimana habet sex dies et .xvi. horas ut .xv. dies finiantur in .viii. hora .xvi. diei et sic de ceteris

---

[47] MS *utris*.

usque ad .xx. Et vigesimus habet horas .xvi. in quibus exspectabis crisim et nullam
medicinam laxativam exhibebis. Similiter in secundo vigesimo dies et horas considerabis tam in opere nature quam in vestro artificio.

[Symptoms]

[29] Preterea vos oportet considerare non solum egritudines, verum etiam sinthomata egritudinum. Dicitur autem sinthoma[48] pravum accidens quod ex qualitate
vel quantitate materiei sepius accidit. Sunt autem sinthomata hec: constipatio ventris
vel urine fluxus nimius, sitis nimia, vigiliarum instantia, falsus sompnus sive oppressio,
dolor nimius.

[1. Constipation]

[30] Ventris constipatio maxime fit in febribus dum calore febrili liquidioribus
partibus superfluitatum consumptis reliquum condensatur et transit in squibala. Tunc
ergo suppositoriis postea clisteribus subvenietis.

[31] Suppositoria sic facietis: accipe mel in sartagine vel in tegula calida subfrixate
[f.125v] et pulverem salis tosti superspargite et movete cum cacia quamdiu spissum sit
et informate inde quasi stuellum, longum in quantitate trium digitorum et rotundum
et ut magis sit mordicativum apponite stercora murium pulverizata et ponite in loco
ubi perflet ventus ut dum infrigdatur condensetur et induretur vel de solo felle taurino
vel de grano solis vel torso caulis intincto in sapone saracenico, vel mercurialem
contritam et super tegulam calidam vel calefactam supponetis. Hec enim mordicant
pudicum circulum et intestina que sunt sensibilia mordicentur. Mordicata moveantur
ad intus habita expellanda.

[32] Clistere prius facietis mollitivum quasi materiei digestivum, deinde mordicativum, nam si a principio faceretis mordicativum, siccitate eius quod intromittitur quo
operante compactionem superfluitatum totum terrestre fieret. Mollitivum ergo clistere sic facietis: malve, herba viole, pruna et viole bulliant in aqua et illa aqua colata
tepida iniciatur. Cum autem clistere intromittitur, facite pacientem, capite deflexo,
natibus elevatis, morari. Os teneat apertum et non loquatur ne a spiritualibus concipi-
entibus flatum nutritiva comprimantur, et habita intro emittant. Intinge caput illius
instrumenti in oleo vel in aliqua re unctuosa et torquendo intromittatis, ne recte
impellendo scindas intestinum. Postquam autem clistere[49] intromiseris obturato pu-
dico circulo, egrum a pedibus eleves atque concuties, ut quod intromissum est
descendat et fecibus misceatur et aliquando super dextrum latus aliquando super
sinistrum facias egrum iacere et ventrem manibus moveat quamdiu poterit tolerare.
Postmodum surgat ad sellam nec dimittas illum multum morari supra sellam, ut ab eo

---

[48] MS *sinthomata*.   [49] MS *clisma*.

quod remanserat in intestinis feces magis dissolvantur et intestina copiosius evacuentur. Vel accipe fenugrecum, semen lini, et malvas, fac bullire in aqua salsa vel salmacina, deinde cola et adde aliquantulum butiri in aqua salsa sive salmacina. Sed prius incorpora butirum vel oleum cum melle et postea misceas simul et trita cola et misce. Vel sulphur [et] polipodium et supradictas herbas fac bullire in aqua salsa et addito melle et oleo et succo mercurialis, ut diximus, misce per clistere. Et hoc est aliquantulum mordicativum propter succum mercurialis et polipodii. Et si vultis facere magis mordicativum clistere, coloquintidam facite in aqua salsa bullire et resolve aliquantulum salis gemme et fellis taurini. Vel de compositis medicinis facite mordificativum clistere, ut de yeralogodion, theodoricon anacardinum vel yperiston, catharticum, benedicta, yerapigra resolutis in aqua salsa sicut facimus epilepticis, apoplecticis, litargicis, quia ista vehementer mordicando intestina [f.126r]materia a superioribus potenter trahunt. Et notate quod in acutis febribus vehementer mordicativum clistere intromitti non debet.

[33] Precipimus etiam ut in nimiis constipationibus nullam laxativam medicinam et maxime dissolutivam detis nisi primo corpore per clistere parato ad fluxum. Si vero fluxus nimius fuerit ventris, datis constrictivis tam cibis et potibus quam medicinis et precedente purgatione expressiva .s. mirto in aqua rosacea vel pluviali dolore existente ab umblico inferius egestione colerica vel sanguinea cum clisteribus et suppositoriis subvenietis. Primo facite mundificativum clistere, postea constrictivum quia ad hoc quod vulnera consolidentur oportet quod prius mundificentur.

[34] Mundificativum clistere sic facietis: ordeum pistatum et bene mundificatum fac diu bullire in aqua communi. Et postea quod liquidum erit in tali aqua proicias. Spissum autem in panno cola et torque et quod exierit retine et ibi resolve aliquantulum mellis rosacei et iterum cola ne alique superfluitates[50] de melle rosaceo opilent clistere. Et hoc tepidum inice, quod diu remanebit et diu retinebit paciens quia nihil mordificativum recipit. Et hoc multum valet, quia aqua ordei mollificat et mel mundificat. Et nota quod istud debet fieri ante prandium intestinis mundificatis a superfluitate prime digestionis et tot diebus hoc facietis donec videbitis illam aquam puram exire sicut intromissa est. Et in die non facietis nisi semel aut bis vel ter, ne frequenti intromissione clisteris rumpantur intestina et eger debilitetur.

[35] Mundificatis intestinis cum constrictivis insistendum est. Que sic facietis: accipe pulverem boli, sanguinis draconis, gumi arabici prius combusti et simphiti et resolve in succo plantaginis vel corrigiole et inice. Vel accipe gallum et rosas et tegulas marinas in suptilissimum pulverem redige et cum predictis succis misce et inice. Vel accipe herbam que dicitur lappula et contere et succum eius cum suptili albumine ovi mixtum per clistere inice. Et quia quandoque paciuntur tenasmon de colera mordicante pudicum circulum et ipsa mordicatio provocat fluxum, accipe sepum caprinum recens et sine sale et resolve sine aliquo liquore et ei resoluto adde oleum rosaceum, et licinium de bombace factum ibi intinge et cum aliquantulum friguerit, suppone. Si

---

50 MS *aliquas superfluitate.*

vero tenasmon de frigiditate fuerit, quod cognosces per muscillentas egestiones et per dolorem aggravativum, non suppones que diximus sed suppone calida, vel tiriacam vel triferam magnam resolutam in musceleo calefacto, et sedeat paciens super lixaturam pulegii, mentastri, frondium lauri, calendule, et tapsi barbasti. Si vero urina denegatur aut modica fluxerit, nisi forte fuerit fluxus ventris, provocabis eam cum diureticis sicut supradictum est. Considerata materia egritudinis ponetis super [f.126v] pectinem brancam ursinam, malvas, paritariam bullitam in aqua et oleo. Hoc idem facietis de gramine bullito in oleo. Similiter fiat de senacionibus et caulibus agrestibus. Si vero multum fluxerit et urina est turbata et spissa, maxime in acutis febribus vel in apostematibus spiritualium, non est ei obviandum. Sed si fuerit discolorata et tenuis et sepe multa mingatur, nisi multus potus et maxime aque frigide processerit, sciatis esse diabetem.

[2. Diabetes]

[36] Est autem diabetes immoderatus transitus urine de nimia calefactione renum. Dum enim renes immoderate calefiunt, tanquam bibuli insaciabiliter suggunt humiditatem ab epate et non permittunt urinam per ebullationem colorari et inspissari. Tunc ergo debetis omnem curam renibus adhibere vel apponere. Accipe ergo succum solatri, vermicularis, summitates rubi, umblici veneris, et aceto apposito vel agresta renes epithimate sicut epati facere consuevimus et quia laborantes hoc morbo siti nimia infestantur bibant aquam decoctionis dragaganti et gumi arabici et utatur diadragaganto.

[3. Thirst]

[37] Siti nimia interdum infestantur laborantes que aliquando est a nutritivis, aliquando est a spiritualibus aut ex nimia siccitate et eorum succensione aut ex fervore et compressione ut in apostematibus. Quando vero a nutritivis, aut vitio assu[m]ptorum aut propter eorum quantitatem immoderatam aut qualitatem distemperatam aut propter caliditatem et siccitatem; quando vicio asumentium, aut propter eorum nimiam inan[i]tionem et siccitatem aut propter nimium calorem et habundantiam colere.

[38] Si ergo sitis fuerit propter spiritualium succensionem sine apostemate, infrigdabitis aera sicut superius percepimus, ut frigidi aeris inspiratione relevetur. Secundum illud .G. alleviat frigidus aer inspiratus nihil iuvans. Sicientes ex ventre subvenietis sirupis et cibis frigidis quia licet hec ad spiritualia perveniant. Fumositates tamen a se emittunt infrigdantes et humectantes spiritualia. Valent etiam si in panno lineo ligaveris psillium et in aqua frigida posueris quamdiu resolvatur in quandam muscillaginem. Deinde humectabis linguam, palatum et que attingi poterunt. Idem facies de semine lini vel de semine citoniorum vel dragaganto.

[39] Si vero sitis fuerit ex compressione spiritualium ut ex apostemate, non debes aerem infrigdare vel aliis frigidis subvenire, quia hec congelant humorem, impediunt

saniem, sed unctionibus et cathaplasmatibus maturantibus subvenietis et in potu dabitis aquam ordei quia apostemate converso in saniem sitis cessabit.

[40] Si vero sitis fuerit de quantitate assumptorum, ut dixit Ypocras, bonum est ut superdormiant, quia hiis sitis fit propter indigestionem dum grosse fumositates a cibis resolute non habentes exalationem circa os stomachi [conculcantur et moventur et per motum actualiter multum calefiunt. Unde calefit os stomachi][51] et ysophagus et lingua arescit. Ergo qui sic exercitantur superdormiant calore revocato ad interiora, virtus digestiva quod primo so[m]pno explere non potuit perficit in secundo. Contra talem sitim valet potata aqua calida decoctionis masticis, anisi et se[f.127r]minis feniculi. Valent et electuaria que procurant digestionem accepta post cibum, ut est diaciminum et dianthos.

[41] Si vero fuerit sitis de qualitate assumptorum que acumine suo immoderate desiccant os stomachi et ysophagum, ut faciunt alba piper, sinapis et forte vinum, utile est frigidam aquam potare.

[42] Si vero sitis fuerit de nimia inanitione et siccitate nutritivorum, ut ex fluxibus ventris sive per se sive per catharticum, datis constrictivis ut zuccaro rosaceo cum aqua rosaceo, cibis et potibus infrigdantibus obviabitis, et dabitis diadragagantum, triasandali.

[43] Electuarium ad restaurationem humiditatis: recipe dragagantum, gumi arabici, succum liquiricie, semen citoniorum, sebesten, semen bombacis. Hec contrita bulliant in aqua et colature aqua addatur zuccarum et fiat siropus vel loco aque ponite succum qui egreditur a cucurbitis obvolutis pasta et decocta in furno. Hoc idem facietis de citro vel cucumeribus vel melonis palestinis et ultimo pone quando coctus est sirupus psillium ligatum in panno. Et notate quod sirupi qui ad humectandum vel qui fiunt de succo herbarum non debent multum decoqui, quia in multa decoctione amittunt vires suas. De succis facimus sirupum contra yctericiam ut de succo scariolarum, portulace, solatri et zuccaro.

[44] Si vero sitis fuerit de habundantia colere, datis divisivis et predictis remediis adhibitis tam ex cibis et potibus quam sirupis. Potissima cura erit per purgationem secundum illud: tamdiu purgentur donec non sicient.

[4. Insomnia]

[45] Vigiliarum instantia sinthoma est valde molestum infirmo quod fit maxime ex febribus acutis cerebro desiccato immoderate cui fomentis obviabis unctionibus et emplastris. Fomentum sic facies: malve, herbe viole, mirta, cassialigna bulliant in aqua tepida, de aqua illa tepida laventur pedes et crura. Sive vas concavum repleatur tali

---

[51] Supplied from the Winchester MS.

aqua et paciens ibi teneat crura usque ad genua et cavete ut fomentum tepidum sit, quia multi facti sunt alieni propter multum actualem calorem fomenti. De eodem etiam fomentabis frontem et timpora, brachia et manus, et membris extensis ungite volas manuum et pedum et loca pulsuum in brachiis, frontem et tempora de populeon et oleo rosaceo et violis, lacte mulieris lactantis feminam quod humidius est alio. Vel facite emplastrum ad sompnum provocandum: accipe semina utriusque papaveris, portulace, jusquiami, et de opio scrupulum .i. et hec bene contrita confice cum lacte mulieris, oleo violarum et albumine ovi et extende super pannum et naribus pacientis appone et diu odoret. Et postmodum timporibus et fronti applica et aer domus in qua infirmus iacet sit frigidus et obscurus. Et quia de aere fecimus mentionem, damus generale preceptum, ut medicus ante omnia prevideat ne aer quem inspirat infirmus corruptus sit et fetidus, quia nunquam in tali domo poterit convalescere et volumus ut mane et sero fenestre domus aperiantur et hostia per unam vel per duas horas, ut aer depuretur et renovetur. Et quia vigiliarum instantia frenesim futuram minatur si aliqua iam [f.127v] est alienatio, totum caput abrasum unctionibus supradictis ungetis et ca[m]phoram resolutam in forti aceto naribus intromittatur, ut facta mordicatione narium sternutatio provocetur et materia que superiora petebat repellatur, quia alia obtarmica ut in aliis egritudinibus intromettere non audemus.

[5. Lethargy]

[46] Si vero falsus sompnus sive opressio aggravaverit egrum, quod est signum litargie presentis vel future, laboretis ad cerebrum excitandum et materiam repellendam. Fiant ergo fricationes in volis manuum et pedum de sale et aceto calefacto. Infunde manum in aceto. Deinde accipe salem aliquantulum pistatum, non tamen multum, et inde fricate et noli statim extergere, immo dimitte salem supra pedes ut faciat mordicationem. Lavabitis etiam de aqua salsa calefacta. Si constipatus est, facies clistere morditivum ut supra docuimus. Sternutationem provocabitis. Accipe euforbium, elleborum et adde castoreum et suptilissime pulverem [istorum] in panno lineo ligatum naribus applica et percute digitis pannum, ut fumus ille resolutus subintret nares, vel pulverem per calamum naribus insuffletur et apponetis etiam sanguissugas naribus et timporibus, ut vero habeant. Ungetis loca illa de vino, quia vinum diligunt. Abradice etiam occipitium et inungite de succo apii et aliquantulo aceto in quo castoreum bullierit. Et in domo lucida collocetur.

[6. Pain]

[47] Si vero fortis et nimius dolor fuerit, facite rosas bullire in aqua et de aqua illa sepe fomentabitis frontem et timpora et supradictas unctiones ungetis, quia alterant discrasiam et repellunt fumositates. Si vero nimius vomitus fuerit de habundantia colere, datis divisivis, eam purgabitis. Si vero de acumine, quod cognoscetis quia parum et sepe vomunt, dabitis acetosa. Comedant lactucas cum aceto, scariolis et poma acetosa. Si vero propter defectum retentive virtutis, quia quicquid accipiunt evomunt, facite rosarum cortices et caduca mali granati, bullire in aceto vel agresta et spongiam sive pannum lineum ibi infusum et aliquantulum expressum superponite stomaco.

[Medications]

[48] Notandum vero est quod ad hostiles morbos inpugnandos artiphicem multiplici medicaminum genere oportet armatum esse et preterea que supra diximus epithimate, cataplasmate et emplastro debet morbis resistere.

[49] Est autem epithima mollius cathaplasmate, ut si acciperes pulverem sandali albi et rubei et misces cum agresta, oleo rosaceo et violaceo et pannum ibi infusum superpones epati et ad infrigdationem adde succum solatri, quia huiusmodi epithimata que epati adhibentur debent fieri inter nonam et vesperas iam peracta digestione, quia aliter multum impedirent digestionem.

[50] Cathaplasma mollius est emplastro et spissius epithimate, ut si accipias malvas, [f.128r] brancam ursinam, semen lini, fenugrecum et facias bullire in aqua et supponas spleni ad ipsum mollificandum. Et notate quod unctiones splenis debent maxime fieri ante prandium, quia post prandium compresso splene comprimitur stomacus et cibus indigestus emittitur.

[51] Emplastrum durius est omnibus, ut si pulverem masticis, olibani, costi, cinamomi et aliorum misces cum cera liquefacta et superponeres stomaco, sicut contra infrigdationem stomachi ad confortandum ut retineat escam. Utimur etiam enchatismate et fricatione et ventosis cum igne.

[52] Dicitur autem enchatisma supersessio, sicut quando facimus bullire herbas in caldario et pacientem facimus sedere desuper, ita tamen quod non attingat aquam.

[53] Si vero species alique ponerentur super ignem et paciens inde reciperet fumum, diceretur suffumigatio, sicut quando storacem[52] calamitum, xilo aloes, ambram ponimus super carbones et mulierem tectam undique facimus per inferiora fumum recipere ad provocanda menstrua que retinentur propter frigiditatem. Et contra exitum ani facimus suffumigationes de pice greca et stercore vaccino desiccato.

[54] Fricationibus utimur quando materiam subcutaneam apertis poris volumus educere aut blanda manus visitatione aut, si materia compacta et frigida est, cum sinapismo, quod fit de pulvere sinapis et aceto vel vino vel de carne marina vel de aliis mordicantibus et hoc facimus in balneo vel in aere calido.

[55] Ventosas cum igne sic ponetis: accipite stuppam vel aliquantulum lini et ponite in aliquo instrumento vel ligno perforato vel cucurbite et superponite membro

---

[52] MS *thoracem*.

pacienti. Cum candela accendite stuppam et statim superponite ventosam quia ignis trahet aera qui est in ventosa ad nutrimentum sui et quia vacuitas sine aere esse non potest trahitur ventosa et heret membro superposito et herens suggit ventositatem subcutaneam. Nichilominus unguentis et oleis laboramus subcutaneam materiam alterare atque consumere. Et quia de oleis mentionem fecimus ideo qualiter fiant olea videamus.

[Oils]

[56] Fit autem oleum aliquando de herba, aliquando de floribus, interdum vero de lignis. De herbis sive radicibus earum sic facietis oleum. In oleo comuni aliquantulum calefacto ponite herbas vel radices aliquantulum contritas et dimi(ti)tte adminus per .viii. dies et cotidie movete herbas marcescentes in vase. Ultimo facite aliquantulum bullire ad ignem, deinde colate et ipsum usui reservate.

[57] De floribus autem sic facietis: Accipite rosas sive violas et replete vas usque ad mediocritatem, deinde effundite oleum ut sit repletum usque ad summum. [f.128v] Deinde vas obturatum soli exponatur adminus per .xl. dies et omni septimana semel aut bis moveantur flores. Ultimo colentur et usui reserventur. Et si vultis quod sit valde clarum, illud oleum colatum effundite super aquam tepidam in vase vitreo et quod supernataverit cum bombace collige et per expressionem in alio vase recipias. Hec facies bis vel ter et erit clarissimum. Vel aliter admodum aque rosacee ponas flores et oleum.

[58] De fructibus et seminibus sic facietis: de baccis lauri, amigdalis et semine sinapis. Accipe baccas lauri, amigdala et semen sinapis. Accipe baccas lauris per .ii. dies vel tres. Dimitte eas ad umbram ut aquositas earum consumatur. Et deinde facite bullire in aqua et deponite ab igne et quod supernataverit colligite. De amigdalis sic facietis: [amigdalas] mundatas et contritas ponite in olla rudi sine aliquo liquore. Et super- ponite caldario bullienti ut vapore aque resolvantur amigdale. Deinde torqueantur per pannum et quod inde exierit effundatur super aquam tepidam et, ut diximus, cum bombace colligatur. De semine sinapis sic facietis: terite semen sinapis et ponite sub cinere calido. Prius tamen aspergite semen de oleo comuni. Deinde exprimatur per pannum et quod exierit reservetur. Et hoc oleum multum valet contra artheticam passionem de frigiditate factam.

[59] De quolibet ligno sic facietis: Facite frustula de ligno et ponite in olla perforata in fundo sine aliquo liquore et illam ollam fabricate super aliam que sit posita sub terra et ignem undique accendite et sic paulatim ligna resolventur in oleum quod cadet in inferiori olla.

[Restoratives and convalescence]

[60] Postquam tractavimus de causa sana efficiente, preservante et curante. Agendum est de nutriente et resu[m]ptiva que exhibetur convalescentibus. Morbo igitur superato paulatim oportet dietam ingrossare, nec quolibet indiscrete uti, sicut quidam faciunt, unde vix convalescit, quia membra de precedenti pugna debilitata inmutare non possunt et inde per indigestionem superfluitates generate morbum efficiunt recidivum, et accidit eis quod dicit Ypocras: Plerumque male habentes secundum principia bene reficientes et nichil addentes in fine rursus abstinent.[53] Et ideo volumus ut per aliquot dies faciatis convalescentes tali uti dieta, ut nec in quantitate nec in qualitate sit peccatum. Valet aeris inmutatio maxime in estate ut sint in aere frigidiori et puriori. Si vero totius illius aer sit corruptus ut ex paludibus vel stagnis, volumus ut faciatis a matutinali hora usque ad terciam [f.129r] accendi ignem in domo in quo morantur ad aerem desiccandum et depurandum. Si vero non propter ista convaluerint, scias reliquias malorum humorum esse in causa .s. in corpore quas te oportet educere unde natura repit et paravit tibi viam in egritudine. Laudamus etiam ut aliquando aliquantulum sanguinis detrahatur, quia multociens sanguis de precedenti putredine in febris convalescentia remanet aliquantulum, unde minus prius membra depurantur, fumositates corrupte evaporant et membra relevantur. Aliquando ducite eos ad balneum et eis procuretur temperatum balneum, ut dum ingrediuntur balneum ungatur eis epar de oleo rosaceo et violaceo et universum corpus unguatur et fricetur donec in sudorem vertatur, quia superfluitates quas natura eicit ad exteriora in fumositates evaporant et in sudorem erumpunt. Deinde balneentur et ingredientes aquam tepidam aliquantulum morentur. Deinde egrediantur bene obvoluti lintheamine, ne possint infrigidari, et bibant sirupum rosaceum vel violaceum vel zuccarum rosaceum cum aqua frigida et aqua rosacea. Odorent et spargant superficiem etiam in volis manuum et super loca pulsuum et parum exterius sudent, ne membra humiditatem quam sucxerunt ab aqua emittant pariter et amittant.

[61] Aliquando facite convalescentes consueta attingere opera et ante eos de hiis sermo fiat, ut incipiant delectari et tam in egritudine quam in convalescentia coetaneos facite esse presentes qui de consuetis habeant sermonem, verbi gratia si sint pueri, advocate pueros qui coram eis commedant et faciant merendinas suas, ut facere consueverant et sic irritent appetitum. Ludant coram eis troco vel alio consueto ludo. Si milites sunt et nobiles, fiat sermo de accipitribus, de canibus et de equis. Senes senem visitent et eis confabulentur, quia dum senes vident iuvenem robustum corpore, extensa cervice, rubentem genis, nobilitantem gestu, credite quia valde macerantur intrinsecus et interdum dum hec fiant medicus sit absens. Deinde ingrediatur ad eos hilari vultu et leta voce dicens: He quanta dixistis, quot letacitates protulistis a modo de nobis non curatis, cito dimittemus vos eis cum gaudio et prosperitate. Et sciatis quia hiis verbis multum gaudebit infirmus. Dum convalescentes consueta opera attingunt, querite si per ea et post ea melius se habent, quod si fuerit, paulatim addetis.

---

53 *Aphor.* II, 32.

[62]   Quia ergo iam finem vestrum consumastis et mea precepta servastis, tempus est de petenda licentia. Unde consulo ut consideretis eum qui egro existit familiaris et a principio favorem adquiratus ei familiarius habeatis, ei vos et vestra exponite, quia in eo de remuneratione vestra eger habebit tractatum. Quod quantum vobis sit utile vos videbitis. Ad ipsum hanc sermonem habebitis. Omnipotens sui misericordia per ministerium nostrum dignatus, hunc dominum ad quem vocati sumus pristine reddere sanitati et nos aliis habemus ewangelizare [f.129v] precepta magistri nostri. Rogamus ut per vos nobis detur licentia et sic honesta dimissio. Et si aliquando nobis indiguerit quod ex humana fragilitate consuevit evenire omissis cunctis in eius auxiliis nos ipsos precipitemus et preteriti exhibitio sit nobis argumentum futuri. Accepto ergo munere cum gratiarum actione, repleta bursa cum gaudio et delectatione, primo a domino, deinde ab universis, si fieri potest, petita licentia. Vade in pace.

The O.F. Translation in MS London, BL Sloane 3525

[f.209vb] [2] O tu, mires, quant tu vendras al malade, tu requerras Nostre Seignor bonement et doucement que il te soit en aide, car nule paine ne vaut rien senz l'aide de Dieu. Et por ce di je que devant ce que tu i viegnes, que tu enquieres [f.210ra] del messagier combien il a que il amaladi et coment la maladie li prist, si que quant tu i vendras, que par l'orine et par le poux puisses demostrer al malade s'enfermeté et donques avra li malades esperance que tu le garras bien aprés Deu.

[3] Mes sachés, devant ce, s'il a esté confés ou non. Se il n'a esté confés, fai le confesser, car Dex envoie souvent as genz grant maladies por lor pechiez. Car se tu gardes s'orine et son pous et sa maladie et puis li dites que il se face confés, donques se despereroit li malades de santé, ce seroit maus. Puis vendras al malade, si parleras doucement et belement et a ceus qui seront entour li, car granz cortoisie et grant enseignement est de biau parler. Einsi conquerras tu l'amor del seignor et des autres genz. Eindemantiers li dois tu loer ses mesons et ses chambres et ses afferes et de ce s'esleecera li malades.

[4] Endementieres le prendras par le braz senestre et puis si li garderas son pous. Se li braz est charnuz, si empresse plus tes doiz el pous. Se li braz n'est charnuz, legierement le prendras sanz estraindre et garde que il ne gise pas sor celui coste. De la senestre main soztendras le braz et se il bat durement, si senefie chaude maladie et durable qui durera longuement.

[5] Garde que li [f.210rb] malades ne soit trop foibles et puis si voiés s'orine. Et si s'orine est vermeille, si senefie chaude maladie. Adonc selonc l'orine et selonc le pous poez jugier sa maladie et li prometroiz santé.

[6] A sa mesniee diroiz qu'il est mult malades, car se il en eschape, tant seroiz vos plus prisiez et se il moert, il vos porteront tesmoing que vos vos desperates de sa santé. Entre ces choses que je vos amonest, vos di que vos ne regardoiz sa fille ne sa feme ne sa pucele, que li malades ne s'en corrost, et por ce soiez simples.

[7] Et quant tu venras a mengier, pren en bon gre quant qu'il te donront. Quant tu avras mangié et tes mains lavees, va a ton malade, se li di que tu as estez bien conreez et bien serviz. Et il se delitera molt en ce.

[8] Quant tu verras tens que li malades ert plus a repos, se li doiz doner a maingier, se ce est en fievre tierceine ou en cotidiene ou en quarteine autretant de tens cum il a devant l'acesse. Autrement en vendroient dur mal, que quant la maladie vendroit et troveroit la viande crue dedenz le gisier, tant seroit la maladie plus grevaine a soffrir et de l'autre part nature atendroit a la maladie. Einsi fetierement de la viande avendroient malveses humors et si seroit la [f.210va] maladie enforciee et la nature

seroit veincue, car nature ne puet mie rester encontre grant maladie et la viande de cuire. Por ce, si la maladie li prent tart, se li fetes maingier par matin ou au mains trois hores devant [l'acesse]. Se la maladie le prent al matin, si le fetes maingier aprés l'acesse, dous ores ou une, de legiere viande.

[9]   Mais dietez le selonc la nature de la maladie et selonc le tens. Plus devez duner a maingier en quarteine que en cotidiene et en cotidiene plus que en tiercene et en tiercene plus que en fievre ague. Ore esgarderons les aages. Plus souvent devez doner as enfanz que as bachelers et plus as bachelers que as veilarz. Regardez lor usage de maingier, s'il ont a custume grosse viande ou non. Si lor donez petit a maingier et clere chose et bien cuisant. Mais totevoes fait a doter que il ne soit serrez ou qu'il n'ait menoison. Se li donez a maingier grosses viandes, que il puisse joruir(?) sicome poires et neffles et cooinz et autres choses.

[10]   Se il est serrez, se li donez legiere chose a maingier sicome prunes maceines cuites en eue et lait d'amandes en tel maniere atorné: traiez le lait des amandes o prunes, si le colez par[f.210vb]mi un drap et prenez cele coleure, si i metez mies de pain. Si metez cuire en un pot de terre, se li donez a maingier. Et quant vos avroiz atorné le lait d'amandes au malade, si le laissiez reposer. Et quant il sera reposez, si ostez la gresse par desus a une penne en sofflant, car totes gresses sunt norrissemenz de chalor.

[11]   Autretele devez vos faire quant vos bevez le chaudel de la geline. Puis se li faites bolie de farine d'orge, si le batez en un mortier tant que l'escorce en soit fors et puis l'esquartelez et cuisiez en eue. Quant il sera cuiz, si l'afetiez au lait des amandes, si le donez au malade. Se vos volez fere tisane, prenez .viii. mesures d'eue et une d'orge, si cuisiez jusqu'al tierz. Quant cele eue sera refroidie, si en donez a boivre al malade. Autretele poez faire d'eue et de miez et de pain d'orge ou d'eue bolie et refroidie(e). Et sachiez que vos ne devez pas doner al malade sirop ne oximel ne eue diuretique quant la viande est dedenz lui, car autrement la geteroit il hors devant que la viande soit deuite.

[12–13]   Selonc les diverses maladies covient les diverses cures et choses qui departient la maladie [f.211ra] est de chaude nature, se li devez doner sirop acceptos et se la maladie est de froide maniere, se li devez doner oximel. Sirop acceptos fet l'en en tel maniere: prenez les dous parz d'aisil et la tierce de çucre, si le cuisiez jusqu'au tierz ou tresqu'a la moitié. Et puis donez ce sirop a dous coillerees d'eue o une de sirop par matin. Et issi faites chascun jor tant que il soit toz gueriz. Oximel fait l'en en tel maniere: prenez miel, si le cuisiez en la paele et si l'escumez. Et quant il sera bien escumez, si i metez les dous parz de miel et la tierce partie de vin aigre. Einsi faites vostre oximel. Compost oximel fait l'en en tel maniere: prenez racine d'ache et de fanoil et de peresil et de raffle et puis les lavez bien. Et ostez les dureillons et metez temprer trois jorz en aisil. Et puis si en traiez l'aisil et colez netement parmi un drap. Et puis fetes vostre oximelles dous parz d'aisil et la tierce de miel. Et se vos volez vostre oximel haster, prenez voz racines, si les batez en un mortier et puis cuisiez en vin aigre et fetes issi come il vos enseigne pardesus.

[14] Donez o cest oximel dous cuillerees d'eue chaude et une [f.211rb] d'oximel al matin. Por ce le done l'en o eue chaude, que la savors abhominable en soit ostee et que la matire de la maladie soit departie. Et issi li donez tant que li signe de la digestion apergent. Et ce porroiz vos savoir par l'acession del malade et par l'orine et par l'acession quant ele ne dure mie tant com ele selt. Par l'orine en dous manieres, car il avient a la foiee que l'orine est coloree, a la foiee descloree, a la foiee clere, a la foiee espesse. Se l'orine est el comencement descoloree et clere et aprés, quant il avra usé de l'oximel, soit coloré et espesse, ce senefie que la maladie soit departie. Et se l'orine est el comencement coloree et espesse et aprés soit descoloree et clere, ce senefie que la matire soit departie et puis se li donez tel medecine encontre tel maladie qu'il espurge. Et icés choses devez faire encontre froide maladie.

[–] Oximel Julien est eissi fez: dis livres reçoit rue, origan, elacterium, alpiados, squille, sommez d'iebles, enterru de seu, polioel, acori, de chascun .iii. onces, anis demie once, racine de madragore once et demie, ireos, folium, espic, reupontic, azarum, amomme, [f.211va] ipericum, comin, de chascun dous onces, crassula, agaric, polipode, epitim, ellebre blanc, de chascun une once, aceti dis sestiers, miel cinc sestiers. Temprez les erbes en l'aisil et puis cuisiez et colez e metez le miel. Avant le cuisiez tant que li aisilz soit la moitié degastez et metez de l'escamonie quant il sera refroidiez selonc ce que vos le voldroiz faire laxatif. Icist oximeax valt a appareiler la matire et a purgier en partie sicome en poacre et en ciracre et en paralisie et valt a curer artetique et a totes gotes froides. Et vaut a ydropsie froide et fet pissier la pierre et purge les rains de gravele et purge tote froide matire en cotidiene et en quarteine et vaut a totes enfleures qui vienent de ventosité et humor froide. Donez en une once.

[16] En chaude maladie fesons nos tele eue diuretique qui depart la chaude maladie sicome en chaut tens et en chaut aage. Nos apelons chaut aage touz ceus qui sunt .xxxv. anz. Nos prenons citrons et melons et concombres et cogordes, si les bat[1] l'en ensemble en un mortier. Et puis le fesons bolir et puis les colons et donons boivre al malade quant [f.211vb] ele est refroidie. En froit tens et en froit esté encontre froide maladie donons la decocion de semence d'ache et de perresil et de fanoil et de brusc. Donons nos a boivre (a) la decoction de lor racines. Se ce est en esté, de froide matire ou en iver de chaude, autretant de chaudes choses come de froides. Nos l'atornons selonc ce que il est forz, se li donons des froides semences et des chaudes. Par ces signes conoissons nos quant la matire de chaude maladie est departie par l'acession. Si l'acession prent ançois que ele ne selt et mains dure, de tant est li malades mains grevez. Et notez que la chalors del cors est comparee a la chalor del feu. Sicome li feus de moilliees busches arses rent greignor chalor que des seches, autresi la chalor de la crue matire est chaude et plus longuement dure que la matire qui est legiere a deffaire. Et puis que la matire est enbrasee (et) ce porroiz vos veoir emprés le cinquisme jor que li malades sera molt malades. Gart li mires que il ne li doint nule purgacion, car issi destorberoit il la nature.

---

1 MS *les bat les bat.*

[17]   Mais ce sache li mires que il le doit fere seignier dedenz le quint jor et quant li sanc en est trez, tant [f.212ra] est li cors plus froiz. Mes a chacune seignié doit l'en regarder le tens et l'aage et les forces et le region. Les aages que enfanz ont et viellart ne doit l'en mie seignier. Les enfanz ne doit l'en mie fere seignier, car il ont poi d'esperit et soutils veines. Les veillarz ne doit l'en pas fere seignier, car se li sanc en estoit tret, li cors refroideroit trop. Nos regardons le tens, car tel tens est que l'en doit petit ou naient traire de sanc, car autrement troi mal en vendroient ou il perdroient sens ou les veines et les arteres secheroient trop. Einsi sorvendroit spasme de inanicion ou (de) sa secherece qui est lime de chalor feroit la matire plus ardant. Molt froit tens doit l'en garder petit ou naient doit l'en traire de sanc por l'atracion de froit air qui mortifie les menbres. Selonc ces choses regardez les regions.

[18]   Et sachiez que au comencement d'iver desqu'a l'aost doit l'en seignier del destre braz, car plus habondent chaudes humors a destre que a senestre. En esté et del comencement d'aost jusqu'au comencement d'iver doit l'en seignier del senestre. Por les maladies del chief seigne l'en de la veine capital; por le mal del cuer et de polmon de la veine coral; por le mal del foie et del gisier de la veine del foie. [f.212rb] Si li frotez le ventreil et si li fetes haucier la destre jambe. Endementieres si li esventez la veine et se li malades se pasme, si li metez al nes eue rose ou autre chose qui rende odor, et tant seigne que li sanc li change si le puet soffrir. Aprés si l'estanchiez et li liez le braz et moilliez tresqu'a l'espaule. Ce deffent le braz d'enfleure. Aprés si li donez a boivre sirop violat ou rosat en eue froide que li malade ne soit raanclez. Et se il est pleins de raancle, si li donez pain destempré o eue d'orge ou o let d'amandes ou pain esmié. Et puis le face l'en gesir en oscur leu, que li esperiz ne li esvanoisse por la clarté [de l'air]. La meson doit estre froide et li air doit estre froiz et en itel maniere: prenez branches de sauz o totes les foilles et foilles de vigne et jagluel, si getez par la meson. Et prenez eue en un pot menuement percié el fonz, si le pendez en haut a une corde et metez un vassel desouz por recevoir l'eue et ce faites souvent tant que li airs soit refroidiez.

[19]   Quant vos avroiz doné voz sirops et vos choses qui departent la matire de la maladie, puis si soiez entendanz se nature i oevre ou non. Et s'ele i oevre, si porroiz veoir au quel jour[2] il terminera. Mais gardez [f.212va] ançois que il termine par sirops et par oingnemenz et par fomentacions que li vilains puisse cuidier que vos l'aiez gari. Car se vos attendiez tant qu'il eust terminé, il diroit que vos ne li avriez de rien aidié. Et por ce si soiez garniz de devant.

[20]   Maintes manieres de terminoisons sunt en fievre ague. Se la matire est en la boche de l'estomac, il avra talant de vonchier et les levres desoz li mangeront et les oreilles li corneront, la dolors li montera el front. Se ces signes li avienent, ce sachiez que il terminera par vonchier. Se la dolors li est el ventre et li ventrelz li enfle et il sente dolor es costez, et maiesmement del nombril en aval, il terminera par menoison. Et se la dolor li est es rains et il aille petit a chambre, sachiez que il terminera par orine. Et se il sent espointures ou menoison el fondement, sachiez que il terminera par

---

2   MS *tour*.

emorroides se il est escustumez d'avoir les. Et se ce est feme, par ses flors, se ele sent dolor en ses reins et en ses cuisses. Et [si] ses tens li viegne et ele sent dolor el front et es temples et sa veue li troble et les narines mainjuent, sachiez que il terminera par le sanc del [f.212vb] nes. Et se la face et toz li cors li mainjue et se il se degrate et soit plus chalz que il ne selt, sachiez que il terminera par suor.

[21] Et issi tost cum vos apercevroiz icés signes, profitable chose est que vos aidiez a la nature de la maladie. Se vos veez le signe de vonchier, si prenez huile et sirop acceptos o eue froide et o eue chaude et si li metez une plume en la boche ou son doi, si vonchera.[3] Einsi sera la nature aidiee. Se vos veez les signes que il termine par aler hors, oigniez li le ventre d'uile violat et puis si li fetes un emplastre de malves et de semence de lin et de fanoil greu et cuisiez tot ensemble en eue et fetes emplastre et li metez sur le ventre. Ice si aidera a la nature. Se il termine par orine, si li donez eue chaude a boivre ou ces erbes aient esté cuites: langue de cerf et politricum et capillus veneris et ces autres erbes diuretiques. Se par les emorroides et eles soient enflees, si les faites seignier ou vos i metez sansues. Se les femes doivent terminer par lor droitures, prennez mauves cuites en eue, si en fetes emplastre, si li metez sor la marriz. Se par le seignier del nes aperent [f.213ra] li signe, prenez les soies del porc, si les fichiez en croiz en un baston, si li frotez le nes tant que il seint. Se par suer termine, covrez bien le malade et prenez eue chaude, se li metez desoz les dras en un pot, par ce suera. Et issi devez vos aidier a nature selonc les signes que vos verroiz.

[22] Et sachiez que selonc le tens de l'an diverses terminoisons attendroiz. En ver determinent les maladies par seignier del nes. En esté par suer et par vonchier. En aost par orine et par menoison.

[23] Et sachiez que vos savroiz la terminoison del malade a la foiee par le conte de troi, a la fiee par le conte de quatre. Se li malades est forz et auques vertuos et la maladie ne soit mie trop griés, ce savroiz vos par accession. Lors devez conter par le conte de trois. Et se vos veez les contraires signes avenir, si contez par quatre.

[24] Emprés ce que la terminoisons soit fete et aucune chose le face renchaoir, o decoctions et o piles et o laituaires covenables (et) si en getez. La remasille de la decocion li dorroiz. Prenez prunes maceines et violes, si les cuisiez ensemble en eue et puis si les colez parmi un drap. En cele coleure metez une once de cassiafitle et demie once de tamarindes et une once [f.213rb] de mirobolanz. Si lessiez estre tote nuit et au matin le colez et donez a boivre. Aprés ce que vos li avrez doné, si li fetes laver sa boche.

[25] Et puis si li fetes maschier une pome ou une poire et puis si li liez bien estroit les mains et les braz et les jambes de bendeaus, ce est por ce que il ne vonche. Aprés ce que il sera menez, si li donez eue de geline a humer por escurer le ventreil. Et puis si li donez a maingier des alerons de la geline. Et ses vins soit tiedes et si se gart come seigniez. Einsi se doivent garder tuit cil qui prenent medecine.

---

[3] MS *boche si vonchera ou son doi.*

[–] Ou nos les purjons o sirop laxatif, le quel nos fesons en cel maniere: reçoit aluisne, comin, vetoine, mente, castoré et soient bolies en vin et en aisil tant de l'un com de l'autre et soit la fumee recoillie el vis et es oreilles. Aprés prenez le jus de la mente et de vetoine et li metez tiede es oreiles. Ou prennez jus d'oignons et metez i comin batu [et lessez] gesir enz par dous nuiz et colez et metez tot tiede es oreilles.

[26] Sirop laxatis est fet en tel maniere: prennez les semences de citrons, de melons, de coordes, de concombres et un pou de[4] polipode et se vos volez pur[f.213va]gier fleume, sandle blanc et vermeil. Si fetes bolir en eue et si metez un pou de çucre destempré o moiel d'uef en l'eue colee devant dite. Et quant tot sera cuit ensemble, si i metez une once de reubarbe. Icist sirops sera tres clers. Si donroiz dous cuillerees d'eue froide et une de sirop, mes gardez que il n'ait viande en l'estomac quant vos li donroiz et ce soit par matin.

[28] Au vespre si li donez laituaire laxatif sicome trife sarrazine ou laituaire de jus de roses. Et se vos i volez metre escamonie treis deniers pesant, si li metez avec treis greins de mastic. Si en aguisiez vos laituaires par le sirop et par tex laituaires garist en le malade de chaudes maladies, par boivre le sirop au matin et le laituaire au soir.

[29–30] Il covient regarder quel [hore] nature ne oevre mie et les causes. Car sovent avient que il est costivez et qu'il ne puet pissier. Et ce avient par la grant chalor de la maladie. A tex maladies aidons nos par clisteres et par supposicions.

[32] Suppositoires faisons nos en tel maniere: nos prenons miel, si le cuisons en une paele, si i metons sel selonc ce que il avra miel, si mellons ensemble et movons tant que il soit espés. Et puis si le laissons [f.213vb] refroidier. Et puis si en faisons tuiaus. Icés suppositoires valent as coutiveures de froides maladies. Autretel poez faire de fiel de tor. Se vos le volez fere plus mordant, si i mellez le miel et le sel avec crotes de soriz, si en metez dous ou treis el fondement. Mes oingniez la avant de douz saim ou d'uile. Autretele poez faire de salgemme ou de la branche de chol moilliee en savon et que plus sunt dedenz, tant vet il plus tost a chambre.

[33] De premiers li feroiz clisteres mollificatis et aprés mordificatis, car se vos le feriez au primerein mordificatif il le serreroit plus. Por ce faisons nos avant mollificatif en tel maniere: nos prenons malves et la foille e la violete, si les boillons ensemble en eue. Et puis les colons et cele coleure getons nos par le clistere el cors. Mes gardez que les nages soient plus haut que la teste et que il tiegne sa boche overte et si ne parolt il mie. Et li chief del clistere soit oinz d'uile ou de saim et si le botez enz cointement en tornoiant qu'il ne blece les boiaus. Et soit einsi que il ne se moeve jusqu'a tant que li ventres soit amoloiez. Et si li fetes froter le ventre et si li soit li fondement estopez de stopes ou de drapel et quan il voudra [f.214ra] aler avant, si gardez qu'il ne soit trop longuement sor la sele. Le mordificatif fesons nos en tel maniere. Prenez fanoil grec, semence de lin o bren et malves, si cuisiez en eue salee et puis colez et metez bolir san sel avec miel et huile. Meslez ensemble et aprés si colez et le getez par le clistere el

---

4 MS *poudre*.

cors. Et se vos le volez fere plus mordificatif, si metez avec saim et fiel de toro mecines compostes sicome beneoite ou de cartatique destempree en eue salee. Et gardez que vos ne doigniez a home mecine trop salee, car perilz, car max en vendroit. Et por ce par clistere, par bones viandes cuisables li devez avant appareillier. Et se ce avient qu'il soit trop menez, vos le devez restreindre par viandes et constrictives et boivres et medicines et par clistere constrictis et mordicatis.

[35]   Mundificatif[5] fesons nos en tel maniere: prennez orge bien netoié de l'escorce. Puis si li fetes bolir en eue chaude com plus porroiz. Espés le colez parmi un drap et puis metez avec miel rosat et puis le colez autrefoiz et le ruez par le clistere el cors. Et fetes li tenir longuement et ce faites devant maingier. Et ce devez vos faire dous foiz ou treis le jor.

[36]   Prenez bol e sanc de dragon et gome ara[f.214rb]bic et consolde la grant. De ces choses fetes poudre seche, si la destemprez o jus de plantein, si li getez enz par le clistere.

[38–43]   Mais por ce que soif sorvient molt a gent qui ont fievre ague, si covient veoir dom ele vient et par quels signes. A la foiee vient soif de la grant secherece del cuer, a la foiee del foie, a la foiee des viandes. S'ele vient del cuer, si devez refroidier l'air sicome nous avons dit pardesus. S'ele vient del foie, par sirops et par froides viandes li devons aidier. Ou prenez sillium, si le metez en eue, si colera l'eue et de cele coleure li metez en la boche. S'ele vient par viandes, si le fetes dormir.

[44]   Et se il a soif par menoison, si li donez çucre rosat ou aucun laituaire sicome dragagant f[r]oit ou vos li fetes un sirop qui reçoit dragagant et gome arabic et jus de requelice et semence de melons et de coordes et de cubebes et icés choses tribléz et cuisiez et colez et en cele coleure metez çucre et gardez que il ne cuise mie trop, car il en avroit mains force. E metez dedenz un pou de sillium lié en un drapel et si fetes cest sirop user al malade. Iceste chose estanche soif sur tote rien.

[46]   Trop veillies fet grant moleste al malade et ce avient [f.214va] de la grant secherece del cuer. Par fomentacions et par oignement et par emplastres li aidons nos; par fomentacions en tel manere: prenez malves et foilles de violetes et mente et semence de chenilliee, si les cuisiez ensemble en eue et de cele eue li lavez les piez et les cuisses et les mains et les braz, et le front et les temples de popelion ou d'uile violat et de lait de feme qui ait femele. Et tel emplastre li fetes a fere dormir: prenez la semence de l'un et de l'autre pavot et de porcelaine et de chenilliee et une drame d'opie. Icés choses batez ensemble et confisiez en lait de feme et huile violat et aubun d'uef. Icest emplastre estendez sor un drap, si fetes au malade recevoir la fumee et puis quant il avra sentie, si li metez au front et as temples, si le metez gesir en oscur leu et gardez que la meson et li airs soient froit. Et sachiez general comandement que li airs soit purs et sains, car s'il n'estoit purs et clers, avisonques eschaperoit li malades.

---

[5]   MS *mordificatif*.

[47]   Se faus dormier sorvient al malade c'est signe de letargie a venir. En ice devez vos le malade esveillier tant com vos poez. Puis si prenez aisil et [f.214vb] sel, si le metez ensemble, si li frotez et les plantes et les palmes. Se il est costivez, si li fetes les choses que nos avons dites devant et si li fetes esternuer. Se il sent grant dolor de la teste, fetes bolir roses en eue et de cele eue li lavez le front et les temples et puis l'oingniez de popelion. La teste, qui sera rese, oingniez de jus d'ache et de silogastoire qui ait esté boliz. Trop vonchier sorvient al malade de cole. Si li donez medicine qui purge la matire. Se ce avient de la violence de la maladie, si le conoistroiz par ces signes: il vonchera et sovent. Encontre le li donez aigres choses et laituaires a maingier et pomes grenates ou pommes aigres. Se ce est par deffaute de vertu, si le savroiz par ce que quant que il mangera il getera arriere. Encontre ce prenez roses et balaustes, si les faites bolir en aisil et en cel aisil metez un drap. Puis le metez al malade sor l'estomac et si li oingniez l'estomac d'uile contrictif (sic) et si use laituaires confortatis.

[57]   Et por ce que nous avons parlé d'uiles si dirons coment il sunt fet et que il valent. Oiles est faiz de diverses choses et en di[f.215ra]verses manieres. A la foiez est fez d'erbes, a la foiee est fez de flors, a la foiee de fust. D'erbes ou de racines le faisons nos en tel maniere en huile comun: un poi eschaufez les erbes et les racines et triblez, si les metez en l'uile et les leissiez eissi .viii. jorz et chascun jor les movez et au chief des .viii. jorz si les faites bolir tant que les erbes voisent au fonz, puis les colez, si en ovrez.

[58]   De flors le faisons nos en tel maniere: prenez roses ou violetes, si emplez un vaissel de voirre demi plain et puis si le paremplez d'uile et puis l'estopez bien, puis le metez .xl. jorz au solail et si le movez chascune semaine une foiz ou dous, si en ovrez et se vos le volez fere molt cler, colez le sor eue tiede en un vaissel de voirre et cele chose qui flote par desus coilliez o coton, si le premez en autre vaissel et insint fetes .ii. foiz ou .iii. tant qu'il soit molt clers.

[59]   De fruiz et de semences fet l'en en tel maniere: prenez baie, si la sechiez .iii. jorz en l'ombre et puis le fetes bolir en eue et puis l'ostez del feu et la lessiez asseour et cele chose qui desus flotera faites bolir en huile, puis en ovrez .

What follows includes some interesting observations on writing about medicine in the vernacular:

> Encontre la maladie qui vient de melancholie na[f.215rb]turel et encontre la maladie del chief qui vient de ceste humor ou de melancolie noient naturel ou de fleume aigre, ja soit ce qu'ele ait duré cent anz, si en puet l'en et doit fere tele cure por le guerir qui m'est aprise et en romanz escrite, ja soit ce que ce soit envuiz et paine de fisique traitier en romanz a clers, la quele oevre ne fust ja fete ne escrite si ne fu li liens d'amors qui toz segrez deslie et totes choses par ferm lien d'amor ralie . . .

The text now continues with instructions concerning conditions deriving from 'melancolie' and 'fleume aigre', with a preliminary consideration of the evidence of the urine. One section begins 'Ces humors funt maladie el chief que l'en apele cephalee' (f.215rb) and it is ailments of the head which seem to occupy the following sections, leading to receipts for 'uile ciprin' (f.215vb), 'huile de camomille' and 'huile nardin' (f.216ra) and an electuary called 'filonium'.[6] Further miscellaneous receipts follow which appear to form part of a digression, the writer recommencing 'Et avons dites les aventures qui puent avenir et des maladies qui avienent a cels qui prenent poison et coment l'en les puet tot secorre. Or volons repairier a nostre matire' (f.218va). There is another allusion to diseases of the head ('Aprés ce que vos avroiz purgiees les humors dont la maladie del chief est fete . . .') and then to the discussion of oils which has already taken place: 'Por ce que par desus avait esté parole d'uiles, a coi il valent et coment en les fait, si en volons encor parler. Se vos volez faire huile de fust . . .' (f.218vb). There is a series of receipts for plasters and then a red rubric as follows: *Icele lessive fetes faire* (f.219va). Quite distinct is a section on weights and measures introduced by (f.219vb) 'Des mesures et des pois medicinarum m'estuet premierement parler; aprés (f.220ra) del pois et des medicines et des especes et des erbes et combien il en soffist a la reçoit de l'Antidotaire Nicolom que l'en dit le petit antidotaire . . . [list of contents], and the weights and measures as follows:[7]

Vint greins d'orge sunt .i.escruple
Trois escruples poisent .i. dragme
Dragme si est pois d'un victorial denier argent
Dragme si est pois la novisme part de l'once
Noef dragmes font une once
Maaille est la moitiez d'une escruple
Miatus est pois de .x. dragmes
Deniers d'or en fisique poise quatre escruples e demie
Doze onces funt .i. livre
Huit onces funt un sestier
Cuilliers poise .iii. maailles
Noiz avelaigne poise .ii. dragmes
[f.220rb] Noiz grosse poise .xviii. deniers
Sestiers de vin ou d'eue poise .ii. livres
Sestiers d'uile poise livre e demie e .ii. onces
Sestiers de miel poise .ii. livres e demie
Muis e pois e mesure de .xliiii. livres

Ici faut li livres des pois et des mesures de fisique. Aprés comence del pois, des especes et des erbes de tot l'Antidotaire (with translation of the *Antidotaire Nicolai* ending on f.244va).

---

6 See *Antidotarium Nicolai* ed. van den Berg, no.49 ('Filonium maius').
7 See the material and discussion in T. Hunt, *Popular Medicine in Thirteenth-Century England* (Cambridge, 1990), pp.59–63.

CHAPTER TWO

Women's Health – 'Trotula'[1]

Of all the legends associated with Salerno and its medical school one of the most tenacious is the ascription of a number of gynaecological treatises to a female physician known as 'Trota' or 'Trotula', variously deemed to have lived in the eleventh or twelfth

1 On women's health in the Middle Ages see, apart from the works of Benton and Green cited below, J. Blondiaux, "La Femme et son corps au haut moyen âge vus par l'anthropologue et le paléopathologiste", in M. Rouche and J. Heuclin (eds.), *La femme au moyen âge* (Maubeuge, 1990), pp.115–37; R. Blumenfeld-Kosinski, *Not of Woman Born: Representations of Caesarian Birth in Medieval and Renaissance Culture* (Ithaca / London, 1990) esp. pp.91–119 'The Marginalization of Women in Obstetrics'; K. Bosselmann-Cyran, *'Secreta mulierum' mit Glosse in der deutschen Bearbeitung von Johann Hartlieb* (Pattensen/Hannover, 1984); V.L. Bullough, "Medieval Medical and Scientific Views of Women", *Viator* 4 (1973), 485–501; *id.* and C. Campbell, "Female Longevity and Diet in the Middle Ages", *Speculum* 55 (1980), 317–25; A. Delva, *Vrouwengeneeskunde in Vlaanderen tijdens de late middeleeuwen met uitgave van het Brugse Liber Trotula* (Brugge, 1983); P. Diepgen, *Frau und Frauenheilkunde in der Kultur des Mittelalters* (Stuttgart, 1963); J.E. Donison, *Midwives and Medical Men: A History of Interprofessional Rivalries and Women's Rights* (London, 1977); A. Eccles, *Obstetrics and Gynaecology in Tudor and Stuart England* (London, 1982); M.H. Green, "Obstetrical and Gynecological Texts in Middle English", *Studies in the Age of Chaucer* 14 (1992), 53–88; *eadem*, "Documenting Medieval Women's Medical Practice", in *Practical Medicine from Salerno to the Black Death* ed. L. García-Ballester *et al.* (Cambridge, 1994), pp.322–52; *eadem*, "Obstetrical and Gynecological Texts in Middle English", *Studies in the Age of Chaucer* 14 (1992), 53–88; M.-R. Hallaert, *The 'Sekeness of wymmen': A Middle English Treatise on Diseases in Women* (Brussels, 1982); M.J. Hughes, *Women Healers in Medieval Life and Literature* (New York, 1943; repr. 1968); D. Jacquart and C. Thomasset, *Sexuality and Medicine in the Middle Ages*, transl. M. Adamson (Cambridge, 1988); G. Keil, "Die Frau als Arztin und Patientin in der medizinischen Fachprosa des deutschen Mittelalters", *Frau und spätmittelalterlicher Alltag: Internationaler Kongress, Krems an der Donau, 2. bis 5. Oktober 1984* (Wien, 1986), pp.157–211; B. Kusche, "Zur 'Secreta Mulierum'-Forschung", *Janus* 62 (1975), 103–23; S. Laurent, *Naître au moyen âge. De la conception à la naissance: la grossesse et l'accouchement (XIIe–XVe siècle)* (Paris, 1989); H. Lemay, "Women and the Literature of Obstetrics and Gynecology", in J.T. Rosenthal (ed.), *Medieval Women and the Sources of Medieval History* (Athens, Ga., 1990), pp.189–209; H. Lüneburg, *Die Gynäkologie des Soranos von Ephesus: Geburtshilfe, Frauen – und Kinderkrankheiten, Diätetik der Neugeborenen* (München, 1984); P. McCracken, "Women and Medicine in Medieval French Narrative", *Exemplaria* 5 (1993), 239–62; Ch. Paschold, *Die Frau und ihr Körper im medizinischen und didaktischen Schrifttum des französischen Mittelalters. Wortgeschichtliche Untersuchungen zu Texten des 13. und 14. Jahrhunderts* (Pattensen/Hannover, 1989); L.B. Pinto, "The Folk Practice of Gynecology and Obstetrics in the Middle Ages", *Bulletin of the History of Medicine* 47 (1973), 513–23; B. Rowland (ed.), *A Medieval Woman's Guide to Health* (Kent, Ohio, 1981); M. Salvat, "L'Accouchement dans la littérature scientifique médiévale", in *L'Enfant au moyen âge*, Senefiance 9 (Paris, 1980), pp.89–106; Cl. Thomasset, "Quelques principes de l'embryologie médiévale", *ibid.*, pp.109–21; Ch. Wood, "The Doctor's Dilemma: Sin, Salvation and the Menstrual Cycle in Medieval thought", *Speculum* 56 (1981), 710–27; A.L. Wyman, "The Surgeoness: The Female Practitioner of Surgery, 1400–1800", *Medical History* 28 (1984), 22–41. Also valuable is J.N. Adams, *The Latin Sexual Vocabulary* (London, 1982).

century.[2] There is nothing intrinsically unlikely about women practising medicine in an age when the licensing of physicians was in the hands of royal officials and neither the Church nor the universities yet exercised control.[3] Nevertheless, whilst Danielle Jacquart has identified some 125 women who practised a form of medicine in some capacity,[4] not one of the 70 or so women bearing the name 'Trota' or 'Trocta' who are recorded in the membership rolls of the confraternity of the Cathedral of Salerno from the 11th to the 13th centuries is described as a physician. However, as John Benton and Monica Green have shown,[5] it is not necessary to abolish her. The first references to her medical activities are found in MSS London, British Library, Sloane 1124 (s.xiii) f.173 and New York Academy of Medicine MS SAFE f.77v where she is described as 'tanquam magistra' ('on a par with a master'). These are the earliest copies of the treatise *De curis mulierum* traditionally attributed to her. Benton made two very important observations about the possible writings of Trota. First, he noted that in the now lost Wrocław MS (c.1200, N.W. France or Norman England) of Salernitan medical writings the excerpts in the compendium *De aegritudinum curatione* which are marked 'Trot' or 'Tt'[6] in fact show no correspondence with anything in the three gynaecological treatises which are often referred to under the title 'Trotula'[7] and, indeed, show no concern with gynaecology, obstetrics or women's illnesses at all. Benton notes, however, that the passages occur in another text, contained in a Madrid MS (c.1200, N. France or England), a collection of Salernitan medical texts, where they form part of a relatively simple, non-theoretical work, identified by the scribe in a marginal rubric as 'Practica secundum Trotam'. Benton concludes that much of the anonymous material in the *De aegritudinum curatione* which recurs in the 'Practica' stems from a now lost *Practica* of the kind exemplified in the works of Platearius and Bartholomaeus and which was written by a woman named 'Trota', with the main sources being Constantine the African and Copho of Salerno.[8] Green is critical of

2   See for a review of the literature E.F. Tuttle, "The *Trotula* and Old Dame Trot: A Note on the Lady of Salerno", *Bulletin of the History of Medicine* 50 (1976), 61–72; C.H. Talbot, "Dame Trot and her Progeny", *Essays and Studies* 1972, 1–14; S.M. Stuard, "Dame Trot", *Signs: Journal of Women in Culture and Society* 1 (1975), 537–42; J.F. Benton, "Trotula, Women's Problems, and the Professionalization of Medicine in the Middle Ages", *Bulletin of the History of Medicine* 59 (1985), 30–53.

3   See Talbot, *art. cit.* On the later exclusion of women from medical practice see P. Kibre, "The Faculty of Medicine at Paris, Charlatanism and Unlicensed Medical Practice in the Later Middle Ages", *Bulletin of the History of Medicine* 27 (1953), 1–20.

4   D. Jacquart, *Le Milieu médical en France du XIIe au XVe siècle* (Genève, 1981), pp.47–55.

5   I am particularly indebted to Professor Green who has most generously made available to me all her findings and on whose work the present introduction is almost entirely based.

6   The compendium is edited by Herschel in *Collectio Salernitana* 2, pp.81–386. It includes material taken wholesale from Platearius's *Practica Brevis*, the 'Liber Aureus' of Afflacius (?), and Bartholomaeus. The excerpts marked 'Trot' (from Wrocław MS ff.52r–111r) are printed by C. Hiersemann, "Die Abschnitte aus der Practica des Trottus in der Salernitanischen Sammelschrift 'De Aegritudinum Curatione' ", diss. Leipzig, 1921.

7   Notably in the misleading print of Georg Kraut, *Trotulae curandarum aegritudinum muliebrum . . . liber* in *Experimentarius medicinae* (Strassburg, apud Joannem Schottum, 1544). An early study was H.R. Spitzner, "Die salernitanische Gynäkologie und Geburtshilfe unter dem Namen der 'Trotula' ", diss. Leipzig, 1921.

8   Benton, *art.cit.*, p.43 n.38 points out (citing Friedrich Hartmann) that the work which De Renzi

Benton's failure to find correspondences between the *Practica / De aegritudinum curatione* and the texts attributed to Trotula and argues that *De curis mulierum*, one of the three treatises customarily attributed to Trotula, has as its principal source the *Practica secundum Trotam*.

How, then, are we to view the three gynaecological treatises traditionally subsumed under the name 'Trotula'? Benton states forthrightly,

> Though the evidence is sparse and subject to dispute, it appears that the name of a real twelfth-century author, Trota, was applied to a set of texts, the *Trotula major* and *minor*, in the thirteenth, and that by a process of back-formation, the diminutive Trotula was then thought to be the proper name of the author.[9]

Such a title 'Trotula' has analogues like 'Angelica', 'Rolandina', 'Rogerina'. Benton stresses that the genesis of the texts has little to do with women:

> Though the treatises of 'Trotula' bear a woman's name, they were the central texts of the gynaecological medicine practised and taught by men.[10]

The meticulous researches of Monica Green,[11] continuing Benton's work, have distinguished a number of stages in the genesis of these gynaecological treatises, namely *Liber de sinthomatibus mulierum*, *De curis mulierum*, and *De ornatu mulierum*, all three of which are presumed to be essentially Salernitan compositions from the twelfth century which originally were discrete works and frequently circulated independently, being combined around the end of the century to form a 'Trotula' ensemble. Green has identified 122 Latin manuscripts representing 142 text copies and 52 copies of 24 different vernacular translations and Latin verse and prose renderings.[12] She shows that the Latin texts existed in 15 distinct versions. Despite its richness, the mass of material yields no explicit indications of date, authorship or localisation, but the indications are that the evolution of the treatises through their various forms occupied more than a century. During this period they became established authorities all over Europe, easily superseding earlier gynaecological works of Caelius Aurelianus, Theodorus Priscianus, Muscio and pseudo-Cleopatra.[13] It is noteworthy that approximately

prints as that of Copho in *Collectio Salernitana* 4, 415–505 shows little correspondence with what is attributed to Copho in the *De aegritudinum curatione* and was probably written by Archimattheus.

9   *art. cit.*, 47.

10 *art. cit.*, 52.

11 M.H. Green, "Estraendo Trota dal Trotula: ricerche su testi medievali di medicina salernitana", *Rassegna Storica Salernitana* N.S. XII,2 (1995), 31–53; "The Development of the *Trotula*", *Revue d'Histoire des Textes* 26 (1996), 119–203; "A Handlist of the Latin and Vernacular Manuscripts of the so-called Trotula Texts, Pt. 1, The Latin Manuscripts", *Scriptorium* 50 (1996), 137–75.

12 See M.H. Green, "Handlist".

13 See M.H. Green, "Recent Work on Women's Medicine in Medieval Europe", *Society for Ancient Medicine Review* no.21 (1993), pp.132–41; *eadem*, "The *De genecia* attributed to Constantine the African", *Speculum* 62 (1987), 299–323 and F.P. Egert, *Gynäkologische Fragmente aus dem frühen Mittelalter nach einer Petersburger Handschrift aus dem VIII.–IX. Jahrhundert*, Abhandlungen zur Geschichte der Medizin und der Naturwissenschaften 11 (Berlin, 1936).

one third of the Latin 'Trotula' MSS come from England, 36 copies being certainly insular, and a further 5 emanating either from England or N. France.

The whole corpus of 'Trotula' texts has its beginnings with the 'Tractatus de egritudinibus mulierum' (inc. 'Quoniam femine non habent tantum calorem. . .'), a modest work citing as authorities Galen, Hippocrates, Dioscorides, Justus, Paul and Constantine, many of the references being already present in Constantine's *Viaticum*.[14] In relatively simple terms the treatise covers menstrual disorders, displacement of the womb, various uterine conditions, infertility, contraception, regimens for pregnancy, and difficulties of birth. It combines fairly popular, unsophisticated, traditional material (from Latin *receptaria*) with elements of the new, theoretical Arabic medicine (especially book VI of the *Viaticum*). The *Viaticum* translation is probably a product of the 1070s or 1080s, so the *Tractatus* can scarcely be earlier than c.1090. The 'Tractatus' now exists in one fragmentary English MS of the fifteenth century (London, B.L. Sloane 783 B) and one thirteenth-century manuscript from England or N. France (Paris, B.N. lat.7056).

The 'Tractatus' was followed by a number of revisions forming three redactions of what Green calls *Liber de sinthomatibus mulierum* (inc. 'Cum auctor universitatis deus in prima mundi constitutione . . .'). The text of the 'Tractatus' is amplified, the vocabulary revised to a more formal level, the contents made more sophisticated. The three extant redactions survive in a total of ten copies. The *Liber de sinthomatibus mulierum* (LSM) draws heavily on Constantine (*Viaticum* and *Pantegni*) and includes references to Galen, Hippocrates, Oribasius, Dioscorides, Paulus and Justinus / Justus (a contemporary of Galen and author of a *Gynaecia*). It is this work that is often identified as 'Trotula maior'.[15]

The second treatise in the 'Trotula' trilogy is the *De curis mulierum* (inc. 'Ut de curis mulierum nobis compendiosa fiat traditio . . .') in two redactions which go far beyond *LSM*'s concentration on reproductive disorders and discuss in a practical manner a range of cosmetics and treatments for dermatological and paediatric conditions and some disorders which are actually unique to men! It is not at all Salernitan in the striking disorder of its contents and yet is the only one of the three 'Trotula' treatises to refer to Salernitan physicians like Magister Mathaeus Ferrarius, Magister Johannes Ferrarius, Copho and Trota. Even more parodoxically, this work, which seems to have such secure Salernitan associations, contains a number of English words and hence suggests the participation of Anglo-Norman intermediaries. Green believes that a major source is the *Practica secundum Trotam*, which survives in only two MSS. The *De curis* became known as 'Trotula minor'.

The final treatise is the *De ornatu mulierum* (three redactions). Essentially it offered a succinct summary of treatments for women's total body care, proceeding in the traditional manner *a capite ad calcem*, taking in hair, face, lips, teeth, mouth etc. A German MS attributes the treatise to 'Reichardus medicus expertus' i.e. Ricardus Anglicus.

---

[14] Cf. *Constantine the African and 'Ali ibn al-'Abbas al-Magusi: The 'Pantegni' and Related Texts*, ed. C. Burnett and D. Jacquart (Leiden, 1994) and G. Bos, "Ibn al-Jazzar on Women's Diseases and Their Treatment", *Medical History* 37 (1933), 296–312.

[15] Printed below pp.116ff.

Having established the complexity of the transmission so far, Green then charts the formation of the 'Trotula Ensemble', which may have been underway by the end of the twelfth century. This represents a gradual process of rewriting (Green distinguishes five stages). The collective attribution to 'Trota', later 'Trotula', is found at a very early stage and derives from the *De curis mulierum*, which has Trota's *Practica* as its principal source. The title of the corpus would then be 'Liber qui dicitur Trotula'. Subsequently 'Trotula' was interpreted not as a title but as the name of the author, which became the norm over the 'Trota' of the internal references. The final 'standardized ensemble' survives in 28 copies and is distinguished by regularized chapter divisions and rubrics (there is a total of 91 chapters). It was the most popular of all the forms of the Trotula texts.

The vernacular verse translation of the first of the Trotula treatises in MS Cambridge, Trinity College O.1.20 appears to be based on the first redaction of the *Liber de sinthomatibus mulierum* which Green records in only two manuscripts: MS Oxford, Bodleian Library, Bodley 361, pp.458–69 and Magdalen College, MS lat. 173, ff.246v–253r. For ease of comparison with the Anglo-Norman verse I print the Bodleian text at the end of the present chapter. It was copied c.1453–9 by Hermannus Zurke of Greifswald for Gilbert Kymer, chancellor of Oxford (1431–4, 1446–53), dean of Salisbury (1449–63) and personal physician to Humphrey, duke of Gloucester.[16] It is not wholly identical with the Magdalen copy which I have used occasionally to correct a reading in Bodley 361. Nor do the readings of the first redaction of *LSM* always agree with the verse translation, which introduces new material. Nevertheless it may be said that the first redaction of *LSM* comes closest to the vernacular verse. The evidence of a number of prose translations (all incomplete)[17] suggests that the Trinity text is a rhymed adaptation of a prose redaction, which was probably made in the first few decades of the 13th century. The manuscripts I have drawn on for the notes are:

1.   S = MS London, British Library, Sloane 3525 (c.1300) ff.246vb–253rb inc. 'Quant Dex nostre Seignor out le mund estoré sor tote creature'. The manuscript's contents have been carefully described by Paul Meyer[18] who states "L'écriture est clairement française et peut être attribuée au commencement du XIVe siècle. La langue est bien celle de Paris ou des environs".[19] There is an important translation of Roger Frugard's *Chirurgia*[20] and of the *De instructione medici*.[21] On ff.178v–179r there are receipts in

---

16   See A.G. Watson, *Dated and Datable Manuscripts in Oxford* 1 (Oxford, 1984), p.15 and L.E. Voigts, "Scientific and Medical Books" in J. Griffiths and D. Pearsall (eds.), *Book Production and Publishing in Britain, 1375–1475* (Cambridge, 1989), p.385. One of the MSS Zurke copied for Kymer is MS Bodley 362, which includes John of Gaddesden's *Rosa Anglica*.

17   For a list of these see Green, "A Handlist of the Latin and Vernacular Manuscripts of the So-Called Trotula Texts" where she lists two MSS of a French translation based on the second redaction of *LSM* (Kassel, Murhardsche Bibl. d. Stadt – und Landesbibliothek, 4o MS med.1 ff.16v–20v and Lille, Bibl. mun. MS 863 ff.122v–125v, 127r).

18   *Romania* 44 (1915–17), 182–214.

19   *Ibid.*, 183.

20   See T. Hunt, *Anglo-Norman Medicine* 1 (Cambridge, 1994), pp.11f.

21   See above pp.59ff.

an English hand only very slightly later than the single hand which is responsible for ff.24–258.

2. **W** = MS London, Wellcome Historical Medical Library 546 (s.xiv med.) ff.46vb–49vb.[22] The text, which is preceded by the red rubric *Or est bon a savoir porquoi fammes ont icelle maladie que l'en apelee fleurs et que [e]les senefient*, is close to the Sloane copy but there are many omissions and the text ends incomplete on f.49vb (rest of column blank). There are occasionally useful complements to the readings of the Sloane MS. There is a very interesting Old French translation (ff.50ra–78rb) of parts of the 'Four Masters Gloss' to Roger Frugard's *Chirurgia* and, as in the Sloane MS, a copy of Aldebrandino of Siena's *Régime du corps*.[23]

Whilst there is no reference in the Trinity text to Celsus or Soranus of Ephesus (paraphrased by Caelius Aurelianus in the 5th c. and translated by Muscio in the 6th century[24]), Galen and Oribasius are cited from the beginning. Oribasius (AD c.325 – c.400) compiled his treatise on gynaecology from the work of his predecessors. *LSM* initially refers to Hippocrates, Galen and Constantine [the African] as sources, though in the French these are amplified to include Dioscorides and Cleopatra.[25] Then later in the treatise there are references to a physician of Lyons, Rufus, Justinus, Paulus. The contents of the treatise are standard, with a natural emphasis on menorrhoea. The nature of man is said to be hot and dry, whereas that of women is cold and moist. To compensate for their lack of heat, women menstruate as a form of purification, which is likened to the 'pollutio nocturna' of men. Menstruation is also likened to flowers on trees which precede the fruit and serve to purge the body of superfluous humours.

Chapter 1 deals with menorrhoea. The menses, or 'flowers' as they are commonly called, are said to affect women from the age of 13 or 14 years up to 50, and exceptionally to 60 (this claim may result from confusion with vaginal bleeding after the menopause caused by uterine carcinoma). Chapter 2 deals with amenorrhoea, the absence of or lapses of menstruation, from constitutional causes, and the application of a whole host of therapies including bleeding (recorded anecdote of Galen). There is also brief consideration of oligomenorrhoea. Chapter 3 is concerned with menorrhagia or excessive bleeding. Chapter 4 on dysmenorrhoea opens with 'suffocatio matricis' and shows an understanding of psychic or hysterical factors. Chapters 5 and 6 continue with retrodisplacement of the uterus including prolapse of the uterus whereby it actually protrudes from the vagina. Suffumigation is a particularly favoured

22 See S.A.J. Moorat, *Catalogue of Western Manuscripts on Medicine and Science in the Wellcome Historical Medical Library* 1 (London, 1962), pp.408–9.

23 See F. Fery-Hue, "Le *Régime du corps* d'Aldebrandin de Sienne: tradition manuscrite et diffusion" in *Actes du 110e congrès international des sociétés savantes* (Montpellier, 1985), Section d'histoire *médiévale et de philologie* 1 Santé, médecine et assistance au moyen âge (Paris, 1987), pp.113–34.

24 See R. Radicchi, *La 'Gynaecia' di Moschione: manuale per le ostetriche e le mame del vi. sec. d. C.* (Pisa, 1970).

25 In the 'Liber philosophorum moralium antiquorum' of the medical writer John of Procida (d.1282) we read under 'Dicta Galieni', that Galen 'didiscit etiam medicinam a quadam muliere dicta Cleopatra, a qua didiscit multas erbas specialiter valentes contra vitia mulierum . . .', see Renzi, *Coll. Sal.* 3, p.141.

technique for restoration of the uterus from retrodisplacement. Chapter 8 deals with myomas of the uterus and chapter 9 with discharges resulting from upper and lower tract infections.

Inevitably, a word must be said about editorial principles. To print the Trinity text as it stands would be quite valueless, since it exhibits many badly garbled passages, constant copying errors, and general inattention to the sense. At what stage in the transmission the miscopying occurred we cannot know. On the principle of never printing something which does not make sense I have emended wherever the text is incoherent. My emendations normally have the authority of the Latin *LSM* and (occasionally *or*) the Sloane prose translation and thus avoid the dangers of creative rewriting. Apart from these emendations for the sense, I have, more contentiously, made emendations for the metre, since the evidence of the surviving copy is that with small, relatively cosmetic changes, the great majority of lines become metrically regular: in the case of decasyllables 4(e + 6 or 3e + 6, occasionally 6 + 4 and 5 + 5; in the case of Alexandrines 6(e + 6 or 5e + 6. Scientific material was committed to verse for greater ease of recitation and assimilation. Modern readers of such texts should, where possible, read them as verse, not silently as if they were prose. The Trinity text is written first in decasyllabics (1–224) and subsequently in alexandrines. I have felt confident in emending for the metre when no violence is done to the sense and content of the line. *LSM* and the Sloane translation have naturally been of considerable service – positive and negative; positive where they suggest what element has dropped out, negative when they suggest that no essential matter is missing. Where the latter is the case, usually in relation to missing lines whose former existence is implied by the rhyme, I have not sought to recreate the line. In short, the Trinity text is heavily emended but not radically changed. The benefit is a text which can be read fluently and efficiently. The alexandrines are almost all marked by a medial caesura, and in the decasyllables the epic caesura is particularly common. The number of radically hypometric or hypermetric lines is very small; such lines are indicated in the notes. So far as conventional elisions are concerned, I have not sought to remove the elided letters and employ the apostrophe. I have, on the other hand, marked hiatus with the *tréma* except where there are alternative ways of reading the line to achieve the full number of syllables.

As explained above, the source is the first redaction of the *Liber de sinthomatibus mulierum*, which may be exemplified in MS Oxford, Bodleian Library, Bodley 361 pp.458-69. A number of divergent readings in the French verse text correspond to variants in other Latin MSS. I have marked all supplementary material in the French text by the use of italics. Conversely, in the Latin text I have indicated material not translated in the French by < >.

The anonymous author employs the first person on a number of occasions (31,100,108,189,252,257,487,507,537,553,692,742,743,772,795,800). Allusions to an unidentified source ('lettre', 'escris') occur at 153,211,562 and there is a reference to 'l'auctor' at 274. Despite the imperfect condition in which his work has survived, his efforts are important evidence of the popularisation of medical texts which took place in the thirteenth century. The translation was itself made in the thirteenth century. Unfortunately, the reference to 'margillois' in line 436 is of little help for dating, since major production of the coins spans the period 1180–1260s. The expansion of their production was closely linked with the economic development of Montpellier,[26] so that it is not surprising to find a reference in a medical text, and it is also the case, of course, that visitors to Sicily from northern territories frequently passed through the lands of the counts of Melgueil.

---

[26] See M. Bompaire, "Les Ateliers de Melgueil, Cahors et Rodez d'après les sources écrites", in G. Depeyrot (ed.), *Trésors et émissions monétaires du Languedoc et de Gascogne (XIIe et XIIIe siècles)* (Toulouse, 1987), pp.12–51.

Bien sachiés, femmes, de ce n'aiés dotaunce,
Ci est escrit por voir de lor scïence
D'enfant avoir et de lor enfanter,
4   De lor secrés tot i est devisé.
Trover poés totes les aventures,
[En]cerchiés sunt les meillors escriptures
De Costentin et del bon Galïen;
8   Diacorides, cil i mist de son sen,
Sa part i mist li sages Ypocras,
Et une dame que out non Cleopatras.
Certeinement eles i troverunt
12   Dont li max vient et coment en garront.

Por ce que femmes nen ont tant de chalor
Que eles puissent degaster lor humors,
Por ce remainent les humors en lor cors,
16   Par la froidure nes poent geter hors.
Li home suent et travaillent fortment,
Por ce s'espurgent, n'ont enfermeté tant.
Mes naturë vout femmes conseiler,
20   Espurgement lor done por aider.
Doné lor a un grant espurgement,   f.216v
Dames l'apellent 'fleur' par engendrement.
Ne poet conceivre par nul engingement
24   Femme nesune sans fleur apparisant.
Arbres ne porte ç'il ne florist avant,
Primes florist, a tous est conoissant.
Herbe ne porte ne grein[e] ne semence

---

7. Although the opening two sections of *LSM* are not translated here, they are represented in S which includes 'Bien sachent que je i met del mielz ke lor besoigne a lor enfermetez que je ai trové des diz Ypocras et Galien et Costentin et Cleopatras . . .' 'Diacorides' is an addition here, though his authority is cited later in *LSM*.

11. MS *troverent*.

14. S has 'desechier', following *LSM* 'exsiccare' [var. 'desiccare'], but MS B.L. Sloane 1610 has 'expurgare' and MS B.L. Royal 12.B.XII 'consumere', a reading which provides the probable source of 'degaster'.

17. MS *craillent f*. There has been some remodelling of *LSM* 'nec tantum laborem valet earum [sc. women] tollerare frigiditas ut per sudorem eos ad exteriora expellat natura ut in viris'.

19f. MS *Par nature uont homes a femmes conseiller / espurgement lor donent por aider*. The emended text is conjectural, following *LSM*.

23. MS *poent*. The phrase 'sans nul engingement' may have arisen by misunderstanding of 'mulieres sine floribus officio conceptionis fraudarentur'.

25. The verb 'porter' is here intransitive, meaning 'to bear fruit / offspring'.

27f. An amplification of 25–6, of which 29–30 are a repetition.

28 Se ains ne floris[t], de ce n'est pas dotance.
Selonc nature arbres ne porte fruit
S'il ne florist, ice conoissent tuit.
Por ce ai jo amené ces semblances
32 Ke femmes ont en fleurs grans conoissances.
A femme vient [i]teu purgatïons
Sicome a home vienent pollutïons.
Pollutïons avienent et tex flors
36 Quant habondance i a grant des humors.

[De menstruis]

Naturelment vient itel purgemens
Quant la femme a ou tresse ou quatorse anz,
A la fiez ou plus tart ou ançois,
40 *Estre ne poent pas totes d'une lois*:
L'une est froide, l'autre est plus chaude,
Ceste est humble, cele est plus baude.
A la femme que est magre bien plus dure,
44 Mains a la crasse, que teux est sa nature:
A la fiez truis qu'a la cinquantime,
A la megre desc'a la soissanteime,
A la maiene dusc'a la quaranteine.
48 [. . .]
Femme ad tous jors [ses] flors solonc nature,
Ne trop ne peu, que tex est sa nature,
Adonc s'en issent les males humors hors,
52 Enfermeté ne remaint mie el cors.
Se ne se espurge de ces males humors,
Nastre en poent enfermetés plusors.
A la fie pert boivrë et manger

f.217r

37. MS *Naturelement*.
38. *LSM* has 'circa .xiiii. annum'; S has 'quant ele a quatorze anz, et a la fiee, selonc ce ke ele est plus chaude, a treze anz ou a doze'; W has 'a .xiii. anz, a la foiz a .xii., quant elle est de plus chaude nature . . .'
41–2. As they stand these lines are octosyllables. Line 42 has no correspondence in *LSM*.
43. MS *m. et p. d.*
44. MS *en s.n.* Cf. ll.50,60.
45. *LSM* has 'Durat autem usque ad .l. annos, si macra est quandoque ad .lx., vel .xl. ut in mediocriter pinguibus, vel usque ad .xxxv. si sit mulier multum pinguis'. Unlike S and W the A-N text omits the age of 35 and the case of women. I take 'truis' as pres. ind. 1 of 'trover' rather than as a spelling for 'tres [que'.
47. MS *mancime*. The missing line 48 presumably referred to the case of fat women.
52. MS *E. nesune n. r. el c.* As it stands in the MS the line is hypermetric. I have emended for the sake of the metre.
53. This does not accord with *LSM*.
54. MS *enfermen*.

56   Et tele hore est que el ne se poet aider.
            A la fïez quant el siet a maison,
            Desire chose que li në est pas bon
            Ou autre chose que est contre sa nature;
60   Tot ce manjue, que tex est sa nature.
            A la fïez li vien[t] dolor al dos,
            Al col, au chief, as ex, au pis, as os;   f.217v
            A la fie li vient le fevre ague.
64   Et tel ore est que froit a . . . resue.
            Quant feme pert ses flors de longement,
            Tous ses maus a, et autres bien sovent:
            Ceste a corpos, ceste dissinterie,
68   Del tot le[s] pert quant a ydropesie.
            A la fie, quant menison la prent,
            Donc les pert ele del tot naturelment.
            Par ce les pert la femmë a la fie,
72   Que la maris li est trop refroid[i]e,
            Et quant les veines que sunt en la maris
            Sunt graisles trop, li trespas est petis;
            Les graisles femmes veines estroites ont,
76   Par ceste chose rien ne s'espurgeront,
            Kar il n'ont voie par ou puissent issir,
            Por ce covient les grans maus [a] soffrir.
            Quant sont espesses les humors congluans,
80   Issir ne poent, por ce sont renuisans.
            Avient por ce que femme poi mangue
            Et mult travaille et par travaille sue.   f.218r
            Ce dit Rufus qui soit de mecinal,
84   Femme movans et quë est en travail
            Ne doit avoir pas grant plenté des flors,

56. MS *ele*. Cf. l.64. There is no reference to the symptom of vomiting, *LSM* 'quandoque provenit vomitus', S 'et si a voncheison'.
60. Both *LSM* and S are more specific: 'Quandoque autem appetit mulier terram, cretam, carbones vel aliquid aliud contra naturam'; 'a la fiee desirre mangier de creie ou de charbon ou ce ou altre desnaturel chose'.
64. The meaning is obscure. The line seems unrelated to the Latin and there is a blank in the MS between *a* and *resue*.
66. *ses* = *ces*.
67. MS *cor por* for *corpos* 'cordis pulsus'. The translator has misunderstood *dissuria* as 'dissinterie'. S has 'dissiure', whilst W substitutes ' a la foit de nuiz'.
70. MS *naturelement*.
75. MS *estroistes*. *LSM* refers to 'vene . . . graciles ut in extenuatis mulieribus'. The reading 'grailes', shared with S, may originally have been caused by eyeskip and we might read 'les megres femmes'.
79. MS *en espesses*.
80. MS *ne ne p*.
83. MS *nifus* is a misreading of 'Ruf(f)us' in *LSM*. S omits it, but W has 'Rufus li bon metres'.
84–6. An amplification expressing the converse of 88–90, which reflect *LSM* (correction needed to MS Bodley 361).

Tant se degastent par travail les humors.
Et derechief cele que mult mangue
88 Et par travail peu se moet et peu sue,
Ceste en a mult par reson et par droit,
Se ce est chose quë estre saine doit.

[Contra defectum menstruorum]

A la fie pert femme son sens
92 Por ce qu'el cors refroidist trop li sans,
A la fie par ce que li sans ist
Par autre liu, sicome avient de fi;
Ore i ad tex qu'e[l] ne[s] seignent sovent,
96 Or est manere qui.l vait escopissant.
Or est un autre qui les pert par irror,
Ou por grant doel ou par trop grant pëor.
Jo les fas sages totes comunement.
100 Sachiés que femme quant les pert longement
Seüre soit de grant enfermeté,
A peines poet un jor avoir sauncté.   f.218v
L'urine est vert ou tornë a rougor
104 Ou de char fresche prent estrange color.
Si cele femme est megre, chose est certeine,
Seignier li estuet de pé sovent – de veine,
Cë est, del pié tot desus la quivillie.
108 *Ceste mecine ai enseignié me fillie.*
Cele se seine e[n] l[e] pé deu senestre
Et l'endemain, s'el puet soffrir, del destre.
Selonc ice que ele porra suffrir
112 Se seinst chescune [tot] a son pleisir.

---

91. The line is hypometric. If *sens* were for *sans*, giving a 'rime identique', it would contradict the meaning of *LSM* 'menstrua deficiunt . . .'
94. Cf. *LSM* 'ut per ficus sive emoroydas vel per nares vel per sputum', reproduced (except for 'emoroydas') by S and W.
95. Correction suggested by *LSM* 'per nares', S 'd'icele que li nes seigne souvent', and W 'cele qui a fi ou nes(t) qui sene souvent'.
97. The return to 'flors' implies that such a reference is the missing element in the obscure and hypometric line 91. S has 'A la fiee les pert femme pour ce ke li sanc al cors refroide . . .'. This might justify the correction 'A la fie les pert femme par tans' (cf. 287–8 tans: sanc), 'par tans' being taken to mean 'for a while'.
100. MS *que quant f. l. p.*
103. MS *Et l'urine . . . et torne.*
104. MS *7 stange.*
109. MS *deus.*
112. As it stands in the MS the line is octosyllabic but might be regularized by emending the first hemistich to 'Si se seigne . . .'

Li seigners doit regarder la pussance
De touz les max, qui n'i ait mesestance.
As febletez [li] mires bien se gart,
116   Kar a tous febles doit bien ovrer par art.

Galïens

En un suen livre reconte Galïens,
Que jadis fist as escolers grant biens,
De une [feme] quë out perdu ses flors
120   Par quatre mois, estre poet par plusors.
Mult devint magre et perdoit le manger,
De nule rien n'avoit le desirrier.
Par quatre jor la comande seignier.
124   Dous livres trait del pié le jor premer,
A l'autre jor en trait de l'autre pié
Une libre, si com li fu ditié,
Et le tier jor dous unches le seigna
128   Del premer pié sicome on li dit a,
Del sanc li trait quatre onces al quart jor,
Aprés cest terme se mist en grant segor.
En peu de terme si rot sa qualité,
132   Char et color sicome avoit esté.

                                        f.219r

Teles i a que perdent lor flors

De teux i a que sovent sont serees,
Perdent les flors, *forment sont cler muees,*
Poisons, pilectes, icestes doivent prendre
136   Od laituare, ce devez bien entendre.

---

113. MS *seigneres*.
114. 'qui' for 'qu'il'. *LSM* speaks of the 'virtus egrotantis' not 'virtus egritudinum'.
116. MS *par sa art*, an addition to the source.
122. MS *el desirrier*.
124. MS *dous leus*.
125f. *LSM* has 'secunda [sc. die] librum .i. de alio pede', followed by S 'le secont jor el altre pié .i. livre'.
126. MS *sicome*.
127. MS *unches*. *LSM* has 'uncias octo', S 'wet onces'.
129. MS *quatre jor*. *LSM*'s 'uncias octo' applies here too.
130. Cf. *LSM* 'restituta est'
131. Cf. *LSM* 'et rediit color et status antiquus'.
134. There is nothing in *LSM* or S which corresponds to 'cler muees' which appears to mean 'become pale'.
135. 'poisons' is an addition to the source. *LSM* has '.v. pilulas'.

Aprés ice si se doivent seigner,
Aprés le quart jor les covient baignier.
Aprés le bai[n]g en mente ou calament
140 Lor convient boivre ice avenaument.
Ces herbes soient bien quites en melie,
L'une moitié d'eue soit une partie.   f.219v
Aprés cest bai[n]g quë on sovent fera,
144 De une leituaire deu deners pesera
Et un dener de castorie pesant
Boillie o ewe et o mel ensement.
Cist letuares est diatesseron,
148 De quatre especes, ja plus n'i avra [on];
Aristelogia si est la premere
Et la secunde gencïene la fiere,
La tierce est mirre, baie soit al quart leu.
152 Quant ert confite, si en boive a son preu,
A un pois ert pesé, ce dist la lettre,
Et le mel cuit, que plus n'i doit on mettre.
   Doner li doit li bons mires poisons
156 De gerapigre, teux doi[t] estre li nons.
Et li doigne gerologodïon,
Kar il i a assés bone poison.
Totes les choses que bien feront pisser,
160 Sicome ache et fenoil, tot poet aider,
Fisalidos, amëos et espis,
Cassïafistre et canele et grumis,   f.220r
Li peresils, savine et quintefoille,
164 Luvesce, anis et satré et cerfoille,
Origanon, polïol et vetoine,
Et ceteca ovesques macedogne,
Totes ces choses seront quites en vin,

138. MS la quarte jor, not in the source. The standard decasyllabic would be restored by emending to 'et al quart j. si l. c. b.'
139. Omits the 'nepita' of LSM (S 'nepite').
142. The line is garbled. Cf. LSM 'ubi .vii. partes sunt aque et octava mellis'. S has 'ou ait les wet parties d'eue et la nuvieme de miel'.
143. MS ceste.
144. The electuary is actually 'dyatesseron' ('made from four ingredients') which in 147 is corrupted to 'dyatesata'.
147. MS dyatesata.
148. MS que ia.
149. MS anstelogia.
151. MS baic.
155. The translator substitutes 'poisons' for LSM 'medicina'.
162. 'grumis' has no equivalent in LSM or S.
166. 'macedogne' denotes macedonia, 'alexanders' or 'horse-parsley' (LSM has alexander). It is not clear what 'ceteca' represents: a possible source in 'centonica' does not seem likely since it is an

168   *Puis en boivra au soir et al matin.*
             Quites seront al tiers en un nuef olle,
             Si estre ne poent totes, ise ne pert une sole.

                              Galïens

             Galïens dist la mere herbe triblee
172   Bone est en vin, *mult vaut la matinee.*
             Si en doit boivre le soir a son coucher,
             A la fïez li covient i baignier.
             Cele herbe quite en euue bevera,
176   Dedens son bai[n]g mult [li] profitera.
             A la fïez en son bai[n]g la quira,
             Quant ele ert quite, dedens se baignera.
             A la fïe vert le doit on tribler,
180   Sor son ventre, soz son nomblil lier.
                Une autre fois la doit quire en recoi
             En un pot chaut, si la methe soz soi   f.220v
             Sor une sele ou chaiere siee –
184   Ens al mileu sera tot drait percié[e].
             De la chalor ist li fu[n]s a droiture
             A la marris sus par la parcëure.
                Un autre fois la mere herbe soit prise,
188   Ce est cele que on apele hernise,
             Ovec les autres que desus ai nomez
             Soit ceste mise, se estre poent troveez.
             Si l'en ne poet totes celes trover,
192   Si mette on celes que l'en poet recovrer.

anthelmintic rather than a diuretic and does not, in any case, appear in *LSM*. The reading may be a miscopying of 'ceterach' (Osmunda regalis L.).

169. MS *s. trescal t.*

170. The meaning is unclear, though it is apparently intended to render *LSM* 'Omnia ista, vel singula vel conmixta' (cf. 190–1). The line is clearly hypermetric. The collocation with 'pert' suggests that 'sole' is to be interpreted as an expression of minimal value.

172. The second half of the line is an addition to the line which sorts ill with the following line.

173–8. These lines are repetitious.

175. MS *en cuue.*

179. MS *verde.*

180. MS *sor son n.*

181. MS *quise.* The detail 'en recoi' is an addition to the source.

182. MS *une p. . . . meche.*

183. MS *ou sor une ch.* The subject of 'siee' ('sedeat') is the female patient.

184. 'percié' refers to the 'sele / chaiere'.

185. MS *Del.* Omitted is the detail of *LSM* 'bene cooperiatur undique ne fumus exeat' (cf. S 'si se coevre bien de dras . . .').

192. MS *recoverer.*

Ces herbes soient totes quites en vin,
Puis si pregne la toie de cossin,
La toië ert d'un petit orrillier,
196   Laine carpie covient appareillier.
De cest vin chaud ert moillie la leine
Dont la cute sera farsie et pleine.

Pudre a faire avoir les flors

Mult valent poudres por fere avoir les flors,
200   *Ki les set fere tost poet avoir secors.*
Prenez la mirre et castorie et flamme
Et centoire, de chescon une drame,   f.221r
De ditaine une et dous de [la] savine.
204   Fete[s] la poudre, cë ert bone mecine.
Boive une drame el bai[n]g quant [ele] ert nue
De l'euë [ou] soit quite sauge et rue.
    Se la marris soit tant fort adurcie
208   Que ces mecines ne puissent faire aïe,
Que nule chose ses flors puissent atraire,
Donc li covient mettre sozpositoire.
Ce dit la lettre: le fiel del tor prenés
212   O autre fiel, entendre ce devés,
Poudre de nitre et d'isope le jus,
Mellez ensemble, pus nen fera on plus.
Leine carpie od le jus seit moillé[e],
216   Aprés ice longuete soit trenchee,
Longe et rëonde; de ce ait conoissance,

194ff. The passage is not so clear as *LSM* 'Inpleatur sacculus lana minutissime decerpta ut fit in modum pulvinaris' (S 'et emplier une taeie d'orellier de line carpie'). In 198 'cute' ('quilt') apparently refers to the 'toie'.
195. MS *une p.*
199. MS *f. a fie les f.*
201. MS *mirte.*
202. S has 'centoine' (*LSM* 'centonicum').
203. The reference to 'savine', common to this text, S and W, is not found in *LSM* (but occurs in MSS Oxford, Bodleian Library, Digby 29 and e mus. 219).
205. 'quant ert nue' is an addition to the source.
206. MS *q. com s. et com r.* *LSM* has 'ubi decoquuntur salvia, ruta', S 'en eue ou la sauge soit cuite et la rue'. I have emended accordingly.
209. MS *fes fl..*
210. MS *c. li m. le s.*
213. MS *Poudre d'isope et de verde le jus.* *LSM* has 'pulvis nitri', S has 'poudre de vitre', W 'poudre de voirre'.
214. MS *p. si en f..* The phrase is an addition.
215. MS *melle.*
217. Omits *LSM* 'teratur ut sit rigida et dura et magna'.

Qu'ele la puise mettrë en sa nassance.

En tel manere et ensi doit en fare,

220   Quë on mette ens cë apele on peissare.

   Un autre funt tot droit a la mesure

D[e] membre d'ome, croes est par [sa] nature,   f.221v

De quievre est fait ou fust en tel manere

224   Qu[e] l'en le met ausi come clistere.

Femme que a peu de ce que [l']on apele flor,

Et ce mauveisement, a peine et a dolor,

Pregne la pulïol ensemble o l'averone,

228   De chescun sa poigné, autretant de vetone;

Ou en ewe ou en vin ces herbes soient quites

Et tant que les dous pars del jus soient esquites

Et la tierc[e] remaigne; par un drap seit colee,

232   Puis le doinst a la femme que a l'enfermeté,

O le fon de la terre en fais cist bevement,

'Gris con' et 'con canu' l'apelent laie gent.

Autre

A ceste enfermeté a autre esperiment:

236   Prenge mentë et rue, polïol ensement,

Des treis une poigné i avra de chescun

Et de roge colés i metés planton un.

Treis drames de saugeme et treis ciés de poret,

240   Tot quirra bien ensemble en un petit potet,

Se li doinst [on] a boivre, [et ce] aprés le bai[n]g,

Ensi porra garrir la femme del mahai[n]g.   f.222r

218. MS *Si qu'ele*.

219. MS *tele*.

223. MS *ou de f. la m.* / *Ou len le met ausi com par deriere*. An addition, the sense of which is 'like a brass or wooden [tube]', possibly arising from a misreading of *LSM* 'etiam' as 'enam'.

224. See *LSM* 'inicitur sicut per clistere'.

225. MS *La f*. The text now moves in to alexandrines.

227. MS *Prendre*. In place of 'averone' (abrotanum), *LSM* has 'antonia', S 'antoine'.

233. MS *de la terce*.

234. On these names see Introduction, p.13.

236. MS *m. rue et poliol e*.

237. MS *Des quatre . . . avera*.

238. MS *plācon*. Read 'planton'? *LSM* has 'plantam caulis', S 'plancon de roge colet', W 'tres plantes de roge cho.'.

239. MS *Quatre d. LSM* has 'salgemme .z. .iii.' (S, 'de la sauge tres .z.'; W '.iii. cimes de sauge'). There is therefore confusion in the translations. In emending I have considered the likelihood that 'quatre' has been introduced through eyeskip to 237.

241. I have emended this obviously hypometric line on the basis of the evidence of S.

Autre

Autre espeirment vus di qui a mult grant secors
244   A cele[s] que lo[n]gtans ont perdues lor flors.
Prenez de reupontic dous deniers bien pesant
[Et] une maille ovec, d'ermose seke autant.
Avec ce covent mettre un[e] drame de poivre,
248   Si en face l'en podre, se li doinst on a boivre.
En mel quit le bevra al matin et au soir,
Par treis jors le fera se sauncté veut avoir.
Le soir soit bien coverte, que ele puisse suer.
252   Autre chose esprové li voil encore mustrer.
De glagol la racin[e] et de luvesce pregne,
De wimavë ovec [et] en un morter fregne,
Et herbe de la nepte si quisez tot en vin,
256   Si li donez a boivre al soir et al matin.
      Une autre chose di, pregne l'en la savine,
De peresil, de l'ache, de chascun la racine,
De fenoil, de luvesce la racine prendra,
260   Trestot quirra en vin et puis se la beivra.
Cerfoil et tanesie, hermoise en bure frit,
[Mete] sor le numblil, tot ensemble li lit.   f.222v

Autre

Uns mires de Lïons fet un' autre mecine
264   A cele que de France estoit clamee roïne.
Prent gingebre et savine et foilles de lorier,
Si tribla tot [petit] ensemble en un morter,
Sor les carbones [vifs] mist ceste medicine,
268   Sor la sele percié fist so[o]ir la roïne.

---

243. MS *espeirement.*
245. MS *ceupoine un drame b.p..* LSM has 'reuponticum', S 'retipontic' (an obvious error for 'reupontic'). I have emended the rest of the line on the basis of LSM 'pondus duorum denariorum et obuli' and S 'deus deniers pesant et maille'.
246. MS *marcele* appears to be a corruption of 'maille', see above.
249. MS *quite.*'En mel quit(e' (S 'si.l solde l'on od miel cuit') is an addition to LSM.
254. The line is suspect, for not only is it hypometric, but 'wimave' (S 'guimauve') has no correspondence in LSM.
261. MS *boire*, an obvious error for 'bure' (LSM 'cum butiro', S 'od bure').
262. Cf. S 'li mete l'on a l'umblil'. 'lit' renders 'ligentur'.
263f. MS *fetet.* LSM has 'Quidam medicus fecit regine Francorum'. S has 'Altre ke li uns (li) mires fist a la reine de France'.
265. MS *preng.*
266. MS *Titriules t. e.*
268. MS *patie.*

Ensi qu'en la nassance la fumee venist,
Bien fu de dras coverte, mult longement i sist.
Dame que tel mecine vodra fere sovent
272   Doit oindre sa nassance de ole rose devant.

[Contra superabundantiam menstruorum]

Quant la feme a trop flors, se torne a grevement,
Solonc l'auctor l'apele de sanc decorement,
Que de la marris sont [trop] overtes les veines,
276   Avient a la fie que recloent a peines.
A la fïez avient icë en conissant,
Que li sanc cliers et rouges en ist hastivemen[t].
A la fï[ez] avient que femme a trop colli,
280   C'est asaver de boire, de manger atresi.
Et de trop grant repos repoet ce avenir
Que li cors ne poet mie bien le sanc recollir.   f.223r
[Et assés] sovent est li sanc trop eschavés
284   Par les coles que issent del fiel quë est troblés.
Les coles funt boillir le sanc et eschaufer
Si que veines nel poent [ne] tenier [ne] sauver.
Il avient derechief par treimains et par tans
288   D'un humor, sausefleume, dont mués est li sanc.
Adonques est tant clier et tant vert devenus
Li sanc, que ne poet estre es veines retenus.
Del sanc qui ist del cors esgardés la color,
292   Se cole [i] est mellé, tornera a jaunor.
S'il avient de fleume, si a blanche color,
Et si c[ë] est de sanc, si tornë a rogor.
Cist max avient [por ce] que li sanc est malmis
296   Par le cors corrumpu, ne poet estre rasis,
Et por ce que li sanc est tot desnaturés

270. 'Bien fu de dras coverte' (S, 'Mais l'on se doit bien couvrir de dras') is an addition to the source.
271. For 'tel mecine' LSM has 'fumigatio', S 'les estuves'.
272. Omits LSM 'ne nimis calefiat', S 'k'ele ne s'eschaude trop'.
273. MS Q. *le fera.*
274. Cf. S 'Ce ke la feme a trop de ses flors apele l'on fluxum sanguinis selon latin, et en romanz le puet l'on apeler sorondement'. LSM has only the phrase 'menstrua preter modum'.
276. LSM has 'vene ... quandoque crepant', S 'A la fiee crievent les veines'.
277. 'en conissant' remains obscure.
278. MS *et et rouges.*
280. MS *De cest a. de b. et de m.*
281. 'De trop grant repos' corresponds with S, but is not found in LSM.
286. MS *Se que.* 'sauver' is an error for 'soffrir' (S).
287. MS *pai t.*
289. The line garbles the source, where there is no reference to 'vert'.

Nel poet cor retenir, en hainë est tornez.
  A la fiez avient cel mal par avo[rter],
300   Donques covient la femme de la mort acorder.
Quant cist mal vient a femme, si en pert la color
E le manger avec, puis se torne a dolor.   f.223v
Se longement i dure, si vient ydropesie,
304   A peines garist hon de ceste maladie:
Li foies refroidit par le sanc qui li faut
Qui li d[e]voit tenir en son naturel chaut,
En bon sanc naturel ne poet sauce muer,
308   *Ainz converse le sanc en eue retorner.*

Quant tel mal avient por aporter

Quant li mal vient par sanc, itel doctrine fas:
Covient la a seigner de la veine del bras,
Et amont par nature des veines le sanc traire,
312   *Quar la ou a issue doi[t] avoir son repaire.*
Se la cole ist del fel par que[i] cist maux aviengne,
Doner covient a femme par coi cist max detiengne,
Doner covient par quei la cole isse del cors,
316   *Ou desoz ou desus le covient geter hors.*
Triphere zarasine li doit estre donee
Ou rosate novele o bone scamonee,
Ou sirop de violes, *ou bon diaprunis,*
320   *Ou autre letuaire ensi come est escris.*

298. MS *cuer . . . torneez. LSM* has 'nature nobilitas'.
305. MS *la s.*
307f. MS *n. p. foie m.* The correction is based on *LSM* 'succositatem digerere et in humores conmutare', which can scarcely be the origin of S 'ne puet muer sa viande en naturel sanc'.
308. MS *Ancois.*
309. MS *itele.*
310. MS *du v.*
311. MS *Contre mont.* The reading 'contremont' is the opposite of *LSM* 'sursum'.
312. MS *Quar loie qua i.*
313. MS *del chief.* Cf. *LSM* 'colera resudans a felle'.
315. MS *coli.*
318. MS *scamonie.*
319. MS *diaprimist.* The electuary 'diaprunis' is not mentioned in *LSM* or S. The following rubric has *fleumeme.*
320. MS *escrist.*

Pur abundance de fleume

De habundance de fleume [s']avenus est cist maux
Ou de colere neire, *n'i vienge mire faux.*
Purgier devons li cors par chose qui se fine,
324   Gerologodïon, c'est propre me[di]cine.
Avec la feuquerole qui sera quite en vin
Ou avec la cervoise, *cel bevra al matin.*
Quant li cors est purgés dedens des humors veines,
328   Si devons recourer as mecines foreines.
Aprés boive la femme [de] l'ewe quë est tiede
U soit quite l'escorce de la pome gernete,
Ou ele boive l'eue ou soit quite l'escale
332   De la nois gauge ou soit mise la galle,
Ou rosat o la foille de caisne ou d'eglenter,
De ronce, de egremone, de plantein, *de meller.*
Tel chose vaut ense[mb]le et par soi ensemant.
336   Puis li doint [l'en] a boívre autre chose effridant
Sicom[ë] ematite en ewe bien molus
Et poudre de coral, a ce si est salus.
De poume gernetë i mete l'en la flor
340   Et gomë arabic tot poet avoir valor,
O le serpol, o bol et de mirte semence,
De quer de cerf [la] poudre, planteine [. . .]
O le sanc de dragon [. . .]
344   Semence de coïgn *avec la tanesie.*
Verveine, ypolifive, de rara la racine,
Mentastre un poi quites, c'est bone me[di]cine.
Racine de feuke[role] et [de] la corrigiale

321. MS *en cist.*
322. MS *c. novele.* The correction is based on *LSM* 'ex colera nigra', S 'de neire cole'.
327. MS *les humes v.* S has 'Quant li cors est espurgiez de humors dedenz'.
328. *LSM* has 'quedam exterius que constringunt', S 'foreines mecines estreingnant'.
331f. MS *qui soit q. el escale et soit de la / nois gauge ou soit mise lescer.*
332. *LSM* has 'galle, testa nucina', S 'ou gaule ou l'eschale de la noiz gauge'. It is clear that 'lescer' is an error, but nothing in the source suggests an explanation. Equally, there is no obvious or safe solution to the hypometrism of the line as emended.
334. MS *planteine.* 'De meller' is an addition to the source.
335. MS *Tele.*
336. MS *Plus.* *LSM* has 'Postea inter cibaria detur . . .', S 'Puis li doinst l'on a boivre choses construistes entre viandes'. 'Effridant' I take to mean 'cooling'.
337. MS *amente*, a miscopying of *ametite* (for *ematite*).
341. MS *bolle et de moutez s.* S has 'piépol' (= portulaca), rather than 'serpol' (= serpyllum).
342. 'quer de cerf' is for 'corn de cerf' (*LSM* 'cornu cervi', S 'corne de cerf'), cf.510. *LSM* and S add 'centonica / centoine'.
343. *LSM* and S add 'spodii / spondion'.
344. MS *corgn.*
347. MS *cortagiale.*

348   *En ewe de ploue quite ensemblë o sale.*
             Gelines en paste mangut . . .
             Poissons frés a l'aisil . . .
             Poissons de doucë ewe [qui soient] eschardeuses
352   *Et [o des] blanches chars [li sunt mult] profiteuses.*
             Tisan d'orge pilé quit[e] en ewe de mer,
             Refroidé et colé li donés a manger.

Si boive rouge vin bon et loial tempré de euue de mer *ou de ploue* et avec la tisane racine de planteine, entre les dous vaut mult.

Ventuse sans garse por le sanc traire amont [. . .] *Laine carpie moillé* en jus de planteine *et trescié* et mise en la nassance auques parfont *se vaut quant el est bien amont.*

             Le jus de barbion quit en rouge vin ou blanc   f.225r
356   Profite mult a boivre por retenir le sanc.
              Bone est laine carpie en cest jus a moillier,
             Enaprés a la femme sor le ventre lïer.
             Bonë est de parele a boivre la racine
360   [. . .]

Quite en vin ou en ewe mult est bone et se li est bone a boivre l'ewe ou les feves aient esté quites. Et se doit on prendre del lard salé et pudrer de coriande *et de luvesce* ou de la semence et faire emplastre et lier sor le ventre avec lard et soz le nomblil.

349. The reading 'paste' diverges from *LSM* 'coctas in pane', S 'soleies en pain'.
351-2. find no correspondence in *LSM* but are reflected in S: 'Li poison soient de dolce eue qui aient escherdes et blanche char'.
351. MS *d. ewe a escalle.*
353. MS *Et tisane.* S has 'orge sechie', *LSM* 'de ordeo primitus desiccato'.
354. MS *Et r.* The detail of *LSM* 'apponatur acetum' (S 'si mete l'on l'aisil ovec') is omitted. The following lines have been 'derhymed'. 'ou de ploue' finds no authority in *LSM* or S. *LSM* continues 'et si radix plantaginis bullietur cum ptisana, tanto melius' (S 'Se il i a racines de plantein od le tipsan, tant valt mielz'). The next remedy is a truncated version of the source. S has 'Moult valt a cest mal a metre la ventose entre les mameles sanz garse k'ele traie le sanc amont' (W agrees, with minor changes of word order).
355. MS *r.v. ou en b.* For 'barbion' ('semperviva') S has the more standard 'jobarbe'. *LSM* speaks only of 'vino albo' (S 'od le viez vin blanc ou roge').
357-8. Absent from *LSM*. S has 'Contre icest mal bon est a prendre leine carpie et moillier en cel jus et lier sor son ventre'.
359. S has 'Bon est a cuire la racine de la parele en eue ou en vin et boivre le jus'. The final phrase has been lost in the process of derhyming which occurs in the course of the remedy. In the next remedy 'faire emplastre' is intrusive and replaces *LSM*'s 'pulvis absinthii' (S 'la poldre de l'aluisne'). I have emended MS *sor le nomblil* (*LSM* 'sub', S 'desus'). The detail 'avec lard' seems to be an anticipation of 'cum auxungia' in the next receipt, which is here omitted (S has the remedy, but not the detail).

La gote des rains

As reins et sor le ventre soit l'ortie triblee,
Vaut mult a la fïez o viels oint detempree,
Si la foille d'olive soit avec ajostee,
364   Mels vaudra la mecine [. . .]

Prenés des nois assés sicome on les escalle, se en faites poudre, puis li donés a boivre en ewe de mer.

A faire emplastre por la goute

Fetes enplastre de oint et fente de berbis,
Partie sor le ventre, partie as reins soit mis.
Prenés escalles d'oef dont sont issi pouchin,
368   *De cele poudre boive al soir et au matin*

[f.225v] par treis jors en froide ewe tant come vus porrés prendre a vos dous dois.

Por flors vermaux

A la fïez avient a femme uns maux haïz,
Aochement l'apelent qui vient de la marris,
[Avient] quant li marris est trop [amont] monté
372   [Et] por ce faut a femme de men[g]er volenté.
Adonc sovent se palme et li cors refroidist,
Li pox li apetice et mult li afeblist,
Qu'ele [le] part del tot; une fois a si grief

361. MS *soz.*
363. MS *f. de li.* I have emended on the evidence of S ('fueille de l'olive'), though *LSM* has 'folia ulmi' (misread as 'ulivi'?).
364. No obvious element of the source is lacking. In the following derhymed remedy (where the MS has *boirre*) 'nois' corresponds to *LSM*'s 'teste maiorum nucum' (S 'noiz gauges').
365. MS *et de f.*
367. MS *escalle del oef.* The following 'dont sont issi pouchin', found also in S, is an addition to the source.
368. At the end of this receipt *LSM* has 'quantum sublevare poteris de pulvere tribus digitis' (S 'od trois deiz', but 'par quatre jourz' for *LSM*'s 'per .iii. dies')
369. MS *f. versmaux h.*
370. MS *Asolement les a..* The emendation is after S which has 'A la fiee avient un mal a feme ke l'on apele aochement de marriz' and W which has 'oschement'.
371. MS *montee.* In the MS the line is obviously hypometric, though nothing from *LSM* / S is omitted.
372. MS *que veut par fevre.* There is no question of fever in the source.
374. MS *li apeire.*
375. S 'si k'ele pert del tot', *LSM* 'pulsus evanescit, ita quod penitus non sentiatur'.

376   Que ele met par son mal a ses genuls seon chief.
               Donc li torne la buch[e] et si estreint les dens
               Et li pis li sozleve asés amarement.

Galïens

               Galïens nus reconte de feme qui out mal,
380   La parole out perdue, le pox, pres ert mortal,
               Në avoit de sa vie nul essamplor
               Nemais entor le quer un petit de calor,
               Plusor des mires le manaceient de morte
384   Et disoient entre lor dens que ele estoit morte.
               Galïens li plus sages laine carpie prist,
               A sa buche et son niés corteisement le mist.
               Li procein esgarde[nt] que un petit se movoit,
388   Adonc aparceurent que encore vive estoit.
               Cis maux avient a femme par mauveise semence
               Qui est desnaturel, s'i est grant habondance.
               C'est por ce que el se tient de home trop longement,
392   Et a femme veve avent ce plus sovent
               Qui sovent [ert] enseinte et avoit grant usage
               Et orë est sauns home et [en] ad grant dammage.
               As puceles cist maux poet [tres] bien avenir
396   Quant vienent a l'age que home doivent suffrir.
               Quant n'ont conjuge de home en icel temperal,
               Adonques la covient entecer de cel mal,
               [Car] naturë habonde en eles par semence
400   K'ele en vodreit geter par male science.
               Hors de cele semence, quant [est] desnaturee,

377. Whilst S also has 'la bouche li torne', LSM has 'labia distorquentur'.
379. MS *de une qui out un mal*. LSM has 'hunc morbum', S 'cest mal'.
380. MS *pres de mortal* is obscure. I have emended in accordance with LSM which has 'erat quasi defuncta'.
381. An obviously hypometric line.
382. MS *de cali* with 'plusor' following on the same line.
384. MS *d. teux i eust e. l. d.*. LSM has simply 'plures eam mortuam reputabant', S 'plusors des mires'.
386. MS *a son n*. The detail 'son niés' agrees with LSM against S, which omits it.
390. 'desnaturel' renders LSM's 'in venenosam conversum naturam'.
391. MS *ele*.
393. LSM 'que consueverunt uti carnali virorum commercio', S 'ki sovent a esté hantee et sovent enceinte'.
400. MS *Ki l'en . . . maligne science*. The line is evidently corrupt. LSM has 'semen, quod per masculum natura vellet expellere', S 'quant la nature les voldreit geter del cors par masle'.
401. MS *Et lors*.

Par habundance grant s'en ist une fumee
Desca as cornilles qui al quer sont ajostees,
404   Al polmon et aillors, teus sont lor destinees,
A autre leus remonte qui a ce apertenient,
Le parler pert la femme quant teus choses avenent.
Cist maux [a]vient a femme par ses flors que ele pert
408   Et se les flors le faillent *et li hom ne li sert*
Et la semence habunde, lors est plus en apert,
Ci[s] maux avien[t] a femme par ces flors que ele pert.
      La preme medecine qui est a icel mal   f.226v
412   Quant doit faire a la femme, ce tien [jo] a loial.
De bon ole laurin doit oindre piés et mains,
Ce est bone medicine, de ce sui jo certains.
Puis [li] metez al nes choses de froide odor
416   Et contrariouses sicome est de castor
Et de galbeene et leine arse et de piez
Et odors ausi fors autre mettre devez,
C'est por trairë aval la semence et les flors.
420   Ventouses li mete on as hanches [. . .]
Et desus le penil ventuses i metés.
De oile et de oignement de bon odor le oignez
Et dedens et defors oignement i mete on.
424   Et au ceir li donez bon diaciminon.
Diaciminon soit o le jus destemprés
De ache, de calament le sirop li donez.
Gerapigre od le jus de aloigne [. . .],
428   *De aloigne qui soit quite li oignez la nessance.*

---

403. *LSM* 'ad quasdam partes ascendit quo vulgo dicuntur 'corneliers', S 'monte une fume as corneilles'. Green, "The Development of the *Trotula*" (forthcoming) lists the formal variants of this word.

404. The phrase 'aillors' coupled with 'a autre leus . . . qui a ce apertenient' (405) replaces *LSM* 'et ceteris instrumentis vocis', S 'et as altres estrumenz ki apertienent a la voiz'.

410. A repetition of 407. Omitted is the detail that the sickness is worst of all 'quando partes occupat alteriores' (*LSM*), 'com il est halt' (S).

415. MS *de nef.* 'froide odor' seems to be an error for 'fort odor' (see 418, and SW), cf. *LSM* 'gravis odoris'.

416. MS *Et de contralienses.* S has 'contrarioses', though this detail is not in *LSM*.

417. A hypometric line, with some material omitted. *LSM* 'galbanum, pix, lana combusta, lineus pannus combustus vel pellis combustus et similia'.

418. MS *fois. LSM* has 'et similia. Oleis autem et unguentis que sint gravis odoris debet inungi vulva, ut yreleon, musceleon, camomilleon, nardileon', S 'et linge drap ars et fumee de peil ars et de altres choses de fort odor. Oile et oignement doit l'en metre en la naisance ki seient de bon odor com est yrileon et muceleon, nardileon . . .'

425. MS *ale j.*

426. MS *de s.*

427–30 are not in *LSM*. S has 'ou od ierapigre ou od le jus de l'aluisne. Si li doint l'on .i. .z. d'agaric od le vin de bon odor. L'on doit laver la naisance od l'aluisne cuite ou de quinalt ou de centoieire ou de anet ou de kalament ou de nepite'.

Lavés [la] de centoine et [de] bon calament,
De pulïol, de nepte, [i]ce vaut autretant.
A [i]cest mal deus drames valent de jusqïan,
432   De castoire et de cost, de ache, de poivre blanc,
De mirre, de chescon drame une destemprez.   f.227r
Puis un poi od [vin] douz a boivre li donez.
Ce que jo apel drame de trois deners est li pois,
436   Ou de trois angevins ou de trois margillois.
[Justin] li mire rove bon comin a secchier
Por [i]cel mal oster pleinë une quillier,
Tribler et faire pudre et a boivre donier.
440   Enaprés si comande autre chose aprester:
Oint rove de goupil et de chievre meller
Et faire bone emplastre et sor le mal poser
Ou par desuz amettre ausi com[e] pesaire.

Oribaces

444   Oribases comande un autre chose a faire,
Racines de egremoine, le finagrec ense[mb]le,
Rove quire et puis mettre tot chaut en la nassance,
Et si dit que mult vaut la racine paree
448   De la wimauve quite, enaprés bien triblee
Ensemble od le viés oint sur le numblil posee,
C'est bone medicine, si est [mult] esprovee.
         Si la marris avale quant avra eu enfant,
452   Ceste mecine faites que trovums en present.
De l'avo[i]ne molés [et] puis li eschaufés,
En toie d'oriller al ventre li metés.
         Par mainte fois avale le marris de son leu,   f.227v
456   Fors est de [la] nassance, cest dammage fais preu.
[Et] ce avient par ce que ele est trop amolie

---

431. Agrees with S ('.ii. .z.') against LSM '.z. .i.'
432. MS castoires.
433. MS De mine.
435–6. These lines are unique to the verse translation. LSM has 'et bibat .z. .i. pondus trium denariorum'.
437. LSM has 'Justinus medicus', S 'Justinus li mires'. LSM has 'dari' for 'a secchier' (S also).
441. MS r. de carpir. For 'oint' (S also) LSM has 'priapum'.
443. MS com apeser. S has 'metre desus ou enz od le pessaire'. The following rubric reads Ombaces.
444. MS Ombases.
445. MS finagrec (LSM 'fenugrecum'). S has 'fanoil'. The reading 'egremoine' is an error – LSM has 'germandrie/germandree', S 'de germandree'. The present rhyme is faulty (but see 537–8) and may originally have been 'de lin la semence'.
447. MS parce. LSM has 'radix levistici', but this is not in S.
448. Instead of 'racine . . . de la wimauve', LSM has 'radix levistici'.
452. MS medicine.

Et par une autre chose, que bien est refroidie.
Cist amoliemens et cist effroidemens
460   Poet avenir par ço que trop [est] longemens
En aucon leu od lui par desus refroidie,
Por bain dë ewe froyde qui a si en baillie.
La marris amolie, par tel entechement
464   Ist desus de l'enfant quant vient enforcement.
Së ele chiet aval et n'est issue fors,
Espece li metés al nes de bon odor[s]
Sicom[e] basme, espic, foille, storac et roses
468   Et de bones odors totes ces autre choses.
Estuver de fors choses par desus la devez,
C'est laine arse, drap lange, opopanas et peiz.
Se ce avient a femme que ad eü enfant
472   Et la marris li enfle par aconoissement,
Laine en oile ou en vin bien moillie prenés,
Totes les faites plastres, sor son nomblil metés.

A la marris

A la marris cheüe [a]monïac prenés,
476   [Et od le jus d'aluisne mult bien le destemprés].
Le ventre od une penne bonement li oignez.
De gase une poigné aquere comandez   [f.228r]
Et autretant de rue et autretant de armoyce,
480   [. . .]
Si les quisés en vin et puis [si] li donés.
Et eschaufés forment, adonques le metés
Sur le nomblil al ventre, ensi li mecinés
484   [. . .]
Quant li marris abesse et est issu[e] fors,

462. MS *Por boivre.*
463. MS *a. itels e.*
464. 'enforcement de l'enfant' corresponds to *LSM* 'conamen pareidi'.
466. MS *les m.*
467. MS *S. foil e. foilles toras et r.* 'roses' is an addition to the source.
468. MS *et totes.*
470. MS *Ceste . . . et panas des pies.*
471–4. find no correspondence in *LSM*, but are in S: 'Se ce avient a feme quant ele a eu enfant, ou
se la marriz li enfle, pregne l'on leine, si la mete l'on en oile et en vin, et la face l'on plate et si la
mete l'on sor l'omblil'.
478. 'gase' = 'cassia' (S 'cassie').
479. S has 'd'altunesie' for 'arthemisia'.
481. MS *Si li q.*
482. MS *fortment.*
483. MS *medicines.*

Premier[e]ment covient quë on [la] mette el cors,
Et puis se baint en eue la femme, ce commant,
488   Ou soit quite la rose et l'ermoise ensement.
De la poume gernete l'escorce metés ens
Et gales et simac et del cheine les glans.
L'escorce o la foille de cheine ovec metés
492   Et poume de ciprés, si trover le poés.
Totes ces choses valent ensemble ajostés
Ou chascone par soi quant eles sont trovees.
De ces choses ansi li fetes estuver,
496   Car mult li aidera, ce doit espermenter.
  Dïacorides dit que estuver la doit on,
Si que de boisce secche soient li vif carbon.
La femme doit so[o]ir desus les carbons vifs,
500   Les carbons doivent estre en un pot bien assis.
Apparreillé doit estre si quë ele se sié
Desure le carbon *sus la sele par[cié]*.   [f.228v]
De dras tot environ la doit on aörner,
504   Si quë a la nassance puisse le funs entrer.
Ses mangers soit tot f[r]e[i]s, n'ait peivre ne comin,
N'i ait ail ni airon et boive feble vin.
De nul fruit ne mangut, [mes] nus otrïon mesles
508   Et cormes et coöns, pomes egres *et pesches*.

A la marris issue medecine

Mecine est esprové a la marris issue:
Poudre de quer de cierf *que soit beste menue*,
De foille de lorer et de mirre prenés,
512   De chascon un[ë] once, ensemble les metés.
Tot destemprés en vin a boivre li donés,
Donc i va la marris en son leu, nen dotés.
  La marris de son leu se muë a la fie,

487. MS *s. b. apres*.
490. MS *des ch*. Omits 'mirta' (*LSM*; S 'mirre').
492. With S omits 'lenticula' (*LSM*).
494. MS *Et . . . eles en s*.
498. *LSM* 'de sicco buxo', S 'de rose seche'.
504. MS *le feus*.
505. MS *soient tos*.
506. 'feble vin' represents *LSM* 'vinum vetus temperatum cum aqua marina', S 'viez vin od eue de mare'.
507f. The lines end in a mere assonance.
509. MS *Medicine*.
511. MS *f. de olive*.
515. MS *se met*.

516   Si que la femme en est malement entechie,
             Et ne vet pas amont desi al corniliere
             Ne aval ne chiet mie, nequedent est [. . .]
             Estraite de son leu et n'est pas fors issue.
520   [. . .]
             Cist maux en tel manere aparcëu poet estre
             Que la dolors en est el flanc devers senestre.
             De la dolor al ventre espointes poet sentir,
524   Enfle li sa sastine que ne pot transglutir.
             Et si la femme ad froit, li membres tendent tuit,
             [Et] ele tort sovent et li ventres li r[u]it.   f.229r
             A ce [prenés de l'ache o] finigrec triblés,
528   [Et] destemprés en vin a boivre li donés.
               Et prenés agarie, avesques soit triblee
             Semence de planteine avec de la sarree,
             Si en faites la pudre et si donés a boivre
532   Od mel et o vin quit; de son mal soit deso[i]vre.
               Ki vodra la marris en son leu amener,
             Si que nule dur[e]ce n'i pusse demorer,
             Moële de cierf prende et oint d'oie ensement
536   Et cire roge et bure, de chascom uëlment.
             Dous onces i ajoigne, sicome jo comant,
             Puis prenge finegrec et mete tot ensemble,
             Tot soit bien quit [en eue], parmi un drap colé,
540   Avec ole de olive tot ce soit ajosté
             Et les choses qui sont la desure nomees
             Quites a petit feu, puis soient ensemblees.
             Tant qui bien seient quites les quisés lentement,
544   Aprés o le passere metés al naissement.
             Ice profite mult, se fait le mire fis
             A plusors achesons quant vient a la marris.
               A la fiez avient encor de autre manere
548   A la marris un mal qui est de tel manere.
             Dedens ad un' angoisse et un eschaufement   f.229v

---

517. Here 'corniliere' (SW 'cornilles') stands for 'spiritualia'.
521. MS *tele*.
522. MS *les dolors . . . el franc*.
523. LSM has 'tortionem et rugitum ventris'.
524. MS *Enfre*.
525. MS *m. tremblent tuis*.
526. MS *tost s. et volenters*. Cf. S 'li ventres li ruit et ele rote'.
529. Omits LSM's 'aspaltum' (S 'espaute').
530. MS *sentee*.
534. MS *male d.*
536. MS *uielment*.
537. MS *iao i.*
548. MS *tele*.

Ke les dames apelent grant esbolissement.
Si par est eschaufee la marris la dedens,
552   *Semble qu'il i art boische ou [bien] tison ardant,*
Contre cel mal covient que nus fortment pensons
[. . .]
De la cire del mel, del mirre, de chascon
556   Quatre onces i avra et de dous oes l'aubon,
D'oilë un once et creie, lait de femme i metés,
Ensi com on doit fere tot ensemble i metés,
Iceste medicine ensi covient a faire,
560   Dedens par la nassance metés o le pessaire.

A la marris

A la fies nassent clos dedens la marris,
Emfleures et boces, sicom dit li escris.
Icés enfermetés sont de plusors maneres,
564   Par ces covient li mires garder les maneres.
Se li clos est de colre, tel est la conoissance,
De sun fiel est issus par si grant abondance,
Adonques ist cist clos de fevre ou de chalor,
568   Encontre covient faire mecine de froydor.
Ce comande Ypocras nus devons par contraire
Contre les maladies les medecines faire.
  Tel [clos] a la fiez est de froides humors,
572   Ensi come est de fleume et de noires humors,
Adonc enfle li clos et si est dur fortment,   f.230r

---

550. Not in *LSM*, but see S 'ke l'en apele boillement e marriz'.
552. *LSM* 'maximus ardor intus sentiatur'; S 'com s'il i eust breses'.
554. *LSM* has 'accipe opii dragmam .i., adipis anserini dragmas .ii.', S '.i. .z. et d'opie et de sain d'oue'.
555. 'mirre' not in *LSM* or S.
557. MS *et cru l*. *LSM* has 'albugines duorum ovorum et cretam et lac mulieris', S 'les albuns des .ii. oes et creie et let de feme'.
559. MS *et ensi*.
564. It looks as if 'maneres' has been repeated at the rhyme through eyeskip, though cf. 571–2.
565. MS *colere*.
567. *LSM* has 'tunc febrem facit vel cancrum', S 'donc est ou crancre ou fievre', W 'est chaut et o fievre'.
568. MS *c. medicine faire de f*.
569–70. Not in *LSM* or S.
571. MS *Tele a*. 'froides humors' assumes a reading 'frigidi humores' (found in some Latin MSS) rather than *LSM*'s 'grossi humores', S 'de grosses humors'.
572. *LSM* 'Si grossi humores ut flegma vel colera enim in causa sint . . .', S 'A la fiee est il de grosses humors com d'enfleure et de noire cole'.

            Les hanches et les quisses vont ape[san]tissant.
            Teus clos i a qui nassent de grant ventosité,
576   Ensi come est de copp ou d'autre enfermeté.
            A la fïez avient quë el [en] pert ses flors,
            Ke tel clou nast dedens, [si] a donc grans dolors.
            Se li clos est devant, tel est la conoissance,
580   Ke la femme ad dolor en[tor de] sa naissance.
            De sei meïmes naist encore autre querele,
            Icil qui la conoissent chaudepisse l'apelent.
            Quant cil clos en la buche de la marris est nees,
584   Es hanches, el nomblil [si] ad dolor assees.
            Par derier vers le dos si li clo est fermés,
            La femme ad mal el dos et desoz les costés.
            Par itel clou covient un autre mal venir,
588   La femme est costivee, qu[ë] il ne peut issir.
              Se de sanc est li clou ou de la ruge cole,
            Adonques covient nus une autre parole.
            La femme suffre un mal que ad nun fevre ague,
592   Le matin et le soir de grant dolor l'argue.
            Par itel mal soffrir a bien sovent dolor,
            Encontre ce covient [avoir] feël aideor.
            [Tot] al comencement encerchier nus covient
596   Dont li cloux est nascus et de que[l] part il vient.   f.230v
            Së il est que li cloux cest chalor li ameine,
            La femme covendra adonc seiner de veine,
            De la veine du pé covient le sanc atraire,
600   Ce comande li mestres dans Galïen a fere,
            Galïens li plus sages maistres disoit, de main
            Se [l'on] la femme seine, le seinie est en vain.
            Il mostre par semblant que nuist ceste seinie
604   [A] femme que el marris ad nule maladie,
            Kar [la] seiné de main [a]trait le sanc amont
            Et cë est l'acheison par quei les flors perdront.
            Por ce l'ad comandé aval del pé seiner
608   Tant come ele porra suffrir et [en]durer.

574. MS *li vont.* Cf. S 'les hanches li endurcissent et apesantissent'.
580. MS *sa conoissance.*
581. MS *un autre.*
582. LSM 'stranguria'.
584. LSM 'circa umbilicum et nares', S 'al nonblil et as naches', clearly suggesting the Latin 'nates'.
585. MS *vers de dors.*
586. MS *si li deut* l.c. Cf. LSM 'est dolor sub costis', S 'a dolor desoz les costes'.
590. MS *Aidonc.*
592. MS *Ke le m.*
595. MS *n. c. encerchier.*
601. MS *m. quisoit*

Se ele ad tant de vertu quë ele est si hardie,
En un jor li covient dous fois ceste seignie.
Et si elë est feble, une fois est li drois,
612   [. . .]
Se li doint on a boivre [deus fïez] enseur jur
Tel chose que li puisse tolir ceste chalor,
Sicome de morele, de ce boive le jus,
616   Cassïafistre et manne, et encore i ad plus
[Come] jus de planteine triblé o barbïon.
Oile que l'en apele rosat *et silïum*
Et autres choses froides a boivre li donés
620   Et emplastre ensement sor le nomblil metés.   f.231r
    Tel seit que li poisse tolir ceste chalor
Et pres de la marris li soit [bon] conforteor
Sicome est de plantaine et jus de barbïon,
624   Semence de conconbre avec le psilïon.
Aprés mellés [a ce] porcelleine et morele,
[Et puis] ole rosat *avec de la canele.*
    Aprés ce li covient tel emplastre a ssufrir
628   Ke soit de tel manere qui le face amollir,
Ausi come de bure quit ovec la litose
Et finegrec ensemble et mauve et tele chose.
Tot [ce] soit quit od oint de owë ou de geline,
632   En ceste manerë est covenable mecine.
Et del meliliton od l'aubon de dous oès.
Aprés ceste mecine passere face on luès,
[Et] de totes ces [choses] ensemblë ou par soi
636   Li poés medicine mult bien faire, ce croy.
    Dïacorides dit que mult profiteroit
Së ele siet en eue ou le spic quit seroit.
    Paulus enseigne [a feme] a faire un grant maistrie

---

613. MS *enseur le j.*
614. MS *Tele.*
616. MS *mauue et encorei ili ad p.*. The line is repeated in 621, as 617 is in 623, largely as the result of the similarity of two successive therapeutic measures in *LSM*.
617. MS *ovec b.*
618, MS *Et mel.* 'silium' may have arisen as a misunderstanding of *LSM* 'et similia' or else as an anticipation of 'psillii' in the next therapy, see 624.
624. 'semence de conconbre' is not in *LSM*.
626. 'avec de la canele' is an addition.
628. MS *tele. LSM* recommends 'maturativa' (S 'choses qui le clou facent meurer').
629. corr. *la litose* to *titolose* ('crow garlic', Colchicum autumnale L.)? *LSM* has 'semen lini coctum cum butiro', S 'linuis cuit od burre'.
632. MS *medicine.*
634. MS *medicine.*
638. MS *ele fiert el pie avec le s.* Cf. S 'moult valt a seeir en une ewe ou espic soit cuit'.
639. *LSM* has 'docet fieri quoddam pessarium', S 'un macine chaude'.

640   Al mal de [la] marris ke trop est endorcie
        Et a ce encor quant ele est trop enversee
        Et la ventosité, coment en soit ostee.
        De veël la moële que un home doit prendre avant,   f.231v
644   Oint de tesson avec sis onces bien pesant,
        De moële de cierf autresi i metra,
        Sis drames bien pesant la mesure sera.
        [. . .]
648   [Et] del seim de ces dous dosse deniers pesant,
        Et saffron et mastic et miel ensemblerum
        Od le lait de la femme tot cest destemprerum
        Et od ole mul[t] bone ensemble mellerois,
652   Aprés o le pessare dedens le lanceroys.
        Emplastre covenable de tot cest poés fere
        Par meus afait[i]er et par santé atraire.

                              De la marris

        Derechif se li cloux est de froyde nature
656   Et des humors espesses, donc convient autre cure.
        Cel medicine estoit sus adonques poser
        Ke la dedens le puisse departir et oster.
        Finigrec, mellilot, od le mecinement,
660   Et les legiers mangiers li doinst on ensement
        Et de boire sotil et delïé manger
        Ke les groses humors puissent atenvïer.
            S'en esgarde qui puisse amendement trover,
664   Donc le face en emplastre que la puisse crever

641. MS *encore*.
642. *LSM* 'contra . . . ventositatem eiciendam a corpore'.
644. MS *Oint de chascon*. *LSM* has 'adipem melote' (S 'oint de taisson'), other versions of the *LSM* have 'adipis caponis' and 'taxonis' (with 'melote' corrupted to 'meliloti'). The measure in *LSM* is given as 'pondus .xviii. denariorum'. In a versified form of this chapter, *Coll. Sal.* 4, p.22 we read "Anseris hec adipem recipit gallique, crocumque, / Ana sex dragmas'.
648. 'ces dous' refers to *LSM*'s 'adipem anserinum et gallinaceum'. For 'dosse deniers' *LSM* has 'ana dragmas .iiii.'
649. Omits *LSM*'s 'ysopi' (S 'd'isope').
650. MS *la lait*.
651. *LSM* and S specify 'oleum rosaceum' / 'oile rose'. Our text is probably corrupt.
652. MS *pesans*.
657. MS *sus os a*.
658. MS *la p*.
659. MS *melle avec la medicine*. *LSM* has 'accipe fenugrecum, mellilotum, semen lini, semen rute'. Our text omits *LSM*'s 'semen lini, semen rute' (S 'linuis et mente') and following instructions.
663. MS *nul a*. This line bears no relationship to *LSM* 'Vel si ad saniem velimus converti apostema', S 'Se l'on veut ke il tort a cuiture'. 'Qui' stands for 'qu'il'.

De l'ermoise quite et finegrés ensement
Et de ferine d'orge et ausi de forment,
Et de la feve quite li ajostent li sage,   f.232r
668   De la fiente ausi quit de colombe ramage.
            Si li cloux est crevé et la palus s'en tret
        A la vessie droit, donc li doinst on de let
        De l'anessë a boivre et del chiefre ensement,
672   Semence de conconbre avec par avenant.
        Encore i ajostés semence de melon
        [. . .]
            A la marris ausi [et] dedens la nassance
676   Avient a la fiez une grant mesestance
        Par les aigres mecines com plaies et malanz,
        Et d'avorter ravient tele chose ensement.
        Ce poet on bien conustre par le palu de cors,
680   Quë ele en voit issir et qui ist del cors fors,
        Par [les] dolors qui sont, par les enpointes grans
        Que la femme sustent en la marris dedans.
        Si malan et les plaies sont de [la] purreture
684   Qui des veines s'en issent par aucone aventure,
        Se la palus que en ist torne a aucon verdor
        Et cele purreture soit d'orible püor,
        En la nassance mettre covient premerement,
688   En la marris avec, tel medecinement
        Ke la nassance puisse neitir et entemprer,
        Ensorquetot encore a la dolor oster,
        Sicome de morele et de plantein le jus,   f.232v
692   Ole rosat ensemble, aubon de oef ne refus,
        Od le let de la femme, o jus de porcell[a]ine,
        Autre froide mecine que [tut] seit en certaine,
        Coördes deit manger la femme por chalor,
696   Porcelleine, autres choses qui sient de froydor.

665. MS *lermoise quite* is an error for 'linuis quit' (S), but the line then becomes hypometric.
666. MS *fortment*.
668. MS *Et . . . de la c.*
674. LSM has 'fiat ei clistere de ptisana et melle' (S 'clistrere li face l'on de miel tipsan').
677. MS *medicines*.
681. MS *de grans*.
683. MS *Li*.
684. MS *de les v.*
685. LSM 'nigredinem', S 'neiror'.
687. MS *c. m.*
689. MS *moistir*.
691. MS *planteine*.
692. MS *Od r.*
694. MS *A autre f. medicine*.
696. MS *le f.*

En l'aue ou soit quite la flor de eglenter,
En l'a[ue] rose, en mirre le face [l'on] baignier
Ou en l'eue [de] flor de [la] poume gernate,
700   O lentilles, o gales et o autre barate,
O les foilles de caisne avec del casteg[n]er,
De coïgnier la foille o cele de mellier.
    Se veines sont purries, pregne sanc de dragon
704   O mirrë o encens o bol erminicon,
U croc o *spodïon*, o aristelogie,
Autant vaut licïum o bonë acacie,
Tels choses valent mult, s'en en fait [un] pesaire,
708   Ensemble appareillee clistre rest bon a fere.
    Se dedens li mangue la nassance quisant,
Pregne litarge et canfre et [le] croc ensement,
Baies o aubun de oef et [puis] ole rosat,
712   Pa[r] clistere o pessaire en [le] cors li enbat.
    Dïacorides dit, li mires qui ne faut,
Poudre de finigrec od sanc d'owe [mult] vaut   f.233r
A la durece grant de l[a] marris oster,
716   S'il est qui tel pessaire sace bien atorner.

Del marris

Ce nus dit Ypocras, que tot le bien enseigne,
Femme ne poet concoivre ou tels teces aveigne:
Femme quë est trop crasse ne fait conceivement,
720   Cele quë est trop megre le pert bien ensement;
Femmes que sunt trop crasses par ce perdent l'esploite,
Ke de la marris est la bouche trop estroite,
Et par ce ne poet [mie] la semence ens entrer,
724   [Et] par ceste raison poet laissier le porter.
    A la fïez [li] rest la marris ensi grans
Que ne poet la semence [si] retenir dedens.
Ne la poet retenir marris par la sentence.
728   Et mult homes refunt qu'espandent la semence,

698. MS *r. et en m.*
701–2. These are additions to the source. S has 'ou foille de cassie ou altres choses de tel maniere'.
705. MS *Veroc . . . et o a.*
706. MS *v. bucilion.*
708. MS *clastre.* Corr. 'clistere est'?
712. MS *Paclistere a puissance.*
714. MS *od saim d'owe chaut.*
725. LSM has 'matrices ita lubricas', S 'la marriz si esluant'. W 'escrilourge' is for 'escolourgeable' or 'escolourgeant'. Our text obscures this reference to the endometrium.
726. MS *Que ele n.*

Nature ont froide et secche, ne ja n'engendr[er]ont
[. . .]
  Cil qui vodra saver se la femme est baraigne
732   Ou par l'enfermeté de l'home se contaigne,
Dous poes covient a prendre, mettre bren a chascon,
Donc doit mettre del date de l'home dedenz l'un,
Del date de la femme en l'autre remetés:
736   Si coupe est en la femme, donc [bien] le conoistrés,
El dat de li verrés vermelles a fïance
Et autretant de l'home se par lui est faillance.   f.233v
Si l'un d'els n'i a coupe, donc lor est bien aidans
740   Li mires par mecines si qu'il avront enfans.

Por conceivre

Femme que voit conceivre de ver prengne collions,
[Et] si en face pudre, ensi le comandons,
Et si la boive en vin, par fai la conseilons,
744   A la fin de ces flors gisë o son baron.
Por masle conceivre fai secchier la nassance
Et la marris del lievre, cë est bone semence,
Et cele pudre a boivre as masles la doinst on.
748   A la femme de lievre portë on l'un coillon,
Le coillon tranglutisse, ce li doi[t] [bien] plaisir,
A la fin de ses flors o masle doit gesir.
Pregne la femme le[i]ne, lie sor son nomblil,
752   Mollie en let d'anesse, se veut ou fillie ou fil,
Et quant ele vora gesir o son baron,
 La leine i soit liee, car fere le doit on.
Pudre de [ui de] chaine boivë ovec le vin

729f. *LSM* has 'Quidam autem viri testiculos habent frigide et sicce complexionis et isti raro aut nuncquam possint generare quia semen eo inutile est generationi'.
734. MS *d. on . . .en l'un.*
735. MS *Et del d.*
737. Omits *LSM*'s 'et cantabrum fetidum'.
738. MS *la f.*
739. MS *Si lon.*
740. MS *medicines.*
745. MS *Par . . . cercher.*
746. MS *Od.* *LSM* has 'testiculos verris' (S 'coiz e ver'), but other MSS have 'leporis'.
750. MS *ovec m.*
751. MS *lu la sor.*
752. The second half of the line is an addition to the source.
753. MS *quam.*
755. MS *P. de canure.* To emend the text in accordance with *LSM* 'Accipe corticem quercus et pulveriza' would produce a hypermetric line. I follow S 'Face poldre de vi(f) de chesne', which may

756   A la comencement des flors et a la fin.
                Pregnë et ait le femme le foie et les collions
            Del premerain porcel que ja trover porons,
            Le foie et les coillons doit on primes sechier,
760   Si en face [l'on] pudre [a] qui avra mester.
            Donés a boivre a home qu[i] engendrer ne peut,   f.234r
            A la femme autresi que conceivre ne peut.
            Costentin nostre maistre ce defe[n]t as meschines
764   O estroites nassance[s] et o marris petites,
            A hom carnelement ne doit pas approcher,
            Kar së ele conceit, el morra de leger.
            Mes par ce quë aucone de tel nature estoit,
768   Ne remandroit pas seine si hant de home n'avoit,
            Chascone de eles face tel medicine ou quiere
            Que ne puisse conceivre par aucone manere.
            A la mustoile masle tollés li les coillons,
772   Lassés l'ent aler vive, ensi le comandons.
            La femme en pel de quir en son sein les avra,
            Nen porra conceivre tan[t] come el les avra.
                Galïens, cil qui dit tante bone sentence,
776   Nus reconte en un livre des enfans la nassance,
            Q'ausi come li fruit en l'arbre en aventure
            Est el cor a la femme li enfes par nature.
                Se femme [q']est enceinte a mester d'espurger,
780   Ce nus dist Ypocras, autresi de seignier,
            El ne le doit pas fere devant les quatre mois,
            Li seines et li autre li resont [b]en de fois.
            Entre le setime, ce dit [il], et la quart

have shared its reading with the exemplar used by the verse translator. W has simply 'Autre poudre face de chene'.
757. MS *Aloine et aile f.*
758. LSM 'testiculos primi porcelli que solum scropha ediderit', S 'les coiz del premier porcel ke truie a sol'.
759. MS *sacer.*
760. MS *faces.*
761. MS *Sen d. . . . que engendireut.*
763. MS *melines.* Another example of final assonance instead of rhyme.
766. MS *ele.*
767. MS *tele.*
771. S omits the contraceptive measures.
773. MS *en un poi de q.* LSM has 'in asinina pellicula'. W is defective after 756.
774. MS *ele.*
775–8. These lines telescope the latin to little more than a reference to Galen's comparison.
776. MS *une l.*
777. MS *Ce ausi . . . est en l.*
779. MS *Se la f.*
781. MS *Ele.*
783. MS *en la q.*

784   Puet on doner mecine et seignier a regart,   f.234v
               Al quint et al septime tot mesurablement
               Solonc ce que porra suffrir le verament.
                   Quant la feme est enceinte de novel, tot de voir,
788   Ne li remembrés chos[e] que ele ne puisse avoir,
               Kar plusors mainte foiz ont perdu [lors] enfans
               Kant eles oent ce dont tant sunt desirans.
                   Quant aproche li termes, au baign sovent se ploit
792   Et dë ole d'olive oindre son ventre doit.
               Entor icel termine la femme manger doit
               Bon manger et soluble et que legier soit.
               Si li piés sunt enflés, jo lo que li oigniez
796   De bon ole rosat ou d'aisil le baigniez.

Ke ne se poent delivrer a l'enfanter

               Auquetes ont grans ventres a lor enfanter,
               Auquetes ne se poent tel ore delivrer.
               Cest a chescon avient par diverse manere,
800   Mes jo en mostr[er]ai conoissance legiere,
               Kar estrange chalor lor vient a fondement
               Et trop de nature, que lor greve fortment
               [. . .]
804   Cele femme devom en tele ewe baignier
               Ou soit quite la mauve, finigrec et linués
               Et de orge quit ovec ole de viole oignés
               Ses flans et sa nassance, ses quises a raison.   f.235r
808   [. . .]
                   Les femmes qui la servent en son liu doivent estre
               Que ne voient son vis par devant ne sun estre,
               Kar teux i a assés que vergoine ont mult grant
812   Quant il les covient estre en tel efforcement.
                   Si ce est que li enfes mestorne ledement
               Ke [le] bras ou [la] jambe en est issus avant,
               A tel bosoign covient que femme soit eslite

---

796. MS *o i doisse*. After this line there is a large cut in the source material which is accurately reproduced by S.
797. LSM has 'Sunt autem quedam mulieres que in officio partus angustiose torquentur et quedam se expedire non possunt, quod quidem ex diversis causis contingit'.
801. *LSM* 'circa anteriora'.
803. A number of lines in the source are omitted.
806. MS *quit quit . . . de huc*(?) *oignies*. LSM has 'Ungantur venter et latera et coxe et vulva e oleo violaceo'.
808. A number of lines in the source are omitted.
815. MS *bosoigne*.

816   Que soit de tel manere que la main ait petite.
       La verveine covient a loier sor le ventre,
       Ou soit mort ou soit vif, faite[s] le issir del [ventre].

A la marris

       Puis que nes est li enfes par aucone aventure
820   Avient que la dedens remaint la vestëure.
       A geter le covient del cors menuement,
       Covient que l'en li face esternuer sovent,
       Et son nes et sa boche li covient a tenir
824   Que fus në aleine ne puisse fors issir.
       Lessive de cendre froide soit aportee,
       De semence de mauve la poudre ert ajostee,
       Une drame de pudre a boivre li donés,
828   Si la fetes vomir si fere le poés.
           En l'ongle de cheval ou en poissons salés
       Ou en fente de chate la femmë estuvés,
       Ice fait de la femme issir la vestëure   f.235v
832   Et le sanc enaprés, c'est tot solonc nature.
           Si aprés la vesteure le sanc ne poet issir,
       Faites cest qu'est ariere, ce ert por flors venir.
       Entendés la sentence, ce nus dit Ypocras,
836   Que de ensegner ses clers ne fu [ja] onques las.
       Ki veut savoir de femme de quel enfant est pleine,
       Pregnë en un vassel de la cliere fonteine,
       La femme de son let traie sus une goute
840   Et se il vait au fons, masle serra sans doute.
       Mes si li lait desus la fontaine flotele,
       Donc est la femme pleine voirement de femele.
       Ypocras fu li m[i]res qui onques ne fausa
844   Et ses clers desor tuz loiaument ensegna.
           Femme de masle pleine est bele et coloree

816. MS *tele*.
817–8. These lines telescope and garble the Latin.
822. MS *estuver*.
829. MS *desus p. s.* As it stands the line makes no sense and appears to telescope *LSM* 'fumigetur subtus de oculis salsorum piscium vel de ungula caballina', 'desus' being the residue of 'subtus' whilst 'oculis' remains untranslated.
830. MS *fonte*.
834. MS *et ce ert par f.*
839. *LSM* has 'extrahat mulier guttam sanguinis de dextro latere'.
842. MS *pleinei*.
845ff. The final section amplifies *LSM* 'Ypocras dicit quod mulier que concepit masculum, rubicundam habet faciem et dextram mamillam grossiorem'.

Et cele de femele ad la color faxee.
Quant la femmë est vide, s'ele a bele color,
848   Donc quant de masle est plene, si l'a assés greignor.
Et quant elë est vide, së ele a color pale,
Si de mescine est pleine, adonc l'arra plus pale.
Sor le masle plus grosse a la mamele destre,
852   [Et] sor la femele plus grosse la senestre.

GLOSSARY

Acacie s. 706   gum from juice of green plums or sloes [acacia]

Ache s. 160,258,426,432,527   smallage, wild celery (Apium graveolens L.) [apium]

Aconoissement s. 472   straining, effort

Agarie s. 529   agaric, larch agaric (Polyporus officinalis L.) [agaricus]

Airon s. 506   any piquant herb [acumen]

Aisil s. 350,796   vinegar

Aloigne s. 427,428   wormwood (Artemisia absinthium L.)

Ameos s. 161   various umbelliferae incl. gout weed (Aegopodium podagraria L.) and bishopsweed (Ammi majus L.) [ameos]

Amoliemens s. 459   weakening, softening [remollitio]

Amoniac s. 475   gum amoniac obtained from plant Ferula or Dorema

Angevin s. 436   coin

Anis s. 164   aniseed (Pimpinella anisum L.) [anisum]

Aochement s. 370   choking, suffocation of the womb [suffocatio]

Apessantir v.n. 574   to grow heavy

Apeticer v.n. 374   to diminish, grow faint [evanescere]

Arguer v.a. 592   to afflict, oppress

Aristelogie s. 149,705   birthwort (Aristolochia rotunda) [aristologia rotunda]

Armoyce s. 479   mugwort (Artemisia vulgaris L.) [arthemisia]

Atenvier v.a. 662   attenuate, diminish [attenuare]

Aubon s. 556,633,692,711   white of egg [albumen ovi]

Avenaument adv. 140   appropriately

Averone s. 227   southernwood (Artemisia abrotanum L.) [antonia]

Avoine s. 453   oats [avena]

Avorter v.s. 299,678   miscarriage [aborsum]

Baie s. 151,711   laurel, bay [baccus] (Laurus nobilis)

Barate s. 700?   material; the attested senses (trade, deception etc.) are not appropriate here

Barbion s. 355,617,623   houseleek (Semperviva tectorum L.) [semperviva] (not in the dictionaries, but found in London, Roy. Coll. Phys. MS 227 (s.xiv) f.164r)

Basme s. 467   balm, balm of Gilead (Commiphora opobalsamum (Kunth) Engler) [balsamum]

Baude a. 42   bold, lively

Boce s. 562   growth, boil, ulcer

Boisc(h)e s. 498,552   log [buxus]

Bol, bol erminicon s. 341,704   fine earth containing iron oxide or Armenian bole, copper ore combining the blue carbonate of copper (azurite) and the green carbonate (malachite) [bolus armenicus]

Bren s. 733   bran [cantabrum]

Bure s. 261,536,629   butter [butirum]

Caisne s. 333,701   oak [quercus] **ui de chaine** 755   mistletoe [Viscum album L.]

Canfre s. 710   camphor [camphora]

Calament s. 139,426   calamint (Calamintha Miller spp.) [calamentum]

Canele s. 162,626   cinnamon (Cinnamomum zeylanicum Blume) [cinamomum]

Cassiafistre s. 162,616   purging cassia (Cassia fistula L.) [casia]

Castegner s. 701   chestnut tree

Castor s. 416   beaver

Castorie, castoire s. 145,201,432   castoreum (secretion of the abdominal glands of the beaver) [castoreum]

Ceir s. 424   evening
Centoire s. 202   centaury (Centaurium erythraea Rafn) error for 'centoine' [centonica]
Cerfoil(le s. 164,261   chervil (Anthriscus cerefolium (L.) Hoffm.) [cerefolium / trifolium]
Cervoise s. 326   beer [cervisia]
Ceteca s. 166 ?   an error for setacul 'sea holly' or ceterac 'scale fern'
Chaiere s. 183   chair, seat
Chaudepisse s. 582   strangury, difficulty in urination [stranguria]
Cheine s. 490,491   oak (Quercus L.)
Ciprés s. **poume de ciprés** 492   cypress cone [cypressus]
Cire s. **cire roge** 536   red wax [cera rubea] **cire del mel** 553   bees' wax [mel cereum]
Clist(e)re s. 224,708,712   clyster [clistera]
Clos, clou(x) s. 561,565,567,571,573,575,578,579,583,585,587,589,596,597,655,669
growth, aposteme [apostema]
Coign, coon s. 344,508   quince (Cydonia oblonga Miller) [citonium]
Coignier s. 702   quince tree
Cole s. 284,292,313,315,589   choler, bile [colera]
Colere noire s. 322   black bile [colera nigra]
Colés s. **roge colés** 238   red cabbage (Rubeus olus L.) [rubeus caulis]
Collion, coillon s. 741,748,749,757,759,771   testicle [testiculus]
Colombe ramage s. 668   stock dove
Colre s. 565   choler, bile [colera]
Comin s. 437,505   cumin (Cuminum cyminum L.) [ciminum]
Con s. **gris con** 234 **con canu** 234   fumitory (Fumaria officinalis L.)
Conceivement s. 719   conception [conceptus]
Conconbre s. 624,672   cucumber (Cucumis sativus L.)
Confit 152 pp. of **confire**   to prepare, concoct [conficere]
Congluant a. 79   viscous [viscosus]
Conjuge s. 397   (sexual) association [commercium]
Contrarious a. 416   contrary
Converser v.a. 308   to oblige
Coorde s. 695   various cucurbitaceae [cucurbita]
Coral s. 338   coral [corallus]
Coriande s. prose f.225r   coriander (Coriandrum sativum L.) [coriandrum]
Corme s. 508   sorb (Pyrus domestica L.) [sorba]
Corniliere s. 517 see **cornilles** below [spiritualia]
Cornilles s.pl. 403   unspecified organs near the heart and lungs (? praecordia), ? diaphragm
[vulgo dicuntur 'corneliers']
Corpos s. 67   asthma [cordis pulsus]
Corrigiale s. 347   knotgrass (Polygonum aviculare L.) or bindweed (Convolvulus
arvensis L.)
Cors s. 373   heart
Cost s. 432   costmary (Chrysanthemum balsamita (L.) Baillon) [costus]
Costivé a. 588   constipated [constipatur]
Coupe s. 736,739   fault
Creie s. 557   chalk [creta]
Croc s. 705,710   crocus (Crocus sativus L.)
Croes a. 222   hollow [concavus]
Cute s. 198   quilt, cover [sacculus]
Dat(e s. 734,735   urine [urina]
Degaster v.a. 14   to disperse, get rid of [exsiccare, desiccare, expurgare] v.refl. 86
Den(i)er s. 144,145,435   penny-weight [denarius]
Desoivre a. 532   free from
Diaciminon s. 424,425   medicament made with cumin
Diaprunis s. 319   medicament made with plums

Diatesseron s. 147 an electuary made with four ingredients, see **Flos medicinae** [Renzi, Coll. Sal. 5] pt.2,c.2 ll.1358–60 [dyatesseron]

Dissinterie s. 67 dysentery [dissenteria]

Ditaine s. 203 dittany (Origanum dictamnus L. or Dictamnus albus L.) [diptanus]

Doi s. prose f.225v finger [digitus]

Dosse a. 648 twelve

Drame s. 202,205,239,247,431,433,435,646,827 dragm

Drap lange s. 470 linen cloth

Effridant a. 336 cooling, refrigerative

Eglenter s. 333,697 eglantine / dog rose (Rosa rubiginosa L. / Rosa canina L.) [bedegar]

Egremoine s. 334,445 agrimony (Agrimonia eupatoria L.) [agrimonia]

Ematite s. 337 haematite, native iron oxide [lapis emathitis]

Emfleure s. 562 swelling [inflatio]

Encens s. 704 incense [thus]

Enforcement s. 464 effort of childbirth [conamen pariendi]

Engendrement s. 22 conception

Engignement s. 23 fraud, deception, trick

Enpointes s.pl. 681 pricking sensation [punctiones]

Entec(h)er v.a. 398,516 to affect [contingere]

Entechement s. 463 affliction, infection

Entemprer v.a. 689 to mitigate, reduce

Ermo(i)se s. 246,488,665 mugwort (Artemisia vulgaris L.) [arthemisia]

Esbolissement s. 550 bout of heat

Escale s. 331 shell [testa] **escalle d'oef** 367 eggshell

Eschardeux a. 351 scaly

Eschavé 283 p.p. of **eschaufer** v.a. to heat

Escopir v.a. 96 to spit out

Esforcement s. 812 childbirth

Espece s. 466 spice [species]

Esperiment, espeirment s. 235,243 experiment, proof, test

Espermenter v.a. 496 to try, test

Espis, espic, spic s. 161,467,638 ? celtic spikenard (Valeriana celtica L.) or broom (Ulex europaeus L.) or eryngo (Eryngium campestre L.) [spica]

Esploite s. 721 achievement

Espointes s.pl. 523 pricking sensation cf. **enpointes**

Espurgement s. 20,21 purging, cleansing [purgatio]

Essamplor s. 381 sign, manifestation [signum]

Estreindre v.a. 377 to grind (teeth) [constringere]

Estuver v.a. 469,495,497,830 to treat with vapour bath [subfumigere; stupham facere]

Faillance s. 738 deficiency

Faxé a. 846 pale, wan

Fel, fiel s. 212,284,313,566 gall(-bladder) **fel de tor** 211 ox gall [fel tauri]

Fenoil s. 160,259 fennel (Foeniculum vulgare Miller) [feniculus]

Fente, fiente s. dung **fente de berbis** 365 ewe's dung **fiente de colombe ramage** 668 dung of stock dove [columba silvestris] **fente de chate** 830 dung of female cat

Feuquerole s. 325,347 royal fern, osmunda (Osmunda regalis L.) [filicula]

Feve s. 667 bean (Vicia faba L.)

Fi s. 94 ficus, fig-shaped pile or haemorrhoid [ficus]

Fi(s a. 545 sure, certain

Finagrec, finigrec, finegrec, finegrés s. 445,527,538,630,659,665,714,805 fenugreek (Trigonella foenum-graecum L.) [fenugrecum]

Fisalidos s. 161 ? dropwort (Filipendula vulgaris Moench) or ? meadowsweet (Filipendula ulmaria (L.) Maxim.) [phisalidos]

Flamme s. 201 yellow flag (Iris pseudacorus L.) [flamula]

Fleume s. 293,321,572 phlegm [flegma]

Fleur(s), flor(s) s. 22,32,65,85,119,134,199,209,225,244,273,407,408,409,419,577,606, 744,750,756,833 menses

Foie s. 305,757,759 liver [epar]

Foille s. 467 leaf of trees of the cinnamom family (Lauraceae) [folia]

Fon de le terre s. 233 fumitory (Fumaria officinalis L.) [fumus terre]

Fondement s. 801 anus

Forein a. 328 external

Forment s. 482 wheat [frumentum] **flor de forment** 666 wheat flour

Fregne 254 pr.sbj.3 of **freindre** v.a. to break up

Fumee s. 402 gas within the body, vapour, fume [fumositas]

Fu[n]s s. 185,504 aromatic vapour [fumus]

Fus s. 824 vapour

Fust s. 223 wood

Galbeene s. 417 gum resin, galbanum [galbanum]

Gal(l)e s. 332,490,700 oak-apple, gall-nut [galla]

Garse s. prose f.224v scarification

Gase s. 478 cassia bark [cassiafistula]

Genciene s. 150 felwort (Gentiana amarella (L.) Börner) [genciana]

Gerapigre s. 156,427 hiera picra, a purgative containing aloes

Gerologodion s. 157,324 yeralogodion, a purgative containing aloes [yeralogodion]

Gesir v.n. 750,753 to lie (with)

Gingebre s. 265 ginger [zinziber]

Gise 744 pr.sbj.3 of **gesir** to lie (with)

Glagol s. gladden (Iris pseudacorus L.) [yreos]

Glan s. 490 acorn [glans]

Gome arabic s. 340 gum arabic (Acacia Senegal) [gummi arabicus]

Grumis s. 162 gromwell (Lithospermum officinale L.)

Hant s. 768 sexual association

Hernise, hermoise s. 188,261 mugwort (Artemisia vulgaris L.)

Irror s. 97 anger [ira]

Isope s. 213 hyssop (Hyssopus officinalis L.)

Jusquian s. 431 henbane (Hyoscyamus niger L.) [jusquiamus]

Laine, leine s. 197,417,470,473,754 wool **laine carpie** 196,215, prose f.224v,357,385 lint [lana minutissime decerpta]

Lait, let s. 557,650,670,693,839,841 milk [lac] **let de l'anesse et del chiefre** 671 ass's and goat's milk **let d'anesse** 752 ass's milk

Laituare, leituaire, letua(i)re s. 136,144,147,320 electuary [electuaria]

Lard s. prose f.225r bacon **lard salé** prose f.225r salt bacon [lardum cum sale]

Lentille s. 700 lentil (Lens esculenta Moench) [lenticula]

Lessive de cendre s. 825 lye made with ashes [lexivium de cinere]

Licium s. 706 astringent juice of the buckthorn (Rhamnus petiolaris / lycioides L.) [licium]

Lievre s. 746,748 hare [lepus]

Linués s. 805 linseed [semen lini]

Litarge s. 710 litharge, lead monoxide [litargirum]

Litose s. 629 ? error for **titolose**, 'crow garlic', Colchicum autumnale L.

Loi s. 40 manner, type

Longuete s. 216 strip

Lorer s. 265,511 bay (Laurus nobilis L.) [laurus]

Luvesce s. 164,253,259, prose f.225r lovage (Levisticum officinale Koch) or scotch lovage (Ligusticum scoticum L.) [levisticus]

Macedogne s. 166 alexanders, horse parsley (Smyrnium olusatrum L.)

Maille s. 246 halfpenny weight [obulus]

Maistrie s. 639 skill, device

Malan s. 677,683 sore, ulcer

Manne s. 616 manna

Margillois s. 436   coin minted in Melgueil, see above pp.74f.
Mar(r)is s. 72,73,186,207,275,370,371,451,455,463,472,475,485, 509,514,515,533,546,
548,551,561,583,604,622,640,675,682,688,689, 715,722,725,727,746,764   womb [matrix]
Mastic s. 649   mastic, resin of Pistacia lentiscus L.
Mauve s. 630,805,826   marshmallow (Althaea officinalis L.) [malva]
Mecinal s. 83   medical book
Mecine s. 108,204,208,263,271,328,364,452,509,568,632,634,677,694 740,784   medicine
Mecinement s. 659   medicine
Meciner v.a. 483   to treat (with medicine)
Medecinement s. 688   medicine
Medicine, medecine s. 267,324,346,411,413,450,559,570,636,657,769   medicine
Mel, miel s. 146,154,249   honey [mellis]
Melie s. 141   honey [mellis]
Meliliton s. 633   melilot (Melilotus) [mellilotum]
Mellilot s. 659   see above
Mell(i)er s. 334,702   medlar (Mespilus germanica L.)
Melon s. 673   melon (Cucumis melo L.) [melo]
Menison s. 69   diarrhoea, discharge from bowels containing blood [diarria]
Mentastre s. 346   horsemint (Mentha sylvestris L.) or water-mint (Mentha aquatica L.)
Ment(h)e s. 139,236   mint [nepita]
Mere herbe s. 171,187   mugwort (Artemisia vulgaris L.) [arthemisia]
Mesc(h)ine s. 763   young virgin woman [virgo] 850 female
Mesestance s. 114   suffering
Mesle s. 507   fruit of the medlar [Mespilus germanica L.)
Mire s. 115,155,263,322,383,437,545,564,713,740,843   physician
Mirre s. 151,201,433,511,555,698,704   myrrh [mirra]
Mirte s. 341   sweet gale (Myrica gale L.) [mirta]
Moele de cierf s. 535,645   marrow of deer [medulla cervina] **moele de veel** 643   marrow of
calf [medulla vituli]
Morele s. 615,625,691   black nightshade (Solanum nigrum L.) or deadly nightshade
(Atropa bella-donna L.) [morella]
Mustoile s. 771   weasel [mustela]
Na(i)ssance, nessance s. 218,269,271, prose f.224v,428,446,456,504,560,580,675,687,709,
745,764,807   vulva [vulva]
Naissement s. 544   vulva
Nassance s. 776   birth
Nastre v.n. 54   to be born **nascus** p.p. 596
Neitir v.a. 689   to cleanse
Nepte s. 255,430   catmint (Nepeta cataria L.) [nepita]
Nitre s. 213   nitre [nitrum]
Nois s. prose f.225r   walnut [nux maior]
Nois gauge s. 332   walnut (Juglans regia L.) [nux maior]
Oint s. 362,365,449   animal fat [auxungia] **oint de goupil et de chievre** 441   fat from the
fox and goat **oint d'oie** 535,631   goose fat **oint de geline** 631   chicken fat [adeps
gallinaceus] **oint de tesson** 644   badger fat
Ole s. 651   oil **ole rose** 272   oil of roses **ole laurin** 413   oil of bays **ole de olive** 540,792
olive oil **oile rosat** 618,626,692,711,796   oil of roses
Olive s. 363   olive see note
Olle s. 169   pot
Once s. 129,512,537,556,557,644   ounce [uncia]
Ongle de cheval s. 829   coltsfoot (Tussilago farfara L.) [ungula caballina]
Opoponas s. 470   opoponac
Orge s. 806   barley **orge pilé** s. 353   barley flour, dried barley [ordeum desiccatum] **ferine
d'orge** 666   barley flour
Origanon s. 165   marjoram (Origanum vulgare L.) [origanum]

Ortie s. 361 nettle [viridis urtica]

Palmer v.refl. 373 to faint [sincopim pati]

Palu(s s. 669,679,685 pus, discharge [sanies]

Parceure s. 186 opening

Parele s. 359 dock (Rumex L.) confused with 'paritarie' 'pellitory-of-the-wall' [paritaria]

Peissare, pesaire, passere, pessaire, pessare s. 220,443,544,560,634,652,707,712,716 pessary [pessarium]

Peiz s. 470 pitch

Pel de quir s. 773 hide

Penil s. 421 pubes, groin [pecten]

Peresil s. 163,258 parsley (Petroselinum crispum (Miller) A.W. Hill) or alexanders, horse parsley (Smyrnium olusatrum L.) [alexander]

Pesche s. 508 peach (Prunus persica (L.) Batsch)

Piez s. 417 pitch [pix]

Pilecte s. 135 pill [pillula]

Pis s. 378 breast [pectus]

Plantein(e, plantaine s. 334,342,530,617,623,691 (and following prose) plantain, waybread [Plantago major L.) [plantago]

Planton s. plant, shoot [planta]

Ploue s. 348 (and following prose) rain

Poes s.pl. 733 pots [olle]

Pois s. 153 weight [pondus]

Poison s. 135,155,158 beverage, drink

Poisson s. 351,829 fish

Poivre, peivre s. 247,505 pepper **poivre blanc** 432 white pepper

Poliol, puliol s. 165,227,236,430 pennyroyal (Mentha pulegium L.) or wild thyme (Thymus serpyllum L.) [pulegium]

Pollution s. 34,35 ejaculation [pollutio]

Pome s. **pome egre** 508 crab apple [acria poma]

Po(u)me gernete, gernate s. 330,339,489,699 pomegranate (Punica granatum L.) [malum granatum]

Porcel s. 758 small pig [porcellus]

Porcelleine s. 625,693,696 purslane (Portulaca oleracea L.) [portulaca]

Poret s. 239 leek (Allium porrum L.) [porrum] **ciés de poret** heads of leek [capita porrorum]

Porter sbst.inf. 724 child-bearing

Potet s. 240 pot [olla]

Pox s. 374,380 pulse [pulsus]

Psilion s. 624 fleawort (Plantago arenaria Waldst. and Kit.) [psillium]

Pouchin s. 367 chick

Preu s. **a son preu** 152 to her benefit, advantage

Puor s. 686 stench [fetor]

Purgement s. 37 purging [purgatio]

Purreture s. 686 pus, matter [putredo]

Qualité s. 131 natural condition (of health)

Quer de cerf s. 342,510 deer-horn [cornu cervi] or (342) buckshorn plantain (Plantago coronopus L.)

Quievre s. 223 brass

Quintefoille s. 163 cinquefoil (Potentilla reptans L.)

Quivillie s. 107 ankle [cavilla]

Rara s. 345 evidently corrupt plant-name; error for 'rapa'?

Recloent 276 pr.ind.6 of **reclore** v.n. to close again

Recoi s. 181 **en recoi** secretly, privately

Renuisant a. 80 harmful

Reupontic s. 246 rhubarb (Rheum rhaponticum L.) [reuponticum]

Ronce s. 334 bramble, blackberry (Rubus fruticosus L.) [prunus]

Rose s. 467,488   rose [rosa] **aue rose** 698   attar of roses
Rosat s. 331   rose [rosa]
Rosate novele s. 318   medicament including roses, **Antidotarium Nicolai** 93 [rosata novella]
Rue s. 206,236,479   rue (Ruta graveolens L.) [ruta]
Ruit 526 ind.pr.3 of **ruire**   to rumble [rugitum]
Saffron s. 649   saffron (Crocus sativus L.) or bastard saffron (Carthamus tinctorius L.)
San(s) s. 92,93   blood
Sanc de dragon s. 343,703   dragon's blood, red gum or resin of dragon tree (Dracaeno draco L.) [sanguis draconis]
Sanc d'owe s. 714   goose blood
Sarree s. 530   savory (Satureia L.)[satureia]
Sastine s. 524 ?
Satré s. 164   savory (Satureia L.) [satureya]
Sauce s. 307   fluid [succositates]
Sauge s. 206   sage (Salvia officinalis L.) [salvia]
Saugeme s. 239   rock salt [salgemma]
Sausefleume s. 288   'salt phlegm' [flegma salsum]
Savine s. 163,203,257,265   savin (Juniperus sabina L.) [savina]
Scamonee s. 318   scammony (Convulvulus scammonia L.) [scamonia]
Segor s. 129   safety
Seigner s. 113   bleeder
Sei(g)n(i)er v.a. 106,123,310,598,602,607,784   to bleed v.n. 780   to bleed, be bled v.refl. 112,137
Seim s. 648   animal fat
Seine a. 782   sixth
Seinie, seiné, seignie s. 602,603,605,610   bleeding [minutio]
Sele s. 183,268,502   stool [sella]
Semblance s. 31   comparison, analogy
Seré a. 133   constipated
Serpol s. 341   wild thyme (Thymus serpyllum L.)
Setime, septime a. 783,785   seventh
Silium s. 618   fleawort (Plantago arenaria Waldst. & Kit.) [psillium]
Simac s. 490   sumach (Rhus coriaria L.) [sumac]
Sirop de violes s. 319   syrop of violets [siropus violaceus]
Soluble a. 794   easily digestible
So[o]ir v.n. 268   to sit
Sozpositoire s. 210   suppository [pessarium]
Spic s. 638   see **espis** above
Spodion s. 705   spodium, powder obtained from various substances, including ashes of ivory, by calcination [spodium]
Storac s. 467   styrax, resin from Liquidamber orientalis [storax]
Tanesie s. 261,344   tansy (Tanacetum vulgare L.) [tanacetum]
Tisan(e s. 353 (and following prose)   tisane [ptisana]
Tort 526 pr.ind.3 of **tordre**   to knot [tortio]
Toie s. 194,195,454   case, cover (of pillow) [sacculus]
Tran(s)glutir v.n. and v.a. 524,749   to swallow [transglutire]
Treimains par treimains 287 ?
Trespas s. 74   passage
Tresse a. 38   thirteen
Triphere zarasine s. 317   soothing medical preparation [trifera sarracenica] See **Antidotarium Nicolai** ed. van den Berg no.113.
Unche s. 127   ounce [uncia]
Urine s. 103   urine [urina]
Ventosité s. 575,642   flatulence, morbid wind in body [ventositas]

Vent()use s. prose f.224v,420,421   cupping glass [ventosa]
Vermelle s. 737   worm [vermis]
Ver s. 741   boar [verres]
Verveine s. 345,817   vervain (Verbena officinalis L.)
Vesteure s. 820,831,833   afterbirth [secundina]
Vetoine s. 165,228   betony (Stachys officinalis (L.) Trev.) [betonica]
Veve a. 392   widow [vidua]
Wima(u)ve s. 254,448   marshmallow (Althaea officinalis L.)
Ydropesie s. 68,303   dropsy [ydropisis]
Ypolifive s.345 ? error for 'iposelinon' (wild parsley)?

Proper Names

Cleopatras 10   Cleopatra (female physician)
Costentin 7,763   Constantine [the African]
Diacorides 8,497,637,713   Dioscorides
France 264   France
Galien 7,117,171,379,385,600,601,775   Galen
Justin 437   Justinus
Lions 263   Lyon
Oribases 444   Oribasius
Paulus 639   Paul [? of Aegena]
Ypocras 9,569,717,780,835,843   Hippocrates

Liber de sinthomatibus mulierum[1]
[MS Oxford, Bodleian Library, Bodley 361 (SC 2462)]

[p.458] Trotula maior: De passionibus mulierum, causis et curis earundem sequitur tractatus, et primo prohemium.

<Cum auctor universitatis in primeva mundi constitutione rerum naturas singulas iuxta genus suum distingueret, supra ceteras humanam naturam singulari dignitate consecravit, cui supra ceterorum animantium condicionem rationis et intellectus contulit libertatem et eiusdem volens perpetuam subsistere generationem in sexu disparia ordinans, principium future sobolis propaginem provida deliberatione dispensavit, quia masculum et feminam creavit eos. Et ut ex eis fructus emergeret fecundior eorum complexiones grata quadam conmixtione temperavit, naturam enim masculi calidam et siccam constituens, ne in alterutro nimis abundaret masculus opposita frigiditate et humiditate mulieris ab excessu nimio voluit coherceri. Fortiores autem qualitates .s. caliditate [p.459] et siccitate viro tanquam digniori persone,[2] ut mulieres .s. frigiditate et humiditate debiliores possideret, ut etiam masculus fortiorum qualitatum officio in mulierem ageret et tanquam in agrum sibi commissum semen et funderet et mulier tanquam servitio supposita semen effusum in gremio nature susciperet.>

<Quia ergo mulieres debilioris nature sunt quam viri, ideo plus viris in partu molestantur angustia. Hinc etiam quod frequentius in eis abundant egritudines quam in viris et maxime circa membra officio nature deputata, et quoniam ipse sue conditionis fragilitatem verecundia et rubore faciei confitentur, egritudinum suarum que circa partes secretiores eveniunt medicis non audent angustias revelare. Earum ergo miseranda calamitas et maxime cuiusdam mulieris gratia animum sollicitat, ut contra predictas egritudines earum provideamus sanitati. Ut ergo ex libris Ypocratis, Galeni, Constantini potiora deserperemus,[3] labore non minimo mulierum genera desudavimus, ut et causas egritudinum et curas exponeremus cum causis.>

[13] Quia ergo in mulieribus non tantum abundat caliditas ut pravos humores qui in eis generantur sufficiant exsiccare, nec tantum laborem valet earum tollerare frigiditas ut per sudorem eos ad exteriora expellat natura ut in viris, propter hoc, inquam, ad caloris recompensationem quandam eis purgationem natura precipuam assignavit, per menstrua videlicet que vulgo aput eas flores appellantur, quia sicut arbores sine floribus fructum non auferunt, similiter et mulieres sine floribus officio conceptionis

---

[1] Numbers in square brackets refer to the corresponding lines of the Anglo-Norman verse text. Material not there translated appears between <...>.
[2] MS *parsone*.
[3] for 'decerperemus'.

fraudarentur. Huiusmodi purgatio contingit mulieribus sicut et viris de nocte contingit vi nature pollutio. Semper enim natura ab aliquibus gravatur humoribus sive in viris sive in mulieribus, jugum suum nititur deponere et exuit laborem.

[c.1] De menstruis

[37] Contingit autem hec purgatio mulieribus circa .xiiii. annum aut paulo minus aut paulo tardius secundum quod magis vel minus abundet calor in ipsa. Durat autem usque ad .l. annos si macra est, quandoque ad .lx. vel .xl. ut in medocriter pinguibus, vel usque ad .xxxv. si sit mulier multum pinguis. Si debito et ordinato tempore contingat, huiusmodi purgatione expeditur natura a superfluis humoribus competenter. Si vero plus vel minus exeant quam oportet, emergunt inde multe egritudines, quia inde debilitatur appetitus, tam cibi quam potus, <et quandoque provenit vomitus.> Quandoque autem appetit mulier <terram cretam, carbones vel> aliquid aliud contra naturam. Quandoque ex eadem causa circa collum, circa dorsum vel in capite dolor vel in oculis et quandoque febris acuta aut cordis pulsus aut ydropisis vel dissuria.[4] Hec autem contingunt vel quando deficiunt longo tempore vel quando prorsus amittuntur ut in ydropisi vel dissuria vel cordis morsu. Non nuncquam etiam contingit diarria propter nimiam frigiditatem matricis vel quia vene matricis multum sunt graciles ut [p.460] in extenuatis mulieribus, quia tunc humores superflui meatus liberos non habent per quos possint erumpere, vel quia humores spissi sunt et viscosi et propter conglutinationem eorum impeditur exitus, vel quia mulier deliciose comedat vel ex aliquo labore multum sudat. Quia sicut testatur Ruffus, mulier que [non][5] multum ex[er]cetur multis necesse est ut abundet menstruis ad hoc ut sana subsistat.

[c.2] Contra defectum menstruorum

[91] Aliquando menstrua deficiunt quia sanguis in corpore mulieris propter frigiditatem coagulatur, aliquando quia per alia loca sanguis emittitur ut per ficus sive emoroydas vel per nares vel per sputum. Aliquando deficiunt pre nimia ira vel dolore vel metu. Si autem diu cessaverint, suspicionem inferunt violente egritudinis. Urina vertitur in viriditatem vel ruborem vel etiam in talem ruborem quandoque qualis est color carnis recentis. Si ergo deficiant et mulier sit extenuata corpore, minuatur de vena quadam que est sub cavilla pedis, primo die de pede altero, in sequenti de reliquo, et extrahatur sanguis secundum quod virtus eius postulabit, quoniam in omni egritudine respiciendum est ad virtutem egrotantis et cavendum est ne nimis debilitetur.

[117] Galienus refert de muliere quadam, cui defecerant menstrua per .iiii. menses, que in toto corpore attrita erat et extenuata, et defecerat penitus facultas appetendi

---

4 Some Latin MSS have *dissinteria*, like the verse translation.
5 The correction is essential, though 'non' is also missing in the Magdalen copy.

et ipse detraxit ei sanguinem de predicta vena per .iiii. dies, prima die libros .ii., secunda librum .i. de alio pede et tertio die de primo pede et quarto die de secundo pede uncias .viii. et parvo spatio restituta est et rediit color et status antiquus.

[133] Ad idem: mulier cui venter constipatur sepe et cessat fluxus menstruorum accipiat .v. pillulas cum acutis electuariis <prout ipsa acumen pati poterit,> et postea minuatur, deinde balneetur et post balneum bibat de calamento vel nepita vel de menta coctis in melle ubi .vii. partes sunt aque et octava mellis. Sepe iterandum est balneum et post balneum bibat de dyatesseron pondus duorum denariorum et de castoreo pondus .i. denarii cum aqua et melle. Dyatesseron fit ex .iiii. speciebus: mirra .s., aristologia rotunda, genciana, et baccis sub eodem pondere, et conficiantur cum melle cocto.

[155] Medicina autem quam ipsa accipiat sit yeralogodion, yerapigra. Omnia diuretica conferunt ei ut spica, feniculus, cuminum, apium, ameos, phisalidos, casia, cinamomum, savina, alexander, origanum, pulegium, anetum, betonica, anisum, satureya, levisticus, andra, cerefolium. Omnia ista, vel singula vel conmixta, cocta in vino et potata conferunt.

[171] Galienus dicit quod arthemisia trita et potata cum vino multum iuvat, vel etiam si coquatur in aqua valet, et potetur in balneo. Non modicum etiam iuvat si in ipso balneo decoquatur vel si ipsa viridis teratur et ligetur supra ventrem sub umbilico. Vel decoquatur in olla et mulier superponat olle sellam perforatam et desuper sedeat et bene cooperiatur undique ne fumus exeat et ut interius receptus penetret ad matricem. Valet etiam si ipsa cum supranominatis diureticis, aut quibusdam aut omnibus, deco[p.461]quatur in aqua et impleatur sacculus lana minutissime decerpta ut fit in modum pulvinaris et intinguatur in aqua illa et sacculus ventri superponatur, et hoc frequenter fiat.

[199] Pulvis ad menstrua provocanda optimum: Recipe flamule, cicute, mirre, castoreum, centonicum ana dragmam .i., diptani dragmam .i.[6] Fiat inde pulvis et detur inde dragma .i. cum aqua ubi decoquuntur salvia, ruta, et bibat in balneo. Si autem adeo induraverit matrix, ut hiis adiutoriis non possint educi menstrua, accipiatur fel tauri vel quodlibet aliud fel et pulvis nitri et misceantur cum succo ysopi et ibi intinguatur lana minutim carpta et post[e]a teratur ut sit rigida et dura et magna, ut possit in vulvam intromitti, et postea vulve intromittatur et hoc appellatur pessarium. Item fit etiam aliud in modum virge virilis et est concavum et imponatur medicina et inicitur sicut per clistere. [225] Mulier si pauca et cum dolore emittit menstrua, accipiatur antonia,[7] betonica, pulegium, de unoquoque plenum pugillum et coquantur in aqua vel vino usque ad consumptionem duarum partium. Postea reliquum coletur per pannum et bibatur cum succo fumiterre.

---

6 Some Latin MSS add 'savine', like the verse translation.
7 Omitted as unknown in most of the MSS, though it is in the Magdalen copy.

[235] Aliud: accipe mentam, rutam, pulegium ana pugillum .i., salgemme dragmas .iii. et plantam unam rubei caulis et tres capita porrorum et coquantur simul in olla rudi et bibat inde post balneum.

[243] Aliud: si diu defecerint menstrua, accipe reupontici pondus duorum denarum et obuli[8] et arthemisiam siccam et piperis dragmam .i. et fiat pulvis et bibat inde mane et sero per .iii. dies et in nocte bene cooperiatur, ut sudet.

[252] Aliud experimentum expertum: accipe radicem yreos et radicem levistici et herbam nepite et coquantur in vino et dentur in potu.

[257] Item: coquantur in vino savina, radix apii, feniculus, levisticus, petroselinus et bibat, et tanacetum et trifolium et arthemisia frixa cum butiro ligentur super umbilicum.

[263] Item, quidam medicus fecit regine Francorum:[9] zinziber, folia lauri, savinam, tere simul et pone in olla super carbones vivos, et mulier desuper sedeat in sella perforata et fumum recipiat in interioribus, et redibunt menstrua. Mulier autem que huiusmodi fumigationem frequentat necesse est ut vulvam ungat interius ne nimis calefiat. <Valet etiam ad idem subfumigatio de cinamomo, aneto, flammula, nepita, calamento, menta, sive conmixtis sive simplicibus. Valet ad idem scarificatio et coitus. Nocet autem minutio facta in manu. Comedat cepas, porros, cepulas, sinapis, piper, allia, cuminum, pisces fluviales, aspatiles cum alba carne; bibat vinum album non forte si sit sine febre et sine dolore capitis, quia in omni febre vinum est nocivum.>

[c.3] Contra superabundantiam menstruorum

[273] Abundant quoque mulieri menstrua preter modum, quod contingit quia vene matricis nimis sunt aperte vel quia etiam quandoque crepant et fluit sanguis in multa quantitate – et tunc apparet sanguis rubeus et clarus – vel quia ex multitudine cibi et potus collecta est in muliere multa massa sanguinis et cum non possit intra corpus contineri, prorumpit extra. Vel contingit [p.462] quandoque pre nimia sanguinis calefactione ex colera resultante[10] a felle que facit sanguinem adeo ebullire, ut non possit in vasis contineri, vel quia flegma salsum admiscitur sanguini et attenuat ipsum et facit a venis prorumpere. Si enim sanguis qui egreditur vergit ad citrinitatem, ex colera contingit, si in albedinem, ex flegmate, si in rubeum, ex sanguine. Huiusmodi egritudines emergunt propter humores interius corruptos, quorum corruptiones nature nobilitas dedignatur sustinere. Quandoque contingit propter aborsum[11] ex quo plurimum mors sequitur. Ex hiis causis mulieres decolorantur et macrescunt et si diu

---

8   Many Latin MSS have the reading *olibani*. The Magdalen copy has *oboli*.
9   Many Latin MSS have 'Francie'.
10 Common variants are *redundante* and *resudante* (Magdalen MS and others).
11 Some Latin MSS have *diabrosim*.

duraverit, facile in ydropisim convertitur quia epatis substantia[12] infrigidatur pre
nimia subtractione sanguinis per quem deberet in suo naturali calore permanere et
nequit propter defectum caloris succositates[13] [digerere] et debito modo in humores
conmutare.

[309] Si sanguis sit in causa, minuenda est <in manu vel> in brachio, ut sanguis
sursum convertatur. Si colera resudans a felle sit in causa, sumendum est aliquod lene
catarticum quod coleram evacuet ut trifera sarracenica, rosata novella cum scamonia[14]
et siropo violaceo.

[321] Si contingit ex colera nigra vel flegmatis abundantia, sumatur yeralegodion
vel[15] filiculam ponat in vino vel cervisiam et bibat. Post purgationem apponenda sunt
quedam exterius que constringunt. Sumat ergo mulier et potet aquam tepidam in qua
decoquantur cortex maligranati, galle, testa nucis maioris, rosa, folia quercus, bedegar,
rubus, agrimonia, plantago: omnia ista iuvant sive simplicia sive composita. Postea
inter cibaria detur ei ad potandum pulvis lapidis emathitis distemperatus cum aqua et
pulvis coralli, gummi arabici, balaustia, semen mirte, portulace, boli armenici, pulvis
de cornu cervi, plantaginis, centonice, sangui[ni]s draco[nis], spodii, seminis citoniorum. Comedat gallinas coctas in pane, pisces recentes cum aceto, <et panem
ordeaceum.> Bibat ptisanam de ordeo factam primitus desiccato et postea bullito cum
aqua mari[na] <donec crepuerit,> et cum refrigeratum fuerit, <apponatur acetum> et
postea coletur per pannum et detur ad manducandum. Bibat vinum rubeum temperatum cum aqua mari[na], et si radix plantaginis bulli[etur] cum ptisana, tanto melius.
Ponantur ignite ventose inter mamillas ut sursum sanguis trahatur. Iniciatur per
pessarium succus plantaginis. [355] Valet et succus sempervive cum vino albo potatus.
Valet et succus idem super ventrem ligatus. Valet etiam succus paritarie bibitus cum
aqua vel vino. Valet etiam potare succum decoctionis fabarum. Vel accipiantur duo
lata frustra lardi cum sale et desuper aspergatur pulvis coriandri et seminis eiusdem
<et pulvis absinthii> et ligantur sub umbilico. <Fiant duo emplastra de sisimbrio trito
cum auxungia, et unum super ventrem et alterum supra renes pone.> Valet ad idem
viridis urtica trita cum auxungia et ligata supra ventrem et renes et cum ea ponantur
folia ulmi[16] tenera, tanto melius. [365] Item accipiantur teste maiorum nucum et fiat
inde pulvis et detur inde [p.463] in potu cum aqua marina. Deinde fac emplastrum de
stercoribus ovium cum auxungia et superponatur ventri et renibus. Vel fiat pulvis de
testis ovorum et detur in potu per .iii. dies singulis diebus quantum sublevare poteris
de pulvere tribus digitis, et detur cum frigida est.

---

[12] Some Latin MSS have *sima*, 'hollow of the liver'.
[13] Many MSS, including Magdalen, have *succositatem*.
[14] Some MSS have *scariole*.
[15] The Magdalen MS and others have *et*.
[16] Some Latin MSS have *urtice*. The verse translation has misread 'ulivi'.

[c.4] *De suffocatione matricis*

[369]   Contingit etiam mulieribus matricis suffocatio quando .s. matrix sursum extollitur. Et hinc evenit subversio vel debilitatio appetitus et ex frigiditate cordis superveniente quandoque sincopim patiuntur et pulsus evanescit, ita quod penitus non sentiatur. Et ex eodem aliquando mulier contrahitur ut caput genibus conjungatur et etiam vocis officium amittit et labia distorquentur et constringunt dentes et pectus sursum preter naturam elevatur.

[379]   Galienus refert de quadam muliere que hunc morbum patiebatur et amiserat vocem et pulsum et erat quasi defuncta quia nullum habebat exterius signum vite, sed adhuc interius circa cor natura modicum caloris retinuerat. Unde plures eam mortuam reputabant. Sed ipse lanam minutim carptam apposuit ori et naribus et modicum visa est moveri et sic vivam esse cognovit. [389] Hec egritudo contingit mulieri quia multum abundat in ea sperma et quia semen corruptum est in ea et in venenosam conversum naturam. Contingit autem hoc quia viris non utuntur et maxime viduis que consueverunt uti carnali virorum commercio. Virginibus etiam solet hoc contingere cum ad annos nubiles pervenerint et viris possint et velint uti nec eis utantur et quia in eis plurimum abundat semen, quod per masculum natura vellet expellere. Ex huiusmodi semine superabundante et corrupto quedam frigida fumositas dissolvitur et ad quasdam partes ascendit que vulgo dicuntur 'corneliers',[17] quia[18] vicine sunt pulmoni et cordi <et ceteris instrumentis vocis,> inde contingit fieri loquele impedimentum. Et huius morbi principium solet oriri ex defectu menstruorum et si deficiant menstrua et superabundant semina, <tanto morbus est molestior et maxime quando partes occupat altiores.>

[411]   Cura: Primum remedium est contra hanc invalitudinem ut pedes et manus mulieris fricentur cum oleo laurino [et] naribus apponantur aliqua gravis odoris existentia, ut castoreum, ga[l]banum, pix, lana combusta, lineus pannus combustus vel pellis combustus et similia. <Oleis autem et unguentis que sint gravis odoris debet inungi vulva, ut yreleon, musceleon, camomilleon, nardileon.[19] Hec enim attrahunt et provocant menstr[u]a.> Apponantur ventose inguibus et super pecten. Et debet inungi unguentis et oleis boni odoris vulva intus et extra. In sero accipiat dyaciminum cum succo apii vel cum sirupo de calamento vel nepta facto. [431] Vel etiam accipiat succum[20] jusquiami, castoreum, piper album, costum, mirram, apium, de singulis dragmam .i. vel plus. Et distemperet cum vino dulci et bibat dragmam .i. pondus trium denariorum.[437] Justinus medicus precipit contra hunc [p.464] morbum dari cimini coclear .i. et teri et dari in potu. Precipit etiam accipi priapum vulpis vel caprioli et fieri inde emplastrum vel inici per pessarium. [444] Oribazius precipit decoqui radicem

---

17 Many Latin MSS have *corniles*. Others have *canales, collaterales*. The Magdalen copy has *cornelieis*.
18 MS *que quia*.
19 The Magdalen copy has *nardaleon*.
20 The Magdalen copy adds *maratri*.

germandrie[21] et fenugrecum <et semen lini> et succum calidum inici et refert quod
ad idem multum valet radix levistici cocta cum auxungia et ligata super umbilicum.

[c.5] *Contra precipitationem matricis*

[451] Si post partum contingat matricem inferius descendere nimis, calefiat avena
madefacta et humecta et sacelletur mulier inde. Matrix quandoque a loco suo movetur
et descendit, quandoque etiam foras per vulvam egreditur. Et hoc contingit propter
remollitionem matricis ex nimia frigiditate interius abundante. Huiusmodi autem
remollitio et infrigidatio matricis contingit ex frigido aere subintrante per inferius
orificium <quando .s. diu sedet mulier vel super lapidem frigidum vel super aliquid
tale,> vel contingit quandoque propter balneum aque frigide quia propter hoc molli-
ficatur matrix et exit de loco suo in conamine[22] pariendi.

[465] Cura: Si descendit matrix et non exit foras, apponantur naribus mulieris species
bene redolentes ut balsamum, spica, folium, storax et huiusmodi bene olentia et
inferius subfumigetur rebus gravis odoris ut pannus combustus et cetera que supradicta
sunt et fomentetur umbilicus de lana infusa in vino vel oleo. [475] Si vero matrix foras
exierit, accipe ammoniacum et distempera cum succo absinthii et inde inungatur[23]
venter cum penna. Postea accipe cassiafistulam cum rutha, arthemisia equali pondere
et decoque in vino <usque ad consumptionem duarum partium. Terciam da ei in
potu.> Sacelletur venter et umbilicus de frumento tosto. [485] Primo autem omnium[24]
matrix egressa restituatur manu apposita proprio loco et postea mulier intret aquam
in qua decocta sint rosa, balaustia, cortex malagranati, galla, mirta, sumac, glandes,
cortex vel folia quercus, et nuces cypressum <et lenticula.> Deinde fiat ei stupha quia
multum confert. [497] Dyascorides precipit eis fieri stupham de sicco buxo posito[25] in
olla super cineres vel carbones vivos et mulier desuper sedens bene cooperta fumum
recipiat. [505] Dieta eius sit frigida sine pipere et cimino et sine omni acumine. De
fructibus commedat mespila, sorbas et citonia et acria poma, bibat vinum vetus
temperatum cum aqua marina.

[509] Experimentum probatum ad matricem foras egressam: Pulvis cornu cervi et
foliorum lauri ana unciam .i. , mirre unciam .i. terantur et distemperentur cum vino
et detur ad potandum et revertetur matrix in locum suum.

[515] Aliquando etiam matrix de loco suo vel tota de sede sua movetur nec tamen
sursum elevatur versus spiritualia nec per orificium foras descendit, cuius signum est:
dolorem sentit in sinistro latere, distentionem membrorum, difficultas transglutiendi,
tortionem et rugitum ventris habet. Ad hoc accipiendum est apium et fenugrecum et

---

21 MS *germanice*. The Magdalen copy has *g'manie*.
22 MS *conamen*.
23 MS *lungatur*.
24 Omitted in the Magdalen copy and many of the other MSS.
25 MS *posita*.

trita distemperentur cum vino et [p.465] potui dentur. [529] Vel accipe agaricum, <aspaltum dragmam,> plantaginis et .s. satureie et pulverizata potentur cum vino cocto cum melle. [533] Ad hoc autem ut matrix de loco suo non moveatur et ut nulla duricie molestetur, accipe medullam cervine et adipem anseris et ceram rubeam et butirum ana uncias .ii. Deinde accipe fenugrecum, semen lini et decoque in aqua cum predictis ad lentum ignem usque ad plenam decoctionem et iniciatur per pessarium. Hoc enim valde necessarium est contra plures morbos matricis.

[c.7] *Contra ardorem matricis*

[547] Contingit etiam matricem esse ita in caliditate distemperatam ut maximus ardor intus sentiatur quod curari potest hoc remedio: <accipe opii unciam .i., adipis anserini uncias .ii.,> mellis cerei uncias .iiii., olei unciam .i. et albugines duorum ovorum et cretam et lac mulieris et conmisceantur et per pessarium iniciantur.

[c.8] *Contra apostema matricis*

[561] Quoniam etiam in matrice nascuntur inflationes et apostemata diversi generis, si colera exiens a felle causa est apostematis, tunc febrem facit vel cancrum. [571] Si grossi humores ut flegma vel colera enim in causa sint, tumidum est apostema et durum et mulier gravitatem sentit in hanchis, coxis et tibiis. Aliquando ex ventositate nascitur idem apostema vel ex ictu vel ex qualibet alia occasione et ex eo non nunquam deficiunt menstrua.[26] [579] Si autem apostema sit in anteriori parte matricis, dolor sentitur circa vulvam et inde nascitur stranguria. Si vero apostema fuerit in ipso orificio matricis, dolor sentitur circa umbilicum et nates.[27] Si est in parte posteriori, dolor est in dorso et venter constipatur et etiam dolor est sub costis. [589] Si de sanguine vel colera rubea natum sit apostema, adest febris acuta <et sitis> et dolor nimius. Primum ergo querendum que sit causa apostematis. Si de calidis causis processit, expedit mulieri ut detrahatur ei sanguis de vena pedum sicut precipit Galienus, qui etiam asserit nocivum esse si detrahatur sanguis de manu quando mulier patitur in matrice, quoniam minutio illa sursum trahit sanguinem et aufert menstrua. Propter hoc ab inferiori parte detrahendus est sanguis iuxta virtutem mulieris. Et si fortis fuerit mulier et sustinere possit, bis in die trahatur.

[613] Postea accipiat aliqua in potu que calorem[28] mitigant, ut est succus morelle, cassiafistula, manna, oleo rosaceo et succus plantaginis vel sempervive et similia. Et fiat emplastrum quod et calorem minuat et matricem confortat, ut est succus portulace, morelle, sempervive, psillii, plantaginis, scariole, olei rosacei. [627] Postea applicat maturativa ut est semen lini coctum cum butiro, malva, fenugrecum coctum cum adipe anserino vel gallinacio, mellilotum, albumen ovi. De his simplicibus vel

---

[26] MS *membra.*
[27] MS *nares.* Some Latin MSS have *renes.*
[28] MS *colorem.*

compositis fiat pessarium. [637] Dyascorides dicit quod multum confert sedere in aqua in qua spica cocta sit. [639] Paulus docet fieri quoddam pessa[rium] circa duriciem matricis et contra inversionem eiusdem et inflationem et ventositatem eiciendam a corpore. Accipe medullam [p.466] vituli et adipem melote pondus .xviii. denariorum et medullam cornu cervi dragmas .vi., adipem anserinum et gallinaceum, crocum ana dragmas .iiii., masticis, mellis ana dragmas .ii., <ysopi pondus .vi. denariorum.> Omnia ista misceantur et terantur cum lacte mulieris et oleo rosaceo et iniciatur per pessarium et fiat inde emplastrum. [655] Si frigidum sit apostema,[29] si autem de grossis humoribus generatum sit apostema, accipe fenugrecum, mellilotum, <semen lini, semen rute. Coquantur in aqua. De substantia fiat emplastrum et succus pessarizetur. Sepe de substantia utatur balneis et emplastris.> [640] Subtilis sit dieta, ut grossicies humorum attenuetur. Vel si ad saniem velimus converti apostema, apponimus maturativa et que rupturam faciunt in cute, ut sanies effluat, ut sunt fenugrecum, <semen lini,> farina ordei cocta simul in aqua et mundissima farina tritici vel fabe cocte cum fimo columbarum silvestrium. [669] Si apostema crepat et sanies descendit in vesicam, bibat lac azininum, lac caprinum, semen cucurbite, melonis, fiat ei clistere de ptisana et melle.

[c.9] *Contra vulnera matricis*

[675] Contingit autem matricem et vulvam vulnerari et acumine medicine et quandoque ex aborsu, quod cognoscitur per saniem egredientem et per dolorem et punctiones matricis. Si vulnera sint ex putredine et corrosione vene, sanies aliquantulum vergit ad nigredinem cum horribili fetore. Primo ergo oportet apponi mundificativum saniei et mitigativum doloris, ut succus morelle et plantaginis cum oleo rosaceo vel albumine ovi vel lac mulieris vel succus portulace et cetera frigide nature commedat, cucurbita, portulaca, et huiusmodi frigida. Balneetur in aqua ubi decoquatur mirra,[30] rosa, fenugrecum, psidia, balaustia, lenticula, galle et cetera consimilia que superius posita sunt. [703] Si vene putrefacte sunt, detur sanguis draconis et mirra vel thus vel bolus armenicus vel crocus vel aristologia. De huiusmodi singulis vel conjunctis fiat clistere vel pessarium. Nec minus valet acacia cum licio iniecta per pessarium.

[c.10] *Contra pruritum matricis*

[709] Quandoque intus in vulva sentitur pruritus quidam. Tunc acceptis croco, camphora, litargiro, baccis et albumine ovi et oleo rosaceo fiat inde clistere et pessarium. Diascorides dicit quod pulvis fenugreci cum sanguine anseris iniectus per pessarium valet contra matricis duriciem.

---

[29] Many Latin MSS make this phrase the conclusion of the preceding sentence.
[30] The Magdalen copy has *mirta*.

[c.11] Contra sterilitatem mulierum

[717]   Sicut testatur Ypocras, quedam mulieres inutiles sunt ad conceptum quia nimis sunt macre et tenues. Quedam propter nimiam pinguedinem que circumvoluta orificio matricis non permittit semen intra matricem recipi, quoniam constrictum est orificium. Quedam habent matrices ita lubricas ut semen infusum non possint retinere. <Contingit etiam quandoque viri istud qui habet semen nimis tenue et infusum matrici liquiditate sua elabitur.> Quidam autem viri testiculos habent frigide et sicce complexionis et isti aut raro [p.467] aut nuncquam possint generare quia semen eorum inutile est generationi. [731] Si mulier non possit concipere et permaneat sterilis, hoc modo scies utrum vicio eius vel vicio viri contingat. Accipe duas ollas et in utraque pone cantabrum, et urinam viri in una pone cum cantabro et urinam mulieris in reliqua <et sic dimittantur per .viii. vel .xv. dies,> et si sterilitas ex vicio sit mulieris, invenies quosdam vermes in olla mulieris et cantabrum fetidum. Similiter in reliqua invenies si ex vicio viris fuerit. Et si in neutra hoc inveneris, in neutra est causa et beneficio medicine poteris adiuvare ut concipiat. [741] Si ergo velit mulier impregnari, desiccet testiculos verris et inde faciat pulverem et bibat cum vino post purgationem menstruorum et tunc concubat cum viro et poterit concipere. Si velit masculum concipere, accipiat matricem et vulvam leporis et desiccari faciat et bibat vir pulverem distemperatum et similiter faciat mulier de testiculo uno leporis in fine menstruorum et iaceat cum viro suo et concipiet masculum. [751] Item accipiat mulier lanam succidam et intingat in lacte azine et liget super umbilicum et sit ibi donec vir eius concubuerit cum ea. Item accipe corticem quercus et pulveriza et bibat cum vino et in principio et in fine menstruorum. Item accipiant epar et testiculos primi porcelli <que[m] solum scropha ediderit[31]> et desiccentur et redigantur in pulverem et dentur in potu masculo qui non potest generare vel mulieri qui non potest concipere. [763] Constantinus asserit quod virgines que strictas habent vulvas .i. matrices et vulvas angustas non debent viris uti propter metum conceptionis ne moriantur, sed quia non omnes tales continere possunt nostro indigent auxilio in hac parte.

[c.12] Contra fecunditatem[32]

<Mulier ergo si non velit concipere, alligat cum carne sua nuda et ferat secum matricem capre que nuncquam fetum habuit. Invenitur etiam quidam lapis, qui a vulgo 'geth' nuncupatur,[33] qui gestatus a muliere prohibet conceptionem.[34]> [771] Item accipiatur mustele testiculi et relinquatur mustela vivus. Hos testiculos ferat mulier in sinu suo ligatos in asinina pellicula et non concipiet. <Item si aliqua mulier

---

31   The Magdalen copy has *quem solet scropha edere*.
32   In the Magdalen copy part of this section is written in cipher. The rubric runs Ut *mulier npncpnckpkbt* and the entry begins 'Exlkfi .npl. ÷ .t. ⊜ : nc ÷ p: r÷. Alliget cum carne sua nxda et ferat ī bccfm. cbprf.'
33   This phrase is not present in the Magdalen copy.
34   In the Magdalen copy this appears as *cp̄fptkpnfm*.

lesa est in partu et pro timore partus non vult amplius concipere, ponat in secundina sua tot grana cathaputii quot annos vult permanere sterilis. Et si in perpetuum, ponat grana plenam manum et nuncquam concipiet in vita eius quia non tot annos vivet quot ibi grana continentur.>

[c.13] *De hiis que cavenda a mulieribus sunt ne semen vel fetus in utero destruatur.*

[775] Sicut refert Galienus, ita tollitur infans in utero matris sicut fructus arboris. <Sicut enim fructus cum procedit a flore tener est et qualibet levi occasione corruit, cum autem aliquantulum adultus firmius adheret arbori, cum vero maturaverit per se sine vento et impulsione collabitur, sic et cum pri[p.468]mo producitur infans ex semine suscepto, tener est et infirma sunt eius vincula ad matricem. Unde mulier vel motu vel saltu vel casu vel per diarriam vel per dissinteriam vel per minutionem vel laborem vel iram vel dolorem potest fetum amittere statim postquam conceperit. Cum iam vita infusa est puero, firmius coheret nec cito elabitur et cum plene maturaverit nature officio sponte foras producitur.> [780] Ypocras dicit quod si mulier pregnans indiget minutione[35] vel purgatione, non debet purgari nec minui ante quatuor menses neque post sex. Quarto vero et quinto et sexto potest fieri, sed moderate et cum cautela secundum hoc quod virtus eius poterit pati, tamen periculosa est et etiam tunc purgatio. [787] Cavendum est etiam cum mulier incipit impregnari ne nominetur ante eam aliquid quod non potest haberi si ipsa postulaverit, quia multe abortiuntur quando suis non possunt frui desideriis. <Si autem desideret commedere cretam vel argillam, detur ei zuccarum cum fabis tostis.> [791] Instante autem tempore partus sepe balneanda est et ungatur venter eius de oleo olivarum[36] et comedat lenes cibos et digestibiles. Si pedes eius tumuerint, ungantur oleo rosarum vel aceto. <Post cetera cibaria commedat et citonia et malagranata. Si venter eius ventositate distenditur, accipiat semen maratri, apii, ameos, zinziber ana uncias .iiii., masticis, gariofili, cardamomi, radicis rubee maioris ana pondus trium denariorum, cinamomum, nucis maius, castoreum, zedoarium, yrisillirice ana pondus .ii. denariorum, zuccare dragmas .v. Fiat inde pulvis subtilissimus et apponatur mellis cocti quod sufficit. Detur dragma .i. cum vino. Hec medicina aufert ventositatem et aborsum impedit. Maturato autem tempore partus se movet puer vehementius et naturaliter nititur ad egressum, tunc oportet ianuam nature ut latius aperiatur et fetus inveniet egressionis sue libertatem et ita fetus de cubiculo suo .i. de secundina vi nature expellatur.>

---

[35] MS *minutioni.*
[36] Some Latin MSS have *violaceo.*

[c.14] Contra difficultatem partus

[797] Sunt autem quedam mulieres que in officio partus angustiose torquentur et quedam se expedire non possunt, quod quidem ex diversis causis contingit: quandoque quia calor peregrinus supervenit mulieri circa anum,[37] unde ipsa preter modum molestatur; <quandoque quia exitus matricis nimis angustus est; quandoque quia mulier nimis est pinguis; quandoque quia fetus est mortuus in utero nec iuvat egressum motu suo. Et hoc quandoque contingit iuvenili muliericule parturienti[38] in hyeme. Cum enim strictam habeat vulvam, amplius adhuc hyemali frigore limen perstringitur. Quandoque etiam ab ipsa muliere totus calor evanescit et evaporat et sine viribus relinquitur nec sufficit eum ut se expediat.> [804] Expedit ergo mulieri que cum difficultate parit ut balneetur in aqua ubi cocte sunt malve, fenugrecum, semen lini et ordeum. Ungantur venter et latera et coxe et vulva de oleo violaceo <et forti[p.469]ter fricentur et detur ei in potu oxizaccarum. Distemperentur etiam menta et absinthium pulverizata cum vino et detur dragma .i. Provocetur sternutatio cum pulvere thuris apposito naribus. Ducatur lento passu per declivia.>[39] [809] Mulieres que assistunt ei non respiciant eam in vultu quia multe mulieres solent esse ita[40] verecunde in ipso partus visu.

De modo obstetricandi, quomodo cum genituro sit faciendum

[813] Si puer egreditur non eo ordine quo deberet, ut si tibia vel brachium prius exeat, assit obstetrix cum parva manu <et suavi et intincta manu in decoctione fenugreci et seminis lini reponat puerum et convertat in locum suum ad rectum ordinem. Si autem puer mortuus est, accipiatur ruta et arthemisia et terantur simul et bibat succum. Bibat aquam ubi lupini decocti sunt vel absinthium. Piper tritum datum cum vino iuvat. Vel satureia teratur et ligetur super ventrem et exibit fetus sive vivus sive mortuus. Idem facit verbena potata cum vino vel cum aqua vel accipiatur aqua salsa et lac azininum equaliter et detur ad bibendum. Vel scribantur iste dictiones in caseo vel in butiro et dentur ad manducandum .s. sator arepo tenet opera rotas.[41] Vel accipiatur butirum cum melle et vino et detur ad bibendum. Quod si adhuc tardat partus vel si puer mortuus est in ea, bibat lac alterius mulieris cum oleo, et statim liberabitur. Item accipe rutam, arthemisiam, oppopanacum, absinthium, terantur cum oleo et modica zuccara et ponantur super inguina. Vel alligetur radix cucurbite renibus eius et auferatur quantum cito fetus exierit ne matrix exeat.> [819] Post egressum autem pueri si secundina intus remanserit, properandum est ut eiciatur. Provocet ergo mulieri sternutationem et clauso ore et naribus contineat spiritum. Fiat lexivium de frigido

---

37 MS *anteriora*. Many Latin MSS have *inferiora*. I adopt the reading of the Magdalen copy which is reflected by the verse translation.

38 MS *perturienti*.The Magdalen copy has *iuveni mulieri herculem parturienti*.

39 Some Latin MSS have 'Ducatur mulier per domum huc et illuc lento passu'.

40 The Magdalen copy has *ut*.

41 For this charm see Hunt, *Popular Medicine*, p.358 n.100.

cinere et admisceatur pulvis malve dragma .i. et detur ei ad bibendum et statim postea vomat. [829] Bonum est si fumigetur subtus de oculis salsorum piscium vel de ungula caballina vel de stercore cati vel cigni. Ista enim secundinam educunt. <Valet etiam decoquere semen lini et dare ad bibendum. Idem facit bullitum cum vino.> [833] Si autem sanguis post secundinam non exeat, fiant ea que superius scripta sunt ad provocandum menstrua. <Si post partum matrix doluerit, accipe storacem et thus electum ana unciam .i. et de semine racemorum nigrorum uncias .ii., ponantur super carbones vivos et suffumigetur inde et multum confert.> [837] [Ad cognoscendum utrum masculum vel feminam conceperit:]⁴² accipiatur aqua de fonte et extrahat mulier guttam sanguinis de dextro latere et infundat aque: si fundum petit, mas[culus] erit, si supernatat, femina.

[843]   Ypocras dicit quod mulier que concepit masculum rubicundam habet faciem et dextram mamillam grossiorem; [si vero feminam concepit, pallida est et habet sinistram mamillam grossiorem].⁴³ <Item ad eductionem fetus, accipe satureiam et pistetur et superligetur utero et exibit fetus. Item ad matricem constringendam: argillam albam misce cum aceto fortissimo albo ad modum emplastri et pone super umblicum et pectinem et muta bis vel ter in die. Optimum est.>

[Sequitur secunda pars. [p.470] Trotula minor]

---

⁴² Supplied from the Magdalen copy.
⁴³ Supplied from the Magdalen copy.

CHAPTER THREE

Euperiston

In the Old Advocates Library, now housed in the National Library of Scotland, Edinburgh, MS 18.6.9 (olim A.6.13) represents an interesting collection of medical texts copied in the fourteenth century. On p.ii in a seventeenth-century hand three items of its contents are identified ('Dispensatorium Nicholai', 'summa magistri Valteri de Agelon de dosis medicinarum', 'praxis medicinae incerti authoris gallicae') and the volume is said to be 'Ex libris Jacobi Balfourii'. On f.iii a similar hand has written 'Ex libris bibliotheca facultitis [sic] iuridicae Edinburgi'. As there exists no detailed description of the MS, its principal contents may be indicated here.

1. ff.1ra–vb inc. '[A]uree alexandrine duas libras facimus, [A]driani magni unam libram . . .' Tables to the *Antidotarium Nicolai*. Preparations and their quantities are listed in two columns. The initial letter of each entry is missing.

ff.2r–37v inc. 'Ego Nicholaus rogatus a quibusdam in practica medicine studere volentibus . . .' A full text of the *Antidotarium Nicolai*.[1] On f.37v there are nine verses beginning 'Collige triticeis medicine pondera granis' (ThK 234) taken from the *Flos medicinae scholae Salerni*,[2] which are often transmitted with the *Antidotarium*.

ff.38ra–40vb without prologue (ThK 1231 'Quia sufficienter de dispensatione omnium confectionum . . .') lists 'de dosibus medicinarum' (ThK 195) commonly transmitted with the *Antidotarium Nicolai*, beginning 'Carpobalsami uncias duas . . .'

ff.40vb–43vb *Synonyma* frequently transmitted with the *Antidotarium* beginning 'Arthemesia id est matricaria . . .' (ThK 147) and introduced by a prose paragraph beginning 'Expletis autem specierum ponderibus que ad omnium predictarum medicinarum confectionem pertinent . . .' (ThK 544).

2. ff.43vb–48r miscellaneous receipts and preparations in a variety of hands, beginning with 'Contra ventositatem stomachi . . .', 'Contra ventositatem . . .' 'Contra lapidem . . .', 'Electuarium ad restaurandum' and including receipts for 'diaturbit', 'diamacis', 'diarubarbaron', 'diabutirum' and various pills and oils ('oleum benedictum', 'Hoc oleum de secretis philosophorum' etc.). From f.45v the text is written across the whole page and letters have been lost through cropping. The lower half of ff.47r and 48r are blank as is the whole of f.48v.

3. f.49ra excerpt from a medical text beginning 'In causa frigida recipe succcum apii . . .'

---

[1] The most convenient text is that by W.S. van den Berg, *ed. cit.* See also D. Goltz, *Mittelalterliche Pharmazie und Medizin dargestellt an Geschichte und Inhalt des Antidotarium Nicolai* (Stuttgart, 1976).

[2] See Renzi, *Coll. Sal.* 1 pp.482f, ll.1136ff. See also *Pop. Med.* p.60.

4. ff.49rb–51rb [Tractatus de pulsibus], often attributed to Matthew of Salerno, inc. 'Pulsus ut dicit Philaretus est motio cordis et arteriarum . . .' (ThK 1151) ending 'Sed hec vobis de pulsibus ad presens sufficiant'.

5. ff.51va–52va *Die diebus creticis* (rubric partly cropped) inc. 'De creticis diebus tractaturi videamus quid sit crisis . . .' (ThK 370). See MS B.L. Sloane 4 ff.29–30.

6. f.52vb excerpt (incomplete) from medical treatise inc. 'Nota de signis perfecte purgacionis'.

7. ff.53ra–56rb displaced (see 9 below) part of the 'Compendium Salerni',[3] beginning halfway through c.10[4] and continuing to c.74.[5]

8. f.57ra–b excerpt from medical treatise including rubrics *Contra tumorem*, *De venis*, *Ad asma*, *Ad scabiem*, *Contra guttam*, *Contra reuma*, *Contra tercianam*, ending 'Qui vero biberit medicinam'.

9. ff.57va–58vb 'Compendium Salerni' headed *De secretis*, beginning with prologue ('Dupplici causa me cogente socii hoc opus instituere desideravi . . .') (ThK 476), list of chapters, and continuing with c.1–10.[6]

10. ff.59ra–65ra Walter of Agilon's 'De dosibus medicinarum' (inc. 'Medicinarum vero quedam sunt simplices quedam composite . . .') (ThK 860), expl. 'Explicit summa magistri Walteri de Agelon facta de dosis medicinarum'.

11. f.65ra–b Galen, 'De signis mortis et vite' inc. 'Quisquis in die prima uniuscuiusque mensis in infirmitate inciderit . . .' (ThK 1250)

12. ff.65v–68r treatise on the properties of urine as signs of various medical conditions, followed by 'Colores urinarum sunt .xix.' inc. 'Albus ut aqua purissima . . .'.

13. ff.68v Receipts beginning 'Unguentum pro vulneribus, pro gutta artetica, pro inflationibus, pro dolore, pro apostematibus, pro cancro . . .' with some receipts in French.[7]

---

3   Printed by Renzi, *Coll. Sal.* 5, pp.201–32.
4   Renzi, p.206, l.24.
5   Renzi, p.221, l.2.
6   Ending in the middle of c.10, Renzi, p.206, l.24.
7   One of the receipts includes the vernacular items 'souerbarbe', 'butyro de may', another 'fullun', 'heyhove', and 'wermod'. The following receipts are mainly in French: Por une maladye quod vocatur 'tetur wilde': recipe blanc de Espayne plus qe de acun autre et sindre de argent et mellét ses deus ensemble en un morter de araume. Et quant il est bin mellé ensemble, metét oyle de olyve bone et espesse et metét ensemble. Pus pernét vin egre et metét desus et medlét ensemble. // Por amirals, quidam morbus in ano crescens ad modum mamillarum canicule: recipe pecies panni diversi coloris .ix. et de cornu cervi tanquam de panno et comburatur et postea pulverisatur et inunge locum cum oleo olive et tunc asperge cum illo pulvere, et curabitur. // Pur ydropesye: pernét le blanc de porrets et kersons de ewe et fetes potage et gruel et use cel potage, si la qe il seit purgé. // Pro tela oculorum: recipe lukechuste, quidam vermis, et edera terrestris et enplastra super oculos. Vel lukechuste tritum bibat. // Pur la teye de le uyl freindre: pernét un racin de gingivere et pudrét menu et medlét o blan vin et metét en le oyl et il le brusera. // Por oye: pernét fel de levere chaud com il vint hors de levere, si metét en les orailes, si garirad san dote. // Por arson: pernét siw de berbiz ou de bouf et friét et medlét flur de forment, si emplastrét sur quant le fu est treit hors par lyes.

14. ff.69ra–80rb Medico-botanical glossary inc. 'Ambra secundum quosdam est sperma ceti . . .' ending with 'Zair fluxus ventris que fit ab intestino recto'.

15. f.80rb Avicenna on leprosy inc. 'Lepra secundum Avicennam est mala infirmitas proveniens ex dispositione colere nigre in toto corpore . . .' (ThK 816)

16. ff.81r–147r medical compendium inc. 'Euperiston est cest livre apelé, ceo est a dire bien esprové, car i[l] n'y a riens escrit en cest livre ke ne est esprové'.

17. f.147r receipts in French inc. 'Et le men esperment est: pernés l'escorse de sambuc . . .', 'Et pour verms de chival . . ..', 'Verm de homme et d'enfaunt', 'Pour lé worms et lé lumbriz . . .' The verso is blank.

18. ff.149(sic)r–52v A number of receipts, some repeated, for the preparation of 'gingebrat alyn' and 'gyngebrat india' and 'bona conserva de gingebre'.

19. f.153r miscellaneous receipts in different hands

20. f.153v charm 'pour laruns'.[8]

21. f.154r charm and receipts for woman in childbirth, the charm incorporating 'liés a soun ventre sest escrist 'Maria peperit Christum + Anna Mariam + Elizabeth Johannem + Celima Remigium'. Sic peperit ista in nomine Patris. . .'[9] There follows a charm against 'surris qui maungent le blé en graunge'.[10]

22. ff.154v–55r miscellaneous receipts in various hands

23. f.156r–v ['De tonitribus'] a short treatise on divination by thunder inc.'In quocumque signo tonuerit sive in die sive in nocte' which is also found in Oxford, Bodl. Lib. MS Can. misc.517 (s.xv) f.20ra–b where it is described in a rubric as 'Hermes Trismegistus excerptus'.[11]

Following the model of the *Practica Brevis*, it is convenient to divide the *Euperiston* in to Nine Books, arranged as follows:

BOOK I: THE HEAD

1. Headache [*cephalea; cephalargia; soda*] 2–19
2. Delirium [*frenesie*] 20–26

---

8   'Pour laruns: pernés escume de argent e aubun de l'eof et medlés ensemble et fetes l'oyl en la pareye e apelez tous ceus ke vus avés suspesciun, ke il regardent cel oyl et le copable suera soun oyl et le niera et denia(?). Et si il denie le larun fetes .i. agulle et ferrés en le et il le senterat tauntost et dirra le fet. Et sy laruns vous ount emblé hastivement fetes ch[an]ter une messe de la invenciun de la seinte croys, si seyés et oyés la messe, pus pernés foyles de lorrer et escrivés les nouns de ceus dount vous avés suspesiun, sy metés desous vostre chef .iii. noys et gardés vous de pollusiouns. Saun doute vous . . .(?) la terse noyt le larrun.'

9   Cf. Hunt, *Pop. Med.* p.90 nos.37–8; p.92 no.46; p.98 no.89; p.278, no.90.

10 Cf. Hunt, *Pop.Med.* p.134.

11 The MS is a collection of astrological texts which include works attributed to Masha'allah, Thabit ibn Qurra, and Arnald of Villanova. On thunder prognostics see M. Förster, "Beiträge zur mittelalterlichen Volkskunde", *Archiv für das Studium der neueren Sprachen und Literaturen* 120 (1908), 43–52.

---

[12] The word *nectalopas* appears in the OE *Perididaxeon* (15,22) and is explained as one who is unable to see between sunrise and sunset. See note to text below p.151 n.14.

BOOK V: THE FACE

1. Freckles,' lentigo' or facial spots [*lentilles, tecches*] 90

BOOK VI: THE MOUTH

1. Toothache [*dolor dé dens*] 91–95
2. Chapping [*lange, levre, gingive . . . escorcees*] 96
3. Halitosis [*puor de la bouche*] 97

BOOK VII: RESPIRATORY AILMENTS

1. Quinsy [*squinantie*] 98
2. Cough [*tusse*] 99–100
3. Haemoptysis [*emoptois*] 101–102
4. Empyema [*empima*] 103–104
5. Phthisis [*ptisike*] 105–108
6. Pneumonia (peripneumony) [*peripleumonie*] 109–111
7. Pleuresy [*pleuresi*] 112–115
8. Chestpain [*dolor del piz*] 116–19
9. Asthma [*asma*] 120
10. Syncope, lipothymy [*paumeson*] 121–123
11. Palpitation [*cardiake*] 124–126

BOOK VIII: THE STOMACH

1. Bulimy incl. 'canine hunger' [*bolismus, cinorodoxa*] 127–129
2. Thirst [*seif*] 130–132
3. Anorexia [*fastidium, anorexia*] 133–135
4. Stomach ulcer [*aposteme*] 136–138
5. Hardness of the stomach [*duresce de l'estomac*] 139
6. Eructation [*acetouse eructation, soure balkinges*] 140–141
7. Abdominal swelling [*emflure del ventre*] 142
8. Stomach-ache [*dolor de l'estomac*] 143–144
9. Vomiting [*vomit*] 145

BOOK IX: THE INTESTINES

1. Morbid evacuation [*flux de ventre*] 146
2. Diarrhoea [*diarria, diarrie*] 147–153
3. Dysentery [*dissinteria / dissinterie*] 154–155
4. Lientery [*lienteria / lienterie*] 156
5. Intestinal worms [*lumbriz*] 157

The treatise is apparently incomplete. Internal references suggest the compiler's / author's familiarity with the whole, but a few of the references lack textual correspondences. 'Sicum nus dirrum el chapitre de lumbriz' (15) refers to (157), 'Sicum nus avum dit el chapitre de empimate' (105) to (103), 'Sicum nus dirrum el chapitre de cardiake' (122) to (124). But without clear correspondences are 'Sicum nus dirrum el chapitre de flux dé flurs' (122), 'Sicum nus dirrum el chapitre de suffocation del mariz' (122), (re fainting) 'Sicum nus dirrum en son lu' (122), (re 'destemperance dé reins en chalor') 'De cele dirrum la cure el chapitre de cele maladie' (132). This may suggest that the treatise as we have it is incomplete.

Whether the whole treatise is a translation from the Latin is difficult to say. The retention of Latin terms regarding headaches (1) and fainting (121) along with the etymological explanation of the term anorexia (133) might suggest so. In addition to the naming of authorities (see supplement to Glossary), there is frequent recourse to unspecified 'authors' / 'authorities': solonc touz les autors, ke touz les autors accordent, comandent les autors, ceo tesmoynent les autors, les autors dient, de ceste parlent les autors sovent. At the same, the author / compiler appears to assert his own opinions and adduce his own experience, but as we know, such declarations may be present in the sources he is reproducing:

(23)   al comencement est mun cunseil . . . sicum nus avom dit

(29)   autre ke jeo ay sovent usé

(45)   Constantin met en sa Practike e nous l'avom esprové

(52)   pus ceo ke nus avom dit

(63)   ausi mon conseil [est] ke . . .

(81)   E jeo di ke en lu d'oyle de alemandes ameres put hom mettre le jus d'oynon ou de poret e pur anis comin

(84)   meme ceo di jeo de baume

(90)   sicum nus avom dit

(127) et jeo di . . . e jeo le grant bien . . . mes si . . . jeo nel granteray mye

(128) est mun cunseil ke

(147) e nus l'avom esprové

Another feature of the author / compiler's technique is to gloss words and concepts with an explanatory phrase or clause introduced by *ceo est a dire* or *id est*, as can be seen from the following examples:

(20)   pleuresie, ceo est aposteme souz les costes

(22)   spasme, ceo est a dire crampe, de quises e de jambes, ceo est asaver ke si eles seyent estendus, ke il ne les puise nient doubler, ou si eles seyent doublés, ke il ne les puise nient estendre

(99)   cynoglosse .i. lange de chien

(112) Quatre tens sont de pleuresie, ceo est a dire comencement, anoytement, estat, declineson . . . declination, ceo est a dire la departye de la maladie

(120) Encuntre asma, ceo est a dire destresce d'aleyne

(122) de inanition, ceo est a dire ke le corps est void

(126) colagogue, ceo est a dire medicine ke espurge colre

(127) cinorodoxa, ceo est a dire joye de chien

(131) E ceo ke curra hors serra muscillage, ceo est a dire ke il serra espés ou viscous ausi cum glette

(133) anorexia, si est dit de *a*, ke est a dire 'sanz', e *orexis*, ke est a dire 'appetit', sicum 'sanz appetit'

(156) sanz change de la viande, ceo est asaver quant la viande vient hors a la chambre foreine tant e tel qu'el est reçu en l'estomac

The MS has been quite heavily annotated in a number of fourteenth-century hands, with supplementary receipts of a brief kind added to appropriate sections. The text of the *Euperiston* has been written out with blank spaces left between sections as if to invite such additions. On a number of occasions (see below) the user is directed to turn the page, back or forward, to locate a specific receipt. The added receipts occur as follows:

f.81r   Ad capitis dolorem . . . / A dolour de la teste de veyle goute . . . / A dolour de teste de freyd enchesoun . . .

f.81v   Pour ague garir . . .

f.82r   Pour tote manere de playe . . .

f.82v   A dolour es orayles . . . / Verm en les orayles . . . / Pour sonis des orrayles . . . / A dolour de chef . . . / Pur le vertin de chef . . .

f.83r   A dolour de la teste ke vent de fellun ou est enflee . . . / Pour sonis des orayles . . .

f.84r   Pour ague . . . / Et pur se ke frenesie est e vent de apostume . . .

f.85r   Pur frenesie . . .

f.87v   pointing hand beside 'E sachét ke de melancolie sont diverses especes'

f.90v   Pour goute kayve . . . / Pernés une taupe vive . . .

f.91r   Pour goute kayve: boyvera piganum id est ruta agrestis . . . / N[ota] esprove. Pur epilencie, goute kayve . . .

f.93v   pointing hand beside 'Ausi veét ci verray esperment esprové'

f.97r   Et si vous volés ke homme ne syt yvre la journee . . .

f.99r   [Pour] ceus ke dorment . . .

f.101v In dei nomine, amen. Pur ouster la mayle . . . / Pour oster la mayle et apostume des [oes] . . .

f.102r Pour oster la mayle des oes . . .

f.102v Pour flux de lermes . . . / Emigreine . . .

f.103r added remedy for redness of the eyes

f.103v Pour oes malades . . .

f.104v Oes dolens. Pur oes ke at maile et feylun et anguses . . . / Unguentum . . . / Pour cop de launse dount ses oes sount estonis et oscurs . . .

f.105r N[ota] pour oes reverses . . . / Pur oes reverses et prurit et ueb . . .

f.107r Pour sonis des orrayles . . . / Pour sonis de orayles

f.107v A dolour des orrayles . . . [three receipts]

f.109r Encountre sonis des orrayles . . . par Water de Zorbery . . .

f.109v Dur oye . . . / Pour sonis des orrayles . . .

f.110v Ad sanguinem stringendum et ad fluxum . . .

f.111v Encountre flux de playe . . .

f.112r Sy flux dé narils de saunk seyt trop . . . Et si se faud . . .

f.115r Pour dolur de dent . . . / Contre [dolur] dé dens . . . [two receipts] / Pour dolour de dent persee ou nent persee . . . / Et si vuus vollés trere hors . . .

f.115v Dent dolour conjuresoun: conjuro te, dencium dolor, per .iii. magos Caspar, Melchisar, Belchisar mus aptanas lot yot midrak, ut non abeas potestatem manendi in dentibus nec in maxillis, per Christum dominum, sanat te Deus, Dey filius qui pro te passus est, sanat te Deus, Dey filius qui in te fusus est, Pater Noster et Ave ter dicitur. Et si il faut, pernés le oynoun rouge.

f.116r   N[ota] (beside 'Destemprét ferine de furment ovek let de titimal') Ou pernés aus et blaunk pey[v]re, miel et tenés et bevés tot chaud et serra tot garry.

f.116v   Dolour de dent persee et nent persee . . . / Item si se la faut . . . / Pour dent dolour . . .

f.117r   Pur dolour de dent . . . / Pour dolour de dent ja ne seyt si rajous . . . Assayé ay.

f.118v   Pernés spigornelle . . .

f.119r   Latin receipt in the gutter

f.119v   Pour squinancie et apostume et felun en gorge . . . / Apostume et fellun . . .

f.120r   Toute maneire tousse . . . / Ou pernés gingivre . . .

f.124v   drawing of front quarters of a dog beside 'Pernét chaels esvoeglés . . .'

f.128r   Encountre distresse de glette . . .

f.132r   Si angoyse ou paumesoun ou dolour de quer aver [corr. avent] a homme ou a femme . . .

f.132v   Pur cardiake et dolour . . .

f.133r   Vees de la foile avaunt de ma mein de paumeisoun et de cardiake . . . [i.e. receipt on f.132r] / Et donés pur cardiake . . . / Pur cardiake et joye (?) . . .

f.137r   Pur apostume . . . / Pur apostume . . . / Ou le apostume seyt . . . / Si vus volés ke il brise . . . tornés [i.e. the receipt is rewritten on f.137v]

f.137v   Pour apostume . . . / Pour apostume . . . / Et si vous volés ke l'apostume brisse et pointure i seyt ou aunguse ja ni seit il si dur . . .

f.138r   Pur apostume . . . / Pur apostume . . . / Et pur remuer apostume . . . / Apostumes et angoyses . . . mettés la foyl de gaunt de gobil . . . / Pur apostumus et felouns . . . / Et si totes choses faylend . . .

f.140r   Pur dolour en l'estomak et trencheysun . . .

f.140v   Pour vomit . . .

f.141r   Flux de fleume . . . / Pur flux . . .

f.141v   Pour trenchesun et flux . . .

f.143v   Pour flux unde sit . . .

f.144r   Sy flux seyt owe fevre ou owe chalour . . . / Pour flux onde [sic] sit . . .

f.144v   Pour flux . . . / Flux de saunk . . . gaunt de gopil . . . / Pur tre[n]cheson . . . / Sy flux de saunk . . .

f.145r   Pour flux de saunk . . . / Et sy le flux seyt trop viole[nt] . . . / Pur flux . . . / Pur flux de ventre . . . tornés pur chaude meneysoun [i.e. f.145v]

f.145v   Pour chaude meneysoun: pernez un poume costarde . . . / Pur pisser . . . / Pur hastivement pisser . . .

f.146r   Pour flux . . . / Pour flux de chalour colre sy il seyt enflé et trenchesoun . . . / Pour flux unde sit . . .

f.146v   Pour lombris et trencheysoun . . .

f.147r   N[ota] et le men esperment est . . . et meme se vaut pur ydropik . . . / Et pour verms de chival . . . / Pour lé worms et lé lumbriz . . .

Euperiston

[f.81r] *Euperiston* est cest livre apelé, ceo est a dire bien esprové, car i[l] n'y a riens escrit en cest livre ke ne est esprové. Premerement dirrum de la teste e pus d'autres membres.

[BOOK I: THE HEAD]

1.

[1] Premerement de *dolor de la teste*. Dolor de la teste a la foyz est en tute la teste e donc est apelé *cephalea* ou *cephalargia* ou *soda*. A la foiz est en milu de la teste e donc est apelé *emigranea*. Ausi avient en divers lus de la teste solonc les quatre complexions, car dolor de sanc est el front, de colre en la destre part, de fleume est par deriere, e de melancolie est en la senestre partye.

[2] La cure de dolor de la teste est, si la materie est de sanc soulement, ke le pacient seit seiné de la veine capitale en la contrere partye de la dolor. E sachét ke i covient ke le pacient se garde de trop manger ou boyvre e nomément de vin. E mult li vaut dormir sovent. La cure de dolor ke avient par certain tens e par certein houre est itele, ceo est asaver ke le pacient se garde de longes pensees e de ire e de cumpaynie de femme. E sachét ke Avicenne dit par l'autorité de Philagorie ke mult vaut a destrure dolor de la teste ke le pacient seit seiné de la veine en le front ou de la veine ke est dedens le [f.81v] levre par aval ou mettre ventouses en le col e desouz la teste e poy aler e lesser viandes ke enflent. E sachét ke acetouses choses nusent a cely ke ad dolor de la teste par encheson de l'estomac.

[3] La cure de dolor de la teste de freid encheson de materie de melancolie quant la dolor est forte: Pernét milium e broillét desure une chaude tuyle e pus metét en un sachel. E raét la teste e metét le sur la teste. Autre esprove: pernét libram semis de anis e metét en eawe chaude en treis sachels e metét un sur la teste e un autre desur l'oraylle, la ou la dolor est. Autre esprove: escorchét un jefne moton e metét la pel chaude sur la teste un jor e une nuyt. Si la dolor ne cesse mye uncore, lavét la teste oveke cette eawe: quissét la racine de cucumbre savage en eawe e en oyle e de ceo lavét la teste. Pus enbruét la teste oveke ces oyles. Pernét oyle de camomille, oyle de pulleole ana libra semis, oyle muscellin unces .iii. Medlét ensemble e de ceo chaud enoynét la teste e enbruét e de ces oyles metét en l'orayle de cele part ou la dolor est. E plongét l'orayle leins, [f.82r] pus surmetét la pel de moton. Si la dolor aviengne de l'estomac, lavét les narilz sovent oveke oyle de camomille tedve e en dolor de chaud encheson oveke oyle violette tedve. Si la dolor seit plus par devant, fetes cest emplastre esprové: pernét cyre blanche e malaschét oveke oyle de camomille e pus l'estendét e surmetét al front chaud e sove[n]t changét. E ceo est la cure de dolor de la teste ke est de freid, sanz materie ou oveke materie de melancolie ou de fleume ou de ventosité ou de fumosités.

[4] A dolor de chalor soulement sanz materie: enoynét la teste oveke oyle roset. E si il ne assuage mie, pernét demi livre d'oyle roset e jus de jubarbe e de morele ana quartroun .i., de blanc vin egre unces .ii. Medlét tut ensemble e moillét leins un linge drap e metét al lu dolent.

[5] La cure de dolor de la teste de vent ke eyt percé dekes al cervel par les orayles ou par les narilz: medlét ensemble oyle de camomille e oyle de anet ana unces .ii., oyle roset uncia semis, e meté[t] enz par la ou le vent entra.

[6] A la dolor k'avient de mauveis fumosités dedenz e pulens e chaus: fetes le patient odorer sovent roses, violes e flur de nenufar e camphre e sandles [f.82v] e lavét la teste oveke l'eawe de la decoction de roses fresches e flurs de nenufar e lavét sovent les narilz oveke eawe rose.

[7] A dolor de la teste ke avient de fumé de souffre: fetes le patient odorer camphre mise en eawe rose e lavét les narilz dedenz de cele eawe.

[8] A dolor de la teste de fu e de fumosité resolee de vin par ont le patient est ausi cum pres de iloeke frenetic Constantin e Alisandre comandent ke le jus de cholet seit bu e l'erbe triblé seit emplastré desure.

[9] A dolor de la teste de playe si i[l] n'i a mye granz flux de sanc par la playe, commune reule est ke le patient seit seiné de la contrere partye de la teste.

[10] A dolor de la teste de brusure de la teste: le patient seit en tenve diete e se garde de vin.

[11] A la dolor de la teste d'opilation del cervel ke vus conoistrét par soniz e siffler en les orayles il covient ke vus usét choses aperitives par fumigations de la bouche e dé narilz e par oynemenz des orayles e laveures entour le lu dolent.

[12] A dolor de la teste de bon odor, sicum de musc: fetes le patient odorer camphre e sandles. [f.83r]

[13] A dolor de la teste de freid odor, sicum de canphre: odorét musc e ambre.

[14] A dolor de la teste ke avient de yveresce: premerement fetes le patient vomir oveke eawe chaude, pus frotét ses pés oveke chaud vin egre e de sel e lavét ses coilz oveke chaud vin egre e quant il a dormi pessét le oveke chous quis e donét li a manger pomes e peyres.

[15] A dolor de la teste ke avient de verms sanz fievre: fetes turtels del jus de centonike .i. *meriswermode* e de ferine d'orge e donét a manger al patient quant il est jun e oveke vin pur. E fetes autres remedies sicum nus dirrum el chapitre de lumbriz.

[16] A dolor de la teste de verms oveke fevre: emplastrét le umbril oveke cest emplastre ke nomément est esprové. E as enfans nomément pernét d'orge libram semis, del jus de tetesoriz libram unam, de vin egre blanc unces .iii. e fetes emplastre e surmetét chaud en yvern e en esté freid. Bien vaudra.

[17] A dolor de la teste ke avient de ceo ke hom chet ou est feru: raét premerement la teste e pus fetes le patient seiner de la contrarie partye. Pus pernét blanche cyre e malaschét al fu [f.83v] e de ceo envolupét tute la teste. Quant vus remuét la cyre e nule brusure ne seit en la cyre, signe est ke la teste n'est pas debrusé. A cele dolor pernét la pel de moton tute chaude e envolupét la teste. Autre: pernet courte leyne ke est apelé en engleis *flockes* e broyllét en une paele sur le fu sanz liqor e metét sur la teste. Si la dolor ne cesse mye, fete[s] le seiner de la mene veine. Pus pernét feves sotilement poudrés e boyllét oveke mel e surmetez sur la leine. Autre a anciene dolor:

Pernét de cyroyne libram unam e malaschét al fu oveke oyle de camomille, estendét sur quir e bien chaud metét a la teste e issi demurge .ix. jors.

[18] Si fevre aperge e l'entendement seit troublé, signifie ke la teste est malade ou ke ele ad aposteme. Donc fete[s] le seyner de la veine capitale e treét la materie aval par clistere. Pernét de violette e de mauve, merculiale, brance ur[sine], flurs de violette ana unces .iii., de cassiefistre munde unce une, d'oyle de violette unces .ii. e fetes clistere. E donét sirup violette.

[19] La diete de ceus ke ont mal [f.84r] en la teste est net payn e bien fourné, vin blanc e sotil, non pas trop fort, tendre char sicum char de aygnel e de porc, gelines e lor poucins, perdriz e faisanz. E le patient eschue char de vache e de boef e de choses ke engendrent ventosité e se garde de fritures e use viandes quites.

2.

[20] *Frenesie* avient en fevre ague. De Avicenne est apelé *karabicus* e Almasor l'apele *sirsen*. Frenesie est aposteme a la foyz en la meule del cervel, a la foiz entre les deus teyes ke envolupent le cervel. E il y a verreye frenesie e nient verreie. La verraye est de ague colre ou[1] de sanc boyllant el quer. La nient verreye avient de acune maladie sicum de pleuresie, ceo est aposteme souz les costes.

[21] Signes de frenesie sont change de pensé, veiles, dormir plein de travail, e la lange est neyre e les oylz lerment e le patient decyre ses dras e cuylle leyne carpie de ses dras e des pareyes. Touz ces signes sont kant l'aposteme est devant el front. Mes si l'aposteme seit en mylu, la reson est corrumpue e le patient [f.84v] ne set ke il fet. Si l'aposteme seyt par derere, le patient ublie ceo ke il veit e ceo ke il fet. Especials signes sont si la frenesie seit de sanc ke la deverie est oveke risee e dormir e roujor des oylz, mes si ele seit de colre, do[n]c verrét les signes avantdiz ovec ire e tenson e tricherie. Signes de frenesie nient verreye sont ke le patient ad le sen changé e ke il veile e pus dort grefment e pus esveile horriblement e parolt hors de reson.

[22] E pur ceo ke frenesie est perilouse maladie desoremés dirrum de la cure. E sachét ke frenesie confermé est incurable e ceo put hom conoystre par quatre choses: par costiveson del ventre, par defaute de l'urine, par veyles, par spasme – ceo est a dire crampe, de quises e de jambes, ceo est asaver ke si eles seyent estendus, ke il ne les puise nient doubler, ou si ele[s] seyent doublés, ke il ne les puise nient estendre. E Ypocras dit par tesmoynage de Avicenne: 'Si une vescie apiert el pouz, certeinement signifie mort'.

[23] La cure de frenesie curable est ke le patient seit seiné de la veine capitale une partye si il seyt fieble, mes si il est fort, seit seyné dekes [f.85r] a paumeson pres de ilokes. E si il seit fort, seit seiné de la veine ke est enmi le front ou de cele ke est el summet del nes. Pus raét la teste e l'enbruét oveke let de femme ke alete pucele. Pus pernét oyle roset e medlét oveke vin egre blanc e enoynét le front e les temples. E le patient seit en oscure meson sanz peinture. E esparpilét par tute la meson foilz de vine e de saus arosees d'eawe rose e de camphre e les foilz seyent cuylliz avant ke le solail

---

1 MS *ou ou.*

leve. E al comencement est mon cunseil ke estupes seyent moyllés en blanc de l'oef ou en jus de morele ou de jubarbe e un poy de vin egre e tedve surmetét el front. E frotét les plansons de[s] pés e de[s] mains oveke vin egre e sel. E aprés l'espace de .xxiiii. houres lavét les pés e les jambes dekes a genoylz e les mayns e les braz dekes a coutes oveke ceste eawe: r[ecevét] de foilz de saus, de foilz de vine blanche, de flurs de nenufar ana manipulum unum, boyllét tut en eawe e lavét sicum nus avom dit.

[24] E sachét ke commune reule est solum les autors ke le patient seit clisterizé al comencement. Pur ceo fetes cest clistere: r[ecevét] de violette, mauve, branke ursine ana manipulum unum, [f.85v] boyllét en eawe e colét e a cele colature ajostét de violes unce une e boyllét dekes a demy livre. E metét enz par clistere lenitif. E pus fetes clistere mordicatif: pernét de foilz de mauve e de merculiale e de branke ursine e de violette ana manipulum unum, de bren libram semis, de mel e d'oyle violette ana unciam semis, de salgemme dragmes .ii. e fetes clistere. Autre plus leger: boyllét eawe e en cele eawe resolét sel e fetes clistere.

[25] Si le patient seit fieble, ne fetes mye clistere, mes fetes suppositories. Et premerement fetes suppositorie lenitif: pernét lard de porc ke est entre le quir e la char unces .ii. e metét en eawe freide, ke il seit dur e espés. E fetes suppositorie. Si li covient aver plus fort, fetes suppositorie de savon e moyllé[t] en oyle violette e souz metét. Autre: pernét fel de tor e enoynét la partye derere. Merveilousement espurge. Autre: pernét l'oyl de mulet salé e souz metét. Autre: pernét alum de plume unce une, poudrét e medlét ke bure e souz metét. Si l'aposteme n'est pas cuylly, ke vus poét conoistre par ceo ke le patient crie assiduelement e veile trop, pernét un blanc chael ke ne veit [f.86r] mie e le fendét parmi l'espine del dos e trehét hors les entrayles e chaud surmetét a la teste par devant. Ou fendét un coc parmy e surmetét. Ou pernét le pomon de moton e surmetét. E quant est refreidé, eschaufét le en chaud eawe. E pus pressét hors l'eawe entre vos mains e surmetét al front. E ceo fetes sovent. Mes el comencement usét repercussifs. Si la lange seit secke ou neyre, mundifiét la lange sovent e raét. Pernét le vin de poumes gernets e medlét oveke eawe tedve e de ceo lavét la bouche e la lange. Pus raét la bouche oveke un cotel de fust e ceo fetes sovent. E pus pur fere le dormir pernét jus de letuse e oyle violette e roset e destemprét a ceo d'opie libram semis e enoynét le front e les temples. Si le patient seit si feble ke il ne pusse estre seyné ou clisterizé, usét les suppositories avantdiz.

[26] La diete est, si le patient est fort, ke il ne manjue ne beive, ou la diete seit mult tenve, sicum dit Rasi. Si ly donét eawe d'orge une foyz ou deus foiz le jor. Si la frenesie assuage e la fevre, donc donét plus grosse diete. E aprés le settime jor donét vin.

3.

[f.86v] [27] De *manie* sont deus especes, ceo est a saver lupine e canine. Lupine est quant le patient regart sicum lou e est irous e saut e parle diversement. Canine est quant le pacient e[st] cumpaynable sicum chien e ke il tense en riant. E sachét ke il y a difference entre frenesie e manie pur ceo ke manie est sanz fevre e frenesie oveke fevre. E sovent avient manie de l'estomac e donc est garrie par vomit. E sachét ke manie e melancolie sont sovent garries par emorroides.

[28] Signe de manie lupine est quant le patient se demeyne cum lou e a la foiz

repose un poy e pus parle trop e si est de neir color e quant il dort ad horrible songes. Signe de manie canine est ke le patient tense e se corouse legerement e pus le ublie meintenant.

[29] La cure de manie est ke le patient seit premerement seiné en la veine capitale e ke il seit ventosé entre les espaules e ke ses quisses seyent fortment liés e acun hom seit devant le patient de ky il eyt poour e honte. Si le patient ne voylle mie prendre medicine, [f.87r] pernét lapis lazuli e lapis armenici ana scrupulum unum, scamonee scrupulum semis, medlét oveke ferine e fetes niweles e donét, car ceo est esprové. Autre ke jeo ay sovent usé: norissét un chapon oveke bren ou ferine destempré ovekes eawe chaude ou² les poudres avantdites e de ceo norissét le chapon par .xv. jors. Pus le quissét dekes la char seit resolee el bru e donét en l'aube de jor dekes a libram semis ou a libram unam al plus, car merveilousement lasche. Bon esperiment encuntre manie: pernét la poudre de diptayne ou la rasure de corn de cerf ou de orobi e donét oveke jus de minte. E si le patient gette escume par la bouche ausi cum cely ke est mors de chen aragé, dedenz .vii. jors murra. E s'il ne gette nul escume, eschapera. Ausi une reule est ke a touz maniacs e melancoliens vaut la cumpaynie de femme pur mundefier le cervel. La dreinere cure de manie est par cyrurgie. E pur ceo seit ars el summet de la teste oveke un fer. Pus seit le fu esteint oveke estoupe de canve moilli el jus de poret [f.87v] ou en rasure de lard e seit surmise dekes a .xx. jors. Quant le fu est esteint, raét la teste un poy ou ele fu arse deke ele seit percee. Pus metét une ventouse sanz garse e sanz fu, ke la fumosité isse hors, car nus l'avom esprové. E sachét ke en la cure de manie mult vaut d'estre seyné dé veines ke sont souz la lange.

[30] La diete seit freide e moiste sicum letuse, purcelane, char de porc e de aygnel e le patient beive mulsa e non pas vin, car vin enaguse manie. Nestpurquant si la maladie seit lente, donét a boyvre un chaud aromatic.

4.

[31] *Melancolie* est une dé quatre complexions e melancolie est une maladie ke avient de cele complexion quant trop habunde. E ceo conoistrét par ses signes: le patient ad poour sanz acheson e ire e tristesce e parle sanz reson e ayme d'estre soul. E sachét ke de melancolie sont diverses especes, car acuns doutent ke le ciel [f.88r] lor chera sur la teste, acuns ke la terre les transglotera, acuns doutent larons e acuns doutent lous. A acuns est avis ke i[l] sont roys ou diables ou bestes ou ke il seyent sanz testes. E acuns quident aver tresor en la main par ont tenent le poyn clos ke a peine le put hom overir. Propres signes sont ke acuns d'eus rient ke ont proprement la melancolie sanguiniene. Acuns plurent ke ont la pure melancolie. Acuns de eus desirent la mort e acuns la doutent. Signe de melancolie ke proprement est el cervel est superflue pensé e ke le patient ayme d'estre soul ou en desert e regart assiduelement vers la terre. La face est neyre e les chevus de la teste. Signe de melancolie ke regne el cors est ke tut le cors ensecchist e devient neir e l'esplen e l'estomac ne sont pas

---

² MS *oue.*

espurgés de melancolie e les flurs cessent e emorroides. Mes[3] la melan[f.88v]colie ke est de l'esplen est signifié par emflure de les costes.

[32] La cure de melancolie avant ke ele seit confermé el comencement asét est legere, ceo est asaver ke le patient [seit] meiné en lu entempré e ke le ayr seit enmoisté de foylz de vine e de sauz e de rose e de violette.

[33] La diete seit jefnes poucins, perdriz, faisanz, char de cheveril. E avant ke il manjue seit bayné en eawe tedve. E aprés le bain versét sur sa teste l'eawe de la decoction de flurs de nenufar, camomille, roses e violette. E le patient eschue cumpaynie de femme e forte suor e feves e vin gros e novel e checune chose salee e de ague savor e quanke ad savor de vin egre. E li donét a manger ceo ke est gras e douz. E sachét ke dormir fet grant bien a melancoliens. Ausi la teste seit conforté ovekes oyles confortatifs, sicum oyle rosette e violette e de camomille e de meme ceo confortét [f.89r] la foye e l'esplen. Ausi al comencement defiét la materie oveke cest sirup: r[ecevét] les racines de fenoil e de ache ana unciam unam, del jus de borage e del jus de buglosse, del jus de fumeterre ana libram unam, nucis mus[cate], folii, cardamomi, gariofili, xilobalsami, carpobalsami, calami aro[matici] ana dragmam unam, ossis de corde cervi, limature eboris, lapis lazuli, epithimi, sene ana dragmam semis, zucure quartroun semis e fetes sirup. Pus espurgét la materie ové diasené e yeralogodion enagusés oveke lapis lazuli. E il covient ke le patient seit occupé en acune chose e ke il oye chansons e estrumenz sicum harpe e viele.

5.

[34] *Lithargie* est aposteme en la partie de la teste par derere. Lithargie avient de fleume soulement a la foyz e donc le patient dort grefment. A la foyz avient de colre e de fleume medlés ensemble e donc dort grefment e pus esveyle ausi cum frenetic. Ausi sicum il est impossible ke le frenetic seit sanz fievre, ausi est impossible ke litar[f.89v]gie seit sanz fevre.

[35] La cure de lithargie est par la premere reule ke vus ne mettrét nule chose ke seit repercussive. Mes raét la teste e enoynét oveke castoreum destempré oveke jus de ache ou de fenoil. Ausi si le patient seit fort e repleni, fetes le seyner de la veine capitale. Autre reule, me[s] ke le patient ne seit pas fort: fetes le seiner el somet del nes. Autre reule est ke le mire travaylle d'esveiller le patient par ont hom tendra un porc par les pés fortment ke le porc crie. Ausi deit corner corns e ferir tabors e si le deit hom apeler par son propre noun e trere hors lé peils de ses narilz. Autre reule: vus ne devét mie enoyndre les narilz. Ausi nule rien del mond ne eveille plus pussantment litargics ke ne fet la fumé des chevus de hom ars. Ausi autre reule: vus nel ferét mye de forte choses, mes ovekes une festue deus foyz ou treis foiz ou [f.90r] plus.[4] Ausi autre reule [est] ke vus le devét froter entor les mains e les pés oveke sel e vin egre tedve. Autre reule est ke il seit clisterizé al comencement e ke vus li facét checun jor suppositorie mordicatif. Ausi fetes le user sirup acetous ou oximel si il ad crue urine. Ausi raét la teste e enoynét ové jus de rue e oyle laurin. Ausi si il seit costivé, fetes

---

3   MS *Mes de.*   4   MS *ou plus.*

clistere de mauve e de merculial, oyle e nitre. Ausi reule est ke le patient seit en cler lu e ou seit grant lumere.

[36] Sa diete seit potage de ferine de furme[n]t e de bru de geline ke issi est fet: quissét une geline oveke os e chars e pus triblét mult bien e colét parmi un drap. E de cel bru e de ferine de furment fetes gruel. Son beivre seit eawe quite ou oveke mie de payn ou mulsa ke est fet d'eawe e de mel. Memes cele diete vaut en fievre cotidiane continue.

6.

[f.90v][37] *Epilemptie* par un autre noun est apelé goute cheve. A la foiz avient de melancolie naturele ke vus conoistrét par ces signes. Le patient est pourous e nomément en oscur lu. E quant il chet a la terre l'escume ly ist hors par la bouche. E a la foiz desire la mort, a la foiz het sey memes. E sachét ke l'epilemptic e lunatic e demoniac sont ausi cum semblables sicum Constantin dit. E pur esprover queldour celi ke chet a la terre seit lunatic ou epilemptic ou demoniac dites cest noun en sa oraylle: *Res cede demon quia essimoloy precipiunt.* Meintenant si il seit lunatic ou demoniac, chera a la tere sicum mort pres de iloec une houre e quant il levera, demandét ly de quele chose ke vus vodrét e il vus dorra e si il ne chet mie kant il[5] oye le noun, sachét ke il est epilemptic. E sachét ke ces sont les signes ke avienent devant epilemptie: dolor de [f.91r] la teste, vertin, oscurté des oylz, grevance en movement. E sachez ke acune epilemptie est de l'estomac e donc est apelé *analemptie*. Acune est dé dereines[6] partyes e donc est apelé *cathalemptie*. Mes cele ke est del cervel est apelé *epilemptia*. E ceo est la difference entre ces especes, ke en analemptie e cathalemptie sent le patient l'accés avant ke il chece, mes si ne fet pas en verreye epilemptie.

[38] E commune reule est ke checun epilemptic de privé encheson deit estre garri par chaudes choses. Mes cathalemptie ke est de chaud sanc e malicious, sicum Constantin dit, deit estre curé par freide choses. Ausi put le mire saver en quel menbre la materie est par ces signes: si la materie [est] el cervel, donc gette le patient escume parmi sa bouche quant il chet; si el estomac, donc vomit; si en les entrayles, donc ad flux de ventre; si en les veyes de l'urine, donc [f.91v] espant sa urine; si en les coylz, donc espand sa nature.

[39] Ausi solom les diversités de la lune acuns sont turmentés par les quatre divers humors, car celi ke travayle de chaude e moiste materie deit estre turmenté el premere age de la lune e en la dreinere. Ke travaile de colre deit estre travailé en la terce age de la lune.

[40] Ausi acun ad l'accés une foiz el jor, acun en la semayne, acun el moys, acun en l'an, acun en les quatre tens de l'an.

[41] Ausi commune reule est ke cele ke plus tart turmente, plus tart est garie. Ausi a la foiz avient ceste maladie as enfans e donc deit hom mettre tute la cure a la norice e en electuaries e sirups e poudres e masticacions e fumigations. E sachét ke entre tutes les herbes ke sont encuntre epilemptie d'enfanz ne vaut nule [f.92r] plus ke ysope

---

5   MS *ill.*   6   MS *est de reinu p.*

queldour l'enfant receve la fumé de l'herbe ou ke la norisse use l'erbe en sirups e en electuaries e en poudre e en quele manere vus volez. Ausi deit hom overer en le cas e autrement hors le cas.

[42] Pur ceo sachét especiale chose ke quant l'epilemptic chet el comencement, trehét hors sanc de quel menbre vus volez, jammés aprés n'avera la maladie. Ausi quant il chet, soufflét la poudre de rue en ses narils ou le jus de l'herbe. Ausi si epilemptie seit de l'estomac ou de la teste, especiale cure est vomit. Ausi checun epilemptic de privé encheson deit manger checun jor [au] matin, kar nule rien les greve plus ke juner. Mes commune reule est, si ceo seit de l'estomac, de juner, nomément si le cervel [est] fieble. Ausi commune reule est ke epilemptics ne deivent mie regarder verre en nule manere, car mult les greve. Au[f.92v]si checun mal odor les greve hors pris ces quatre: odor de rue, castor, armoniac, opopanac. Nestpurquant si i fussent trop usés, grevereient. Par ont castoreum ne deit pas estre pendu al col ne porté[7] en la main. Ausi en epilemptie de privé encheson apperent desouz la lange deus veines vertes ke aukes sont pales e sont apelés *sargiotides* e les deit hom overir en tel cas, car par lor overture epilemptie enviellie solait estre garrie. Ausi une reule est ke bain e foutre nusent a eus pur ceo ke enfieblissent les nerfs. Ausi autre reule [est] ke a touz epilemptics hors pris cathalemptie vaut tiriake donee de .xv. jors en .xv. une foiz al peis de .v. deners ové vin de la decoction de rue. Ausi fetes fumigation de rue deus foiz en la semaine. Autre[8] reule [est] solonc touz les autors ke le coagle de levre delivre epilemptie.

[43] Ausi veét ci bon oyle e[9] chaud ke desoude humors freis en epilemptie e ke desoude e degaste: pernét de laureole e de lancelé ana libram unam, quassét e quissét en une livre de vin e un autre d'oyle dekes le vin seit degasté e oveke cest oyle enoynét la teste a l'epilemptic e l'estomac de analemptic. E cest vaut en dolor de la teste de freide encheson e en parlesie e en spasme de repletion e en freide ar[f.93r]tetike e en opilation de freis humors. E il covient ke la teste seit froté e piné e eschaufé.

[44] Ausi soufflét cette poudre en ses narilz: r[ecevét] piperis, zinziberis, mirte, euforbii, castorei ana dragmes .ii. Fetes poudre e soufflét en les narilz pur fere l'esternier. Ausi fetes le patient porter tutdis rue oveke ly, ke il eyt l'odor de l'herbe. Ausi porte la racine de peoyné al col e nomément enfanz la portent,[10] kar mult prophite sicum Galien dit. Ausi autre esprove: pernét la secundime, de madle enfant a madle, de femme a femme, e quissét en un pot sanz liqor dekes seit de neire color, issi ke il pusse estre poudre. E donét de cele poudre soulement a la quantité de une fecche, en quel liqor ke vus volez ou en nuyle. Ausi la teste seit fortment lié de une forte bende e pus seit coverte de un gros quir e lessét issi [f.93v] par .xl. jors. Ausi seit changé de freide region en chaude region, car mult prophite sicum Ypocras dit en Amphorimes.

[45] Ausi veét ci verray esperiment esprové ke Constantin met en sa Practike e nous l'avom esprové. Si le patient ad pere e mere, donc seit mené d'eus a muster en un jor de quatre tens, premerement c'est asaver mekerdi e pus vendredi e pus samadi e pus le dimayne aprés suant. E fetes un chapelein ou un homme de religion escrivre l'ewangelie ke est secundum Marcum e finist *Hoc genus demonii in nullo eicitur nisi in oratione et jejunio.* E Constantin met cest esperiment pur ceo ke avient sovent a ceus

---

7 MS *parte*   9 MS *e e.*
8 MS *Ausi.*   10 MS *parter.*

ke fure[n]t nes en maveise esposayles. E sachét, tut seit il demoniac ou lunatic ou epilemptic, il serra delivres. E bien vaut as enfans ke ne poent prendre purgation.

[46] E le patient se garde de granz sons sicum de grant cloches e de noyse de gent e [f.94r] de tabours e de veiler e de ire e de poor e de grant freid e de forte chalor. E use viandes ke legerement defient e ne use mie trop de vin e eschue grosses chars e touz pessons e douces choses e grasses choses e chous e ache e gros fruts hors pris stiptics e tutes choses ke sont pleines de vapor sicum mustarde. E se garde de yveresce e d'enflure de vens e de dormir aprés manger. E sa teste ne seit pas lavee d'eawe chaude ou freide. Ausi se garde des oyseus ke vivent en riveres e de char de boef e de vache e de chevre e de levre e de let e de furmage e de tutes choses ke engendrent gros humors. E ne manjue nuls pessons hors pris petit ke sont en eawe curante sicum perches, lus, darz. Mes sachét ke tutes les testes de pessons plus grevent a epilemptics e plus nusent [f.94v] ke les testes d'autres bestes.

[47] Si epilemptie aviegne de l'estomac, defiét la materie oveke oximel squillitic. La materie defié seit purgé oveke ces piles: r[ecevét] yerapigre, yeralogodion ana unce une et demie, pulpe colloquintide scrupulum unum, succi abscin[thii] unciam semis. Fetes piles de ceo e donét sovent en l'an. Nestpurquant si le patient seit fort [. . .]. E pus il covient aprés ke l'estomac est mundifié ke il use assiduelement choses confortatives sicum diagalanga medlé oveke pliris. E il covient ke l'estomac seit void lung tens e ke il use ceste poudre el comencement al manger oveke bru: r[ecevét] anisi, maratri ana unce une, zinziberis, galange, macis, nucis muscate, cinamomi, xilobalsami, carpobalsami, calami aromatici, cassieligne ana unciam semis, gariofili, cubebe ana dragmes .iii., granorum peonie dragme un, panis, zucare unce une,[f.95r] e fetes poudre. E quant l'accés avient, le patient sent la fumé de l'estomac monter, donc seit fortment enbracé de un fort humme. Si il seit enfant, pernét coral e la racine de morele e liét en un drap e li pendét al col en la lune decressante. Ausi enoynét l'estomac checun jor oveke oyle de mastic ou oyle nardin.

[48] Ausi esperiment sicum Alisandre dit de un vilein en Tuscane ke aveit triblé rue savage el champ. E avint ke son servant cheÿ devant ly e il plein de tristor prist aventurousement la rue e la mist en ses narilz e l'autre tut sein leva sus.

[49] Ausi en cathalemptie ke avient de fumosité de acun menbre, sicum dit Haly, seit la materie defié oveke le digestif avantdit. E pus seit espurgé ové la medicine avantdite. E si l'accés avient, seit defendu en ceste manere. Pernét bendes de fort linge drap e me[f.95v]tét en rouge cyre liquifié e pressét aukes hors e liét le menbre fortment. E avant l'accés fetes ruptorie sur le menbre dont vient la fumosité. Pernét cantarides e triblét e poudrét e medlét oveke su de moton e un poy de vin egre e metét sur le menbre e lessét estre par une pose deke le venim isse. Tels manjuent nomément poucins, pertriz, faisans, char de jeune porc non pas gras, char de aignel de un an, oefs humables e les coilz de sengler e de moton.

7.

[50] *Emflure de cervel*[11] put hum conoistre par ceo ke la face est emflee e les temples plus hauz ke ne solayent e les veines sont hautes e les oylz e la face est rouge. Ceste passion a la foiz avient oveke fievre, a la foiz sanz fevre. Ausi a la foiz avient de sanc, a la foiz des autres humors. Si ceo seit de sanc e la passion seit novele, fetes le seiner de la capitale de la contrere partye. Si la passion seit vele, seinét le de meme la partye e de la veine ke est desouz la lange e de la veyne ke est pres del pouz del pé. Si autre humor seit en encheson, fetes cest emplastre: [f.96r] pernét la mie de payn e semence de lin e ferine d'orge e oyle e quissét en eawe e metét sur le lu dolent.

8.

[51] *Scotomie e vertin* en signes se acordent solonc ceo ke Avicenne dit: oscurté des oylz, grevance e soun des orayles. Propre signe de scotomie est quant hom est sicum maniac e touz ses menbres sont fiebles e les nerfs sont mols. Propre signe de vertin est quant al pacient est al vis ke tutes choses ke il veit movent e nomément roundes choses. E sachét ke l'une e l'autre passion a la foyz est del cervel, a la foiz de l'estomac: si del cervel, le[s] signes sont continues, si de l'estomac, ne sont pas continues.

[52] A ces passions fetes cest remedie. Pernét de ladano dragme un, de musc scrupulum unum e medlét oveke jus de sambuc. E fetes de ceo ausi cum une poume. E le patient odoure sovent e mette a ses narilz. Ausi si ceo seit del cervel, fetes le user cest electuarie checun jor: r[ecevét] diagalange vel diasené, pliris cum musco ana libram semis medlét ensemble. Ausi si ceo seit de l'estomac e de freis humors, use cest electuarie [f.96v] checun jor matin e seir: r[ecevét] diacitoniton sanz peyvre, dia-galanga ana libram semis medlét ensemble. Ausi si ceo seit de chaus humors de l'estomac, fetes le user rosate novelle e diacitoniton ana libram semis medlét ensemble. Ausi si la maladie seit de cop ou de cas, raét premerement la teste e fetes le seiner de la veine capitale e le ters jor de la veine ke est derere l'orayle. E pus pernét cyre blanche e malaschét oveke oyle de camomille e metét sur la teste ausi cum un chapel. E cest esperiment est esprové. Autre pernét curte leyne .i. *flocken* e broyllét en oyle roset e bien chaud metét sur la teste. Mes ceo fetes al comencement e pus ceo ke nus avom dit de la cyre e pus fetes ceo ke est esprové. Escorchét un jeune moton e la chaude pel metét sur la teste. Ausi en scotomie e en vertin raét la teste e lavét oveke le [f.97r] eawe de ces herbes: r[ecevét] foliorum lauri, betonice, valeriane, rute recentis ana manipulos .ii. Boyllét les en eawe.

[53] Ausi il covient ke le patient ne rewarde mie parfund fosses ne hautes muntaines ne hautes overaynes sicum clochers. E ke il se garde de superflue manger e boyvre. E eschue yveresce e als e porets e oynons. E beive vin aromatic e entempré. E se gard[e] de chous e de letuses e de choses ke ne defient mie legerement e ke engendrent

---

[11] Cf. 'inflatio cerebri' in *Coll. Sal.* 2, p.142.

ventosité. E se garde d'oysels de rivere e de vin e de tart super e de chalor e de freidure
e de travail. E use pessons de fluvie e perdriz e faisans e poucins de geline e char de
moton e de porc. Sur tute rien se garde de cumpaynye de femme.

9.

[54] *Yveresce* sicum Ysaac dit esteint la force de l'alme resonable e fet hom aver la
manere de beste. E sachét ke acune yveresce est bone e acune est male solonc acuns.
Male yveresce est sicum Avicenne dit ke avient sovent e ke corrumpe la complexion
[f.97v] de la foye e del cervel e amene[12] parlesie e apoplexie ou sodeine mort. Bone
yveresce est solonc acuns ke assuage les vertuz en quiete e fet reposer e ke fet bien
uriner e suer. Por ceo dit Avicenne ke a acuns est avis ke il prophite d'estre yvre deus
foiz el mois. E sachét ke acuns sont tost yvres e ceo est pur fort vin ou pur ceo ke poy
manjuent ou pur ceo ke se governent malement ou pur ceo ke sont plein des humors.
Mes acuns sont tart yvres pur le contrere.

[55] E sachét ke les signes de yveresce sont divers solonc la diversité de[s] quatre
complexions. Car acuns se coroucent e veilent e tensent sicum colerics quant sont
yveres. Acuns rient e chantent sicum les sanguiniens. Acuns suent et tremblent e
dorment sicum fleumatics. Acuns sont tristes e pourus e desirent religion sicum
melancoliens.

[56] La cure de yveresce est ceste. Les coilz seyent lavés de fort vin egre e seyent
frotés fortment. E donét poumes crues ou peyres a manger. E si yveresce dure, donét
[f.98r] cest sirup a beyvre: r[ecevét] succi alborum caulium libram unam, succi
granatorum acetosorum libram semis, aceti albi quartroun un. Boylét aukes e ajostét
de zucre libram unam. E fetes sirup e donét avant ke hom beive vin, car il tarde
yveresce. Sicum Avicenne dit, mult prophite. Ausi fetes le odorer camphre e sandles
e metét sur la teste freide choses repercussives sicum oyle roset medlé oveke vin egre
de vin. E pur remuer yveresce vaut mult ke vin egre seit doné medlé ovekes eawe. Si
le yveroyne seit de chaude nature, raét la teste e surmetét linge dras moillez en oyle
roset e violet ové jus de jubarbe e de morele medlees ensemble. Aprés dormir fetes le
entrer en un bain d'eawe douce e les pés seyent frotés en eawe chaude oveke sel e oyle
violette e vin egre. Ausi fetes le vomir oveke eawe chaude ou en autre manere. Pus
pernét minte e triblét aukes e medlét ovekes eawe rose. Pus colét e donét a boyvre.

[57] E sa diete seit perdriz, poucins, purcelane [f.98v] oveke vin egre ou jus de poume
grenette. Ausi use poumes grenettes, peyres e medles e poumes e coynz. Si le yveroyne
seit de freide nature, donét ly oximel a boyvre devant le bain. Aprés le bain auge
dormir. E pus frotét ses pés oveke eawe chaude e sel e pus donét ly a beyvre vin medlé
oveke alosne e donét ly a manger chous quiz oveke grasse char de porc, car il desoudent
yveresce e defendent les freis humors munter. E si seit nurri oveke fritures e rost e
grasse viandes e ke legerement defient. E sachét ke a ceus ke avient dolor de la teste
aprés ceo ke ont bu vin mult prophite ke il manjuent coynz ou peires ke pussent
cumbatre encun[tre] la fumé del vin. E sachét ke il covient ke ceus ke sont apelé
ptisik[13] ke il se gardent de yveresce sicum dit Constantin.

---

12 MS *a. a p.*   13 MS *aptisik.*

10.

[58] *Apoplexie* est quant les quatre humors habundent trop el cervel. De apoplexie [f.99r] sont treis especes. La grenure e la mene e la menure.

[59] La grenure apoplexie est ke tout le sen de tut e movement oveke grant destourbance de spirituale vertu e oveke grevance de alener. Ceus ke ont ceste maladie dorment grevement e l'escume ist hors par la bouche. Signes de ceste espece sont perte dé .v. sens e le pacient gist ausi cum mort. Ceste espece est incurable, car meintenant ou en meme l'oure occist.

[60] La menore apoplexie est ke ne tout mye tut le sens, mes enfieblist les vertuz d'esperiz, mes le patient put oyr e ver, mes nient parfitement, e si font signe dé mains ou des autre menbres quant ne poent nient parler, mes bien trehent lor aleine. Acuns travaille par .vii. jors, acuns par .viii. jors, acuns par .xiiii. jors, acuns par treis semaynes, acuns par un moys. E ceste espece change sovent en parlesie.

[61] La mene apoplexie est ke ne [f.99v] tout mie le sen ne movement de tut, mes nomément en partye e greve plus ke la menore e meins ke la grenur les spiritualtés.

[62] La cure est de l'une e l'autre si ele seit curable: si ceo seit de sanc, ke vus conoistrét par roujor de la face e par la complexion, par seigner le garrez. Si de sausefleume ou pure fleume e de autres humors, premerement donét oximel pur defier la materie, pus l'espurgét oveke yeralogodion ou theodoricon euperiston ou benedicta ou yera fortis ou piles de euforbe ou pillulis fetidis ke proprement apertiene[n]t a ceste maladie sicum est escrit en *Viatikes* el chapitre de apoplexie. Ausi donét checune nuyt opopiram ou esdram ou aueam alexandrinam ou tiriake ou mitridatum, mes seit destempré ovekes eawe de la decoction de sauge e castoreum. Ausi fetes le esternier ové la poudre de euforbe e de castor e ellebre. Ausi metét les piles diacastorum en ses narilz destemprés en eawe [f.100r] chaude. Ausi fetes emplastre de castor, euforbe, pelestre, mustarde e raét la teste e surmetét. E si fevre surviegne, seit tenue pur haute medicine. E sachét ke el comencement devét fere leger remedies sicum oximel e les opiates avantdites. E pus quant le patient est plus fort, donét plus fortes choses ke espurgent la materie e degastent sicum beverages e les piles avantdites. Nestpurquant se gardent de vin e beivent eawe quite ou mulsam. Ausi une reule est ke en checune apoplexie seit fet clistere mordicatif e laxatif. Ou destemprét sel oveke fel de tor e moillét leinz un suppositorie de gros savoun e dur. Ausi commune reule est solonc touz les autors ke al comencement seit tiriake doné al peys de .v. deners. Ausi autre reule est ke al comencement le ferés vus esternier oveke sueves choses. Ausi en checune encheson fetes suppositorie, clistere, gargarime.

[BOOK II: THE EYES]

1.

[100v][63] *Obtalmia* est aposteme en l'oyl. A la foiz avient de chaude encheson, a la foiz de freide. Mes commune reule est ke vus ni mettrét riens as oylz devant le quart jor. Ausi autre reule est ke il seit seiné de la veine capitale. Autre reule: metét une ventouse e[n] la funtaynele del col. Autre reule: si ceo seit de chaud encheson, seit la diete sicum en fevre continue. Autre reule: ke hom deit user repercussifs mes noun pas violenz. Pur ceo pernét le jus de violette e confisét oveke blanc de l'oef e eawe rose e ferine d'orge e fetes emplastre sur les oylz. Ausi poet [hom] fere del jus de morele ou de jubarbe. Ausi mon conseil, ke vus metét tutdiz un drap ou cotoun entre les oylz e l'emplastre pur la tendresce des oylz. Autre reule est ke vus devét sovent renoveler l'emplastre [. . .] encheson e si grant dolor seit, metés choses ke assuagent dolor sicum mie de pain de furment ové let de femme e eawe rose. E pus usera choses ke desoudent, ceo est asaver de jus de [f.101r] fenoil e de minte.

2.

[64] Si *sanc* habunde en l'oyl, la reule est ke le patient seit seyné de la veine capitale. Ausi veét ci esperiment ke touz les autors acordent: poudrét comin e malaschét al fu oveke cyre e fetes petiz emplastres e les eschaufét e surmetét as oylz. Ausi quissét comin en vin blanc e versét leynz le jus de rue e metét en les oylz. A meme ceo ardét la cruste de payn, e de la poudre de ly e de jus de rue e le vin avantdit fetes emplastre, e metét desur les oylz. Mes sachét ke cest emplastre ne vaut mie al comencement, mes premerement metét en l'oyl le jus de paritarie oveke eawe rose e moyllét leinz un coton e surmetét.

3.

[65] Si les oylz suffrent de *fleume ou de melancolie*, ke vus conoistrét par pallor de la face e emflure, pernét vin egre chaud e metét en un vessel de arem e mirabolans e lessét refreider. [f.101v] E pus pernét cel vert ke aert a cel vessel e metét en l'oyl.

4.

[66] A la foyz avient *grant ardor as oylz* e donc pernét psillium e metét en eawe e quant cel eawe est engelee moillét leinz estoupe e surmetét as oylz, e vaudra. Autre commun encuntre arsure e pointure e roujor e encuntre ceo ke les oylz sont en anguisse par inversion dé palpebres: r[ecevét] thuris, masticis, dragagant, aloes, gumi arabici, tutie, rose ana [. . .] [e] sotilement poudrét e destemprét ovekes eawe rose e let de femme e jus de letuse. E quant il va dormir metés deus goutes en les angles des oylz.

5.

[67] Pur oster *la mayle des oylz*: frotét gingivre sur un keus e ovekes oyle metét en les oylz. Ou quissét la poudre de gingivre en vin e gardét en un vessel de arem e metét en les oylz. Ou poudrét antimonii e ajostét un poy [f.102r] de musc e cele poudre esparpilét sur la mayle. Celes choses font la mayle tenve. Pus pernét .xl. greins de centrum galli e metét en l'oyl pur trere hors la mayle. Ausi pernét un rouge limasoun oveke sa escale e ardét a poudre en treis jors, ostera la mayle. A meme ceo le sanc de pijons de columb plus vaut. A meme ceo pernét greins de furment e metét sur une plate de fer chaud e cel jus ke curra metét en l'oil. Kiran dit ke le let de une jumente mis en l'oyl de homme ke ad la mayle si le garist e oste la mayle nettement. Autre pur clarifier la veue en checune encheson d'opilation de la veue ou de coverture de la purnele fetes cest collirie: r[ecevét] mirre, aloes, olibani, masticis, sarcocolle, castorei, croci, yreos ana [. . .], fetes poudre e destemprét oveke vin blanc e degoutét en les angles des oylz.

6.

[f.102v][68] A *flux de lermes* de veynes par dehors, ke vus conoistrét par dolor entor le front e par prurit .i. *yecche*, fetes emplastre d'encens e ferine d'orge e del jus de rapistre e de nitre fortment triblee e de blanc de l'oef. Si ceo seit de veines dedens, donét al seir diaolibanum. Ou pernét la poudre d'encens e broyllét sur une tiwele en un vessel d'arem issi ke la fumé ne pusse mie issir. E la poudre ke vus troverét par desus el fount del vessel metét en les oylz. Meme la poudre vaut a *chacie des oylz*.

7.

[69] A *la mayle e a la teye e a l'ungle* fetes poudre de asa, amoniac, castoreum, salgemme, lithargire, mes de li seit meins ke d'autres, e metét en l'oyl. Salgemme par sey asét vaut. Ungle est vielle mayle.

8.

[70] Veét ci bon collirie encontre *roujor des oylz*. Quissét poume grenette souz les cendres e quant ele est quite pressét hors le jus e medlét a ceo [f.103r] la terce partie d'eawe rose e un poy de gumme arabic. E gardét en un vessel de verre. Autre pur roujor ke lunges ad duré: vaut aloen cicotrin medlé oveke vin blanc ou vin de poume gernette.

9.

[71] *Nectilopa*[14] est quant la veue est troublé de none e[15] en avant. Cest passion avient de melancolie. Pur ceo est commune reule ke il seit espurgé oveke medicine ke espurge melancolie sicum yeralogodion e autres tels. Ausi seit seiné de la veine capitale ou de la veine ke est a la racine del pouz e del dey pres de ly. Ausi sachét ke pica, ceo est a dire *hnotehech*, arse en un pot e poudree vaut en manger ou en boyvre encontre nectilopam e cardiake de freid encheson.[16] Ausi sicum Constantin dit, metét peyvre lung en la foye de chevre e rostét e ceo ke court hors cuyllét e metét une goute ou deus en les oylz.

10.

[72] A *defaute de veue* de chaud humor ou freid le patient seit seiné de la veine ke est en l'angle de l'oil pres del nes ou metet ilokes une sancsue. Esperiment commun encontre defaute de veue de freid encheson e encontre lermes: pernét les fels de treis oysels ke vivent de ravine e trehét hors le jus de fenoil e de rue e de frasere e oveke ces .vi. liqors destemprét owele medlee de mirre e de aloes e tutie e sarcocolle e colét parmy un drap. E de ceo metét une goute ou deus en les oylz. Encuntre defaute [f.104r] de veue de chaud encheson e encontre flux de lermes e encontre arsure e roujor des oylz fetes collirie en ceste manere: pernét foilz d'egremoyne e de verveine e de fenoyl e de foilz de roses a la quantité des autres e trehét eawe en la manere de eawe rose e de cele eawe metét une goute ou deus en les oyl[z]. Si vus ajostez sarcocole oveke l'eawe, plus vaudra. Ou si vus ajostét oveke l'eawe la poudre de tutie, plus vaudra encuntre flux de lermes. Ausi autre collirie a l'un e l'autre encheson: pernét jus de fenoyl e jus de rue e de poume gernette e ajostét mel e quissét dekes seit espés. E plus vaudra si vus ajostez de fel d'oysels ke vivent de ravine ou de pessons ke vivent de ravine. A meme vaut le fel de levre e le fel d'angule. A meme ceo trehét hors eawe, en la manere d'eawe rose, de la drasche de vin e metet en les oylz.

[73] A ceus ke ont bels oylz e rien ne [f.104v] veyent quissét tormentille en vin blanc dekes a la moyté e donét a eus a boyvre tant soulement e emplastrét l'erbe quite desur les oylz e fetes issi par .v. moys ou .vii. dekes aytant ke il veyent. A meme ceo triblét bien la semence de lin e surmetét as oylz.

> Camphora, sarcocola, licium, celidonia, ruta,
> Mel, aloe, maratrum, tiria, mirra, merum,
> Lac muliebre, liquor roseus, sanguisque columbe

---

14 See *Practica Petrocelli* c.21 in *Coll. Sal.* 4, p.203 'noctilopos, id est qui post solis ortum usque ad occasum videre non possunt'.

15 A superscript insertion after *none*.

16 There follows a set of instructions which are clearly insititious and hint at the way in which the work was compiled: Si cancre [f.103v] seit en la verge de homme, levét la oveke l'urine al patient e quant le lu est ensecchi esparpilét la poudre desure. Encontre cancre de levres ou de autre lu. Lavét le de vin egre e quant le lu est ensecchi esparpilét la poudre desure.

Obscuros oculos extenebrare solent.
Feniculus, vervena, rose, celidonia, ruta,
Ex istis fit aqua que lumina reddit acuta.
Allia, vina, venus, ventus, faba, fumus vel ignis,
Ista nocent oculis set vigilare magis.[17]

11.

[74] Pur *teye des oylz e prurit*, ceo est a dire *yecche*: le jus de la racine de fenoil seit mis en un vessel de arem al solayl par .xxx. jors e en manere de collirie metét en les oylz. Encuntre prurit de l'oyl certain esperiment: medlét trop bon aloen ové jus de fenoil e metét en un vessel d'arem al solail par .xv. jors e pus me[f.105r]tét en l'oyl sicum collirie.

12.

[75] Encuntre dolor des oylz ke avient sovent ové grant ebullissement e grant emflure e sanz emflure, ové sanc e par lermes, e a la foyz par chaud, a touz mals des oylz: quissét mult bien le rouge limason en eawe, si cuyllét la gresse, si oynét les oylz quant vus irrét dormir. E si metét sur les oylz e si il seit de mauveis sanc ou de quiture, tut istera hors.

13.

[76] Sachét ke la fumigation de vin egre soulement estanche *flux de reume* as oylz.

14.

[77] Pur *destreindre lermes des oylz*: r[ecevét] salisgemme dragme un, mente, cuscute ana dragme semis, destemprét en sotil vin blanc e degotét une goute en l'oyl. Ou ardét vertes grapes e egres en un pot de terre e sarcét la poudre parmi un sotil drap. Cette poudre mise en l'oyl destreint lerme e tout roujor. Ou fetes un oynement pur destreindre lermes del jus de mellilote, fenoil, rue e vin e urine d'enfant ovek un poy de aloe. Ceste decoction mult vaut as oylz. Ausi fetes collirie de peivre lung, zucre e spica nardi.

---

[17] These verses are drawn from the Salernitan *Regimen Sanitatis*.In the text and translation published by P.W. Cummins, "A Salernitan Regimen of Health", *Allegorica* 1 (1976), 78–101 lines 5–6 correspond to lines 239–40 and lines 7–8 to lines 235/38.

[BOOK III: THE EARS]

1.

[f.105v][78] Aprés les passions des oylz dirrum de[s] passions d'oraylles. Pur ceo est la premere reule ke en les passions des oraylles n'i metrét freide chose mes tedve. La secunde reule est ke vus ne mettrét nule grosse chose en poudre ne en collirie. La terce reule est ke fort collirie ne demorra mie trop lungement en les orayles.

2.

[79] *Dolor des orayles* a la foyz est de chaud humor, a la foiz de freid. Si de chaud humor, defiét la materie oveke fumigation de l'eawe de la decoction de mauve e de violette e payle d'orge e de aveyne. E donc metét enz une goute ou deus de jus de letuse ou de vin de poume gernette e donc estopét l'oraylle ovekes un coton. Si la dolor seit de freid encheson, fetes fumigation ové l'eawe de la decoction de fenoil, de persil e de aloyne e de anis. Pus metét enz une goute ou deus de jus d'oynuns tedve ou d'oyle de alemandes ameres. Mester Bertelmeu dit de dolor des orayles, si [f.106r] la dolor seit de freid encheson, de glumous humors, de ventosité ou d'emflure dedenz ou dehors [. . .] Si la dolor seit de grans humors e de ventosité, le patient sent grant grevance en la teste. Si la dolor seit de chaud encheson, donét letuses, cicoree e pessons ke ont grosse char, car bien assuagent dolor. Si la dolor seit entour l'oraylle, le jus de poret chaud par sey ou oveke mel degouté leins mult vaut. A meme ceo triblét origanum oveke let de femme e un poy de mel e mult vaudra. A ceus ke ont dolor des orayles e grevement oyent: degotét enz sovent urine de chevre. Ausi triblét la racine de verveine oveke vin egre e usét. A ceus ke grevement oyent e n'ont pas dolor: le jus de blete oveke fel de tor mult vaut. A dolor de cop: moyllét leine en oyle roset tedve ou fresche bure tedve ou gresse de geline liquifié e metét enz.

3.

[f.106v][80] Aprés dolor des oraylles dirrum de *aposteme des orayles.* Pur ceo est la premere reule ke vus n'i mettrét nule chose repercussive. A apostemes en l'un e l'autre encheson metét enz let de femme. Mes en chaude encheson mielz vaut ke vus ajostét un poy d'oyle violette. Emplastre maturatif e mitigatif issi est fet pur freid aposteme: quissét ferine de furment en oyle e mel e vin e metét en les orayles. Si l'aposteme seit mult freid, quissét en jus d'oynun e souz metét. Encuntre chaud aposteme fetes cest emplastre: pernét les [f.107r] summés de jusquiame e un poy de la racine de parele e envolupét en estoupes moyllés en eawe. E quissét desouz les cendres e pus triblét oveke gresse de geline ou d'owe e fetes un oynement de bure e d'oyle e enoynét les oreyles e surmetét l'emplastre. Cest emplastre sur tous emplastres assuage dolor e esteint chalor e fet venir quiture.

4.

[81] *Soniz des orayiles* a la foyz est de chaud encheson, a la foyz de freid encheson. Si de chaud encheson, donc le put hom conoistre par pointure e morsure e arsure des orayles. Pur ceo pernét anis, quassét e quissét en vin de poume gernette e deus goutes tedves me[f.107v]tét en les orayles. E pus estopét les oveke coton. E sachét ke en lu de poume gernette poet [hom] mettre le jus de poumes savages, ceo est a dire *wodecrabben*, e en lu de anis anet. Si ceo seit de freid encheson, ke hom put conoistre par freidure des orayiles, fetes collirie solonc les autors d'oyle de alemandes el quel seit anis quit. E metez deus goutes tedves en l'orayile. E jeo di ke en lu d'oyle de alemandes ameres put hom mettre le jus d'oynon ou de poret e pur anis comin. Macre dit ke aloyne oveke fel de boef assuage soniz des orayles.

5.

[f.108r][82] Encuntre *quiture des orayiles* dient les autors ke i[l] covient ke le patient seit espurgé ovekes oximelle juliani. E pus moyllét une tente de cotoun ou de carpie en terebentine ou en mel e metét en l'orayle. Trop bien vaut.

[83] Veét ci bon esperiment a meme ceo e a sourdesce de checune encheson e pur trere hors pere ou grein ou payle des orayiles: fetes acun vil ou povre mettre sa bouche a l'orayile issi ke sa aleyne entre [f.108v] en l'orayile. Ceste aleyne lasche les yssues e defie la materie e fet tenve la quiture e pus sucche fortment e issi isterad la materie hors. Ausi mult vaut de fere le esternier. Si oreylin est entré en l'orayle, donc comandent les autors mettre enz ameres choses pur tuer le verm. Mes mielz vaut de mettre une poume aromatike bien eschaufé al fu a l'orifice de l'orayile par une nuyt issi ke le tenon de la poume seit osté. Al matin [. . .] trover et le verm en la poume pur l'odor de ly. [f.109r] Autre: pernét pain de siegle tut chaud e metét desouz l'orayle e ceo est esprové. Autre esprové: pernét les tendrons de canve e metét desouz l'orayle. A la foiz court sanc hors des orayles e donc cumandent les autors ke le patient seit seiné.

6.

[84] Encuntre *sourdesce*: dient les autors ke le jus de jubarbe vaut issi ke une goute ou deus seyent mises en l'orayle ovekes owele medlee de gresse de geline rostie al fu. Ausi le jus de camomille tedve medlé vaut a meme ceo en l'un e l'autre encheson. Ausi anciene sourdesce de checune encheson issi est garrie: pernét jus de jubarbe e emplét de ceo un pot e metét desouz la tere par un an. Pus trehét le pot de la terre e donc ceo ke vus troverét ausi cum gresse fetes [f.109v] tedve e metét sovent en les orayles. Meme ceo di jeo de baume. A meme ceo de freid encheson pernét la gresse de heyron e d'angille e sanc d'angille e sanc de bouc e metét en un oynon concavé e metét el fu deke l'oynon seit mol. E pus pressét hors del jus e deus goutes tedves metés en les orayles. Nestpurquant si mester seit, fetes purgation devant. Ausi en la s[e]cunde age de la lune ou la terce metét sancsues a la racine de l'orayile.

[BOOK IV: THE NOSE]

1.

[f.110r][85] *Flux de sanc dé narilz* a la foiz avient a seins, a la foiz a fevros. A la foiz avient de la teste, ke vus conoistrét par dolor de front e des oylz e dé temples. Ausi si il court del destre naril, donc dit hom ke il avient de la foye e donc est grevance el destre flanc. Si il court del senestre, donc court de l'esplen e donc est grevance en le senestre flanc. Si de l'un e l'autre naril, donc vient de l'un e l'autre menbre. Mes si il avient del mariz, put hom saver par la femme si ele est defaute de ses flurs. Pur ceo dit Ypocras en *Amforimes* 'Si femme ad defaute de ses flurs e flux de sanc dé narilz avient, bon est'. Ausi a la foyz court en degoutant, a la foiz par cours e hastivement, e a la foiz court pur brusure dé veines del cervel e des arteries. E tel flux occist sovent. E avient sovent pur dolor de la teste. A la foiz avient pur cas ou pur cop. E flux de sanc des arteries est [f.110v] mult chaud e mult violent, si est conu del flux ke vient dé veines pur ceo ke il est sotil e rouje e chaud. E sachét ke flux de sanc dé narilz a la foiz prophite, a la foiz noun. Il prophite quant il avient a cely ke est mult repleni e [a] roujor e aprés agues maladies e departyes de denz, sanguiniens e colerics en le cervel e la foye e le pomon. Cel flux nust communement quant il y a doute de fieblesce de la foye e de ydropisie.

[86] E sachét ke vus devét estancher checun flux de sanc si tost ke le patient devient fieble. Si le sanc court del destre naril, overét donc la veine ke est apelé basilica del destre bras. Si del senestre, donc overét la salvatelle de la senestre mayn. Si le patient est fevrous, donc ne l'estanchét mye trop hastivement, mes poy e poy en ceste manere: fetes vin egre tedve e lavét le vit e les coylz [f.111r] a l'homme e les mameles a femme e liét les extremités, c'est asaver les jambes e les bras. Ou poudrét roses e medlét oveke ferine d'orge e destemprét oveke jus de plantayne e fetes emplastre sur les temples e le front si il court de la teste, si de la foye, sur la foye, si de l'esplen, sur l'esplen, si del mariz, sur le mariz. Nestpurquant si ceo seit del mariz, mielz vaut ke vus overét la veine desouz la keville del pé e embruét les pés ovekes eawe freide e les jambes dekes a genoilz. Ausi suffumét les narilz. Pernét l'escorce de un oef e ardét ovekes une chandele desouz les narilz. A meme ce vaut la fumee de vin egre e ceo est esprové. Ausi le patient odoure l'estront de asne chaud. A meme ceo pernét le sanc al patient e rostét sur une tiwele e fetes poudre e sufflét cele poudre en les narilz. A meme ceo vaut la poudre d'estront de l'[f.111v]asne en meme la manere. A meme ceo fetes une tente de sotil linge drap e moyllét en enke e pus jetét desur cele tente la poudre de vitreole e d'arnement e metét el nes e ceo est esprové de nus sovent. Autre bien esprové pur estancher sanc hastivement: pernét blanc cauz e leger e sufflét sovent en les narilz. Ausi pernét une mecche e moillét en blanc de l'oef e metét enz. Autre bien esprové: fetes une tente de une esponge e piz liquifié e plungét en vin egre e metét el nes. A meme ceo pernét les peils de levre e blanc de l'oef e la poudre d'encens e medlét e surmetét. E Avicenne dit ke si le patient tiegne eawe freide gelee en sa bouche, estanchera flux de sanc de[s] narilz. E sachét ke hom put vivre a la foiz en flux de sanc dé narilz dekes il eyt seiné a la montance de .xx. livres ou .xxv. e pus moert.

[87] Si flux de sanc seit de playe trenché, pernét lumbriz de terre, ceo est a dire *maddockes*, e ardét sur une chaude tuylle e fetes poudre e esparpilét en la playe. E pus liét la playe [f.112r] fortment ovekes un linge drap, meintenant l'estanchera. Si ceo seit de legere trenché, pernét de sanc dragon dragmes .ii. e fetes poudre e metét en la playe, meintenant estanche le sanc e soude la playe, e ceo vaut a playes d'espeye e autretels e en flux de sanc dé narilz, car il estanche le sanc. Autre sovent esprové: si vostre dey seit trenché d'un cutel, pernét teyle de yreine e surmetét e pus liét ovekes une cince, meintenant estanche le sanc. Le patient manjue viandes ke legerement defient e se gard[e] del contrere e de cri e de freid e de foutre e de travail.

2.

[f.112v][88] *Polipus* est une passion ke avient de reume. A la foiz les humors corunt de la mene partye de la teste e descendent de la teste en les narilz. E a la foiz en les narilz crest une sustance de char sicum une verrue. La cure de cest polipus seit deguerpi a cyrurgiens. Nestpurquant la teste seit premerement mundifié e pus le deit hom trencher e arder. Ausi a la foiz estapit la reume en les pors dé narilz sicum eawe en les pors de un drap. Donc est la reule ke la teste seit premerement mundifié e pus sufflét enz ceste poudre: pelestre, castoreum e mustarde e canele. Ausi vaut une ventouse en la funtaynele del col.

3.

[f.113r][89] *Coriza*[18] est flux des humors a[s] narilz, a la foiz dé chauz, a la foiz dé freis. Si dé chauz, donc sent le patient ausi cum arsures e chaude fumé ke broylle les narilz. Si ceo seit dé freis humors, donc sent ausi cum glace en ses narilz. En chaud encheson est commune reule d'estre seyné. Autre reule est en l'un e l'autre encheson ke le front ne les temples ne pés ne main deivent estre lavés e nel[19] fetes esternier. E le gardét dé choses ke plus desoudent ke degastent. Al comencement del reume fetes fumigation ke vaut en l'un e l'autre encheson ové l'eawe de la decoction de roses e de ladanum. Ausi en chaud encheson enoynét le entor le front e les temples ovekes oyle violette, en freid encheson oveke bure. Ausi a corize de chaud encheson lavét la teste sovent ové l'eawe de la decoction de roses e de morele e autres freides herbes. Si ceo seit de freid humor, lavét la teste oveke l'eawe de la decoction de pulleole, rue, aloyne,

---

18 Cf. *Practica Cophonis* in *Coll. Sal.* 4, p.476 'Decurrit humor flegmaticus ad nares et facit corizam' and *De egritudinum curatione, Coll. Sal.* 2, p.109 'Coriza est strictura narium ex fluxu humorum ad nares, frequenter frigidorum, aliquando calidorum'. In G. Lafeuille (ed.), *Les Amphorismes Ypocras de Martin de Saint-Gille 1362–65* (Genève, 1954), p.63 no.40 the editor cites a note 'Le reume est dit catarrus quant il descent a la poitrine, et il est coriza quant il descent aux narines, et il est dit brauchus quant il descent aux joes'. Cf. though p.68 no.20 and note 'corize est reusme descendant aux yeux'; p.67 no.13 note 'les reumes qui descendent au nez que l'en apelle corise'; p.69 no.23 note 'c'est flux ou decours d'umeurs au nez'.

19 MS *ne nel*.

averoyne. Mes si fevre avient de corize, [f.113v] sicum sovent fet, fetes meme la cure a corize ke vus fetes a la fevre. Le patient se garde de repletion de mangers e de boyvres e de tard soper e de trop dormir.

[BOOK V: FACIAL BLEMISHES]

[90] *Lentilles* e autres tecches en la face a la foyz sont natureles, a la foyz avient aventurousement. Si eles seyent natureles, jammés ne purront estre garries, mes covertes. Ausi les tecches a la foiz avient de chalor del solail, a la foyz de par force de nature ke les deboute hors, a la foiz de retention dé flurs. Si eles seyent par force de nature, donc est commune reule ke vus ne mettrét nule rien dehors avant ke le [f.114r] cors seit espurgé. Si de retencion dé flurs, donc seit la femme seyné de la veine ke est desouz la keville del pé. E pus metét remedies dehors. Encuntre tecches de la face de freid encheson fetes fumigation a la face oveke l'eawe de la decoction de aloyne. Pus enoynét la face oveke savon de France agusé oveke nitre e destempré oveke vin egre. Si de chaud encheson, fetes fumigation de aveyne e pus destemprét amidum e ferine de feves oveke vin egre. Ausi moyllét une estoupe ou un coton en chaud sanc de cok ou de columb e surmetét a la face pur checune manere de tecches. A meme ceo en checun encheson vaut sanc de levre surmis sicum nus avom avant dit e issi demurge desure dekes il chece par sey. Ausi encuntre pan aprés enfantement vaut tiriake destempré oveke jus de fenoil ou vin e surmise. Ausi encontre livor .i. *wanhede* de cas ou de cop pernét bayes de lorer e poudrét e boyllét en mel e fetes emplastre e tedve surmetét. Ceo vaut encontre lentilles e pans de freid encheson.

[f.114v blank]

[BOOK VI: THE MOUTH]

1.

[f.115r][91] *Dolor dé dens* a la foiz est de chaus humors, a la foiz de freis. Commune reule est pur dolor ou aposteme de checune encheson ke le patient seit seyné de la veine capitale. Si ceo seit de chaud encheson, ke vous conoistrét par ague dolor, par la citrine face ou roujor, donc overét la veine ke est desouz la lange. Si ceo seit de freid encheson, ke vus conoistrét par ceo ke la face est blanche ou pale, donc ne overét mie la veine, mes metét une ventouse en la fontaynele del col. Ausi pur ceo ke ceste passion avient de reume deit hom estancher la reume. Por ceo en chaud encheson fetes fumigation en la bouche overte ové l'eawe de la decoction de roses. Ausi tienge en sa bouche vin blanc de la decoction de roses e de morele e de chenilé. Ausi fetes fumigation ové la semence de chenilé. Ausi mult vaut de mascher la racine de plantayne ou de cincfoil. [f.115v] Mes en freide encheson le patient tiegne en sa bouche le vin de la decoction de pelestre, ysope, euforbe ou peivre. Ausi tostét sel e metét en un poket e tedve surmetét dedenz ou dehors. Ausi liét ayl sur le pous del bras

de cele part ou la dolor est. A meme ceo versét le jus de heyre terrestre en l'orayle de
la contrere partye ou le jus de primerole savage .i. *kousleppe*. Ou fetes gargarisme de
vin blanc de la decoction de la poudre de staphizagre e de pelestre. Ou pernét la poudre
d'encens e de mastic e de spike e destemprét oveke blanc de l'oef e estendét sur
cordewan e surmetét as temples. Ou metét minte en ayle percé e tostét desouz les
cendres. E pus triblét en un morter e enoynét la dolente partye. Ou quissét encens en
ayl e surmetét. Ou pernét un oynon e le concavét dedenz e metét leinz la poudre de
peivre, [f.116r] pus l'envolupét en estoupe e quissét en les breses. E triblét e metét al
lu dolent. A dolor de denz ke sont percees de freid humor ou chaud purgét le ové
yeralogodion. Pus pernét poudre de galles percés e destemprét oveke terebentine e
metét el dent e asét vaudra. A meme ceo vaut la poudre de mirre destempré ové jus
de rue e mise enz. Pelestre vaut en meme la manere. Si le verm ne moet pas uncore
n'en ist, pelestre, galle, euforbe destemprét ensemble oveke vin e metét enz. E tutdis
aprés manger espurgét la dent, ke nule purreture ne remaygne.

[92] Si ele ne put estre garrie en tele manere, trehét la hors ovekes un fer. Ou trehét
la hors plus legerement en ceste manere: destemprét ferine de furment oveke let de
titimal e metét el pertus e entor la dent e issi chera par sey. Ou pernét la racine de
chenilé e eschaufét fortment [f.116v] e bien chaud metét en la dent e entor la racine
de la dent. Nestpurquant pernét garde ke il ne touche mie les autres dens, car ausi
cheyereyent.

[93] Pur dolor dé dens e pur neyrs gingives fetes le patient seiner checun ters jor
dedens la bouche sur les veines ke sont entre les dens deke les denz seyent garriz. Donc
pernét pomiz, si en fetes sotile poudre e frotés les dens dekes seyent enblanchis.

[94] Pur trere hors dens sanz dolor pernét la poudre de rouge parele arse ové la
racine e metét cele poudre en une cince de cendal e metét desouz une pere de verre
en un anel de argent. E tuchét la dent e ele saudra hors. Pur dolor dé dens e ronge, le
patient tiegne en sa bouche l'eawe de la decoction de la limure de corn de cerf.

[f.117r][95] Movement dé dens a la foiz est de freid humor ou de chaud, ke vus
conoistrét par les signes avantdiz e de medicines avantdites serra purgé. Si de chaud
humor, fetes le seiner de la capitale. Ou fetes le garser en le haterel. Pus tiegne vin
egre en la bouche el quel seyent quit galla, sumac, aluine e l'escorce de poume gernette.
A meme ceo vaut de laver la bouche dedenz e les denz e les gingives ové la decoction
de roses e de l'escorce de poume de gernette e de foilz de mirte. Mes sachét ke en
checune terre put hom mettre pur l'escorce de poume gernette tan e en lu de mirte
foylz de bux.

2.

[f.117v][96] A la foiz avient ke *la lange ou les levres ou les gingives sont escorcez*, donc
seit le patient seyné dé veines ke sont desouz la lange. Pus pernét gumme arabic e
metét en eawe rose par une nuit e de ceo enoynét al matin ou mester serra. Ou
esparpilét desure la poudre de roses, gumme de ceraser ou de pruner. Ausi si les gingives
seyent nues, pernét ferine d'orge e medlét oveke la poudre d'encens e de ceo frotét les
dens sovent.

3.

[97] *Puor de la bouche* a la foiz est de purreture dé gingives e dé denz, a la foiz de fleume purri en l'estomac. Si ceo seit dé gingives, put hum apercevoir par taster e par veue. Premerement frotét les oveke [f.118r] vin egre e lavét el quel seyent quit mirtus ou mirre oveke balausties. E pus frotét de ceste poudre, c'est asaver encens e galles e roses. E le patient se garde de let e de tutes choses ke viegnent de let. Si ceo seit de fleume purri en l'estomac, donc se garde de checun manere de peisson e de grosse char e des herbes ke engendrent fleume. E fetes le laver sovent la bouche oveke l'eawe de la decoction de comin e d'anis, mel e minte. Ausi tiegne en sa bouche e desouz sa lange checune nuyt ces piles .iii. ou .iiii. dekes seyent liquifiez: r[ecevét] cinnamomi, anthophali, nucis muscate, masticis, ligni aloes, squinanti, rosarum ana dragmam semis, sandali albi, spice, cubebe, cardamomi, gallie muscate ana dragme .i. et semis, camfore dragme une. Fetes poudre e destemprét oveke vin e fetes piles. A meme ceo le patient masche sovent canele e asét vaudra. E ceo tesmoynent les autors.

[BOOK VII: RESPIRATORY COMPLAINTS]

1.

[f.118v][98] *Squinantie* a la foiz est de colre, a la foiz de sanc, a la foiz de fleume. Si est aposteme entor la gorge ke tost occist. Pur ceo est commune reule ke le patient seit seyné dé veines ke sont desouz la lange, car ceo est la parfite cure. Mes a la foyz devient la lange si courte ke hom ne put atteindre les veines e donc le deit hom seiner de la capitale. Ou metés petites ventouses entre le col e les jowes a la racine de l'orayle. Ausi al comencement fetes clistere ou suppositorie mordificatif. Ausi al comencement usét gargarimes repercussifs e el meyn [f.119r] maturatifs e en la fin mundificatifs. Repercussif est fet ové diamoron destempré oveke l'eawe de la decoction de figes e de grapes quites en un fourn e fetes de ceo liqor mundificatif oveke let de chevre e la colature de bren de furment. Cest maturatif debruse l'aposteme. Ausi emplastres deyvent estre diverses solonc divers tens. Ausi commune reule est ke vus ne mettrét mie repercussifs par dehors, mes choses ke departent e attrehent. E ajostét acune chose confortative ou aukes pontike e attrehét de la materie al comencement. Pur ceo metét emplastre de ferine de furment e de jus de ache e de vielle gresse de porc ou jus de minte ou poudre de roses. E en le mein tens de la maladie fetes cest emplastre maturatif: r[ecevét] de racine de lilie e racines de wimauve, branke ursine ana manipulum unum, quissét en eawe e colét, e medlét les herbes ovekes libram unam de fresche bure e de[20] figes blancs e fetes emplastre. En la fin pur debruser e mundifier fetes emplastre de leveine e de oyle e de sel. [f.119v] Ou pur enmeurer e debruser l'aposteme sicum dit Alisandre vaut diacelidonion, ke est fet de la poudre des arundes arses destempré oveke vielle gresse de porc. Encuntre squinantie de fleume: fetes gargarisme de oximel medlé

[20] MS *dis.*

ové l'eawe de la decoction de pelestre e la racine de radich, squinant e cassiafistre. A meme ceo valt l'estront de chien destempré oveke ptisane ou mulsa e mis en un drap sur le lu dolent. Ou gargarize a meme ceo: maschét furment e medlét oveke leveyne e figes secs e fetes emplastre. A meme ceo donét ly a boyvre arnement destempré ovekes eawe. Acuns dient ke spigornele vaut bue ov columbine.

2.

[120r][99] *La tusse* est une maladie ke avient de reume. Pur ceo est commune reule solonc les autors ke la reume seit estanché. Mes si ele seit de chaud encheson, donc seit le patient seyné. Si de freid encheson, metét une ventouse entre les espaules. Por abatre la reume pernét treis greins de blanc encens a la quantité de une chiche e le patient les trangloute al seyr. Ou fetes le user cest sirup: r[ecevét] radicem lilii, marrubii albi, ysopi recentis, eupatorii, capilli veneris, calamenti, origani, pulegii, thimi recentis, camedreos ana manipulum unum, liquiricie mundate, maratri, anthos, uve passe ab arillis mundate, caricarum, pistacearum, seminis altee ana unce une, mellis, zucre ana libram unam e fetes sirup. Ausi anoynét le piz de cest oynement: r[ecevét] amigdalarum dulcarum, dialtee, butyri ana unces .ii., olei, pulegii unces .ii., storacis liquide, adipis anatis, adipis anseris ana unces .ii., cere nigre unce une e fetes un oynement e enoynét le pis. En chaud encheson fetes le user matin e seir sirup de blanc popy ke issi est fet: quassét la semence e quissét en eawe, colét e a la colature ajostét zucre [f.120v] e fetes sirup. Ausi donét piles de cynoglosse .i. lange de chien une foyz en la semayne ou deus ke valent en l'un e l'autre encheson a la quantité de une chiche. E le patient les tiegne desouz sa lange deke seyent resolés. Fetes les issi: r[ecevét] mirre unces .vi., thuris unces .v., opii unces .iiii., cinoglosse unces .iii. Confisét ovekes eawe rose. Ausi les autors dient ke suffumigation d'orpiment vaut si le patient seit gras e moiste, mes si il seit megres e seit [. . .] le defendét.

[100] Ces sont les choses ke valent pur la tusse e pur le pis: daucus, valeriane, filipendula, gelofré, gentiana, gallia muscata, mellilotum, calamente, mirre, sisimbrium, mauve, popi, origanum, anetum, averoyne, sticados, noys mugette, pistacee, centorie, serpillum, gingivre, dragagant, gumme arabic, penides, enula, yreos, macis, peivre, peucedanum, scordeon, sparage, senecion, satureye, basilicon, ysope, maroil, betoyne, diptayne, licoriz, fenugrec, meu, policarie, junevre, lovache, parele e autres plusors.

3.

[f.121r][101] *Emoptoici* sont cels ke gettent sanc ou escopent. E ceo avient a la foiz de la teste e ceo conoistrez par ces signes: grevance en la teste e emflure dé veines en les narilz. A la foiz avient del pomon e ceo signifie cler sanc e escomous ové tusse. A la foiz avient de brusure de la veine de l'estomac e donc est le sanc neir ou cler oveke vomit. A la foiz avient dé procheins menbres sicum de la gule e les jowes.

[102] Veét ci electuarie ke merveilousement vaut a ceste maladie: r[ecevét] olibani dragmes .iii., amidi dragmes .iiii., consolide maioris dragmes .viii., dragaganti, boli ana

dragmes .vii., sanguinis draconis, opii ana dragmes .ii. Temprét oveke diacodion ou jus de plantayn ové bol, dragagant, amidoun e ypoquistidos e donét a boyvre. Ou fetes une decoction dé choses avantdites ové mel e eawe la terce partie e quissét dekes l'eawe seit degasté. Si ceo seit del pomon ou de la teste, frotét la pere ke est apelé emathides desure un keus ové jus de plantayne dekes il seit tut vermail e donét a boyvre. A meme ceo vaut athanasia ou acharistum. A meme ceo donét cest especial [f.121v] sirup: pernét le jus de plantayne e boyllét al fu e colét e clarifiét e ajostét zucre e fetes sirup. Mes en la premere decoction metét la racine de licoriz. A meme ceo donét la decoction de sanigle a boyvre. E ceo est esprové.

4.

[103] *Empici* sont ceus ke escopent quiture par la bouche. E sachét ke ceste maladie, ceo est asaver *empima*, a la foiz est de aposteme del piz ou del pomon. E sachét ke il avient sovent ke pleuresie change en empima e donc y a grant dolor dé costes e grevance de alener e destresce del piz e forte fevre e aspresce de la lange e secke tusse e change de reson e veyles. E sachét si l'aposteme aprés ke il est debru[f.122r]sé ne ert mye mundifié dedenz .xl. jors, ke le patient tornera en ptisike. Ausi a la foiz aprés emoptois vient empima e donc put l'aleyne e ceo est malveis signe e ausi cum incurable. Nestpurquant a la foiz avient ke la selive est medlé de quiture e l'aleyne ne put nient. Pur ceo est commune queintise ke hom gette la selive desur charbons e si ele put, sachét ke le pomon est blescé. Autre: jetét la selive en eawe e si rien auge al font le pomon est blescé. Mes a la foiz avient ke la quiture est medlee ové la selive e donc les departirét ovekes une verge tenve de coudre ou de figer e la quiture ira al font en la departye.

[104] Encuntre ceste maladie donét al matin diadragantum e al seir diapenidion. E ke il ne passe mie en ptisike, fetes le user cest electuarie: r[ecevét] fenugreci, liquiricie ana unce une, amili, seminis lini, assi, amigdalarum, prassii ana unces .ii., dragaganti, gummi arabici ana unciam unam et semis, piretri unciam semis, mellis quod sufficit. Donét al matin e al seir ke ptisana quite oveke licoriz e fetes emplastre de figes e [f.122v] de la racine de wimauve oveke ferine d'orge. Le patient se garde nomément de ire e de cri e de poudre e de fumé.

5.

[105] Ore dirrum de *ptisike* ke degaste le cors. Signe de ptisike est fievre continue, salive medlé oveke quiture, le cors est tenve e sec, les extremités sont courvés, les chevus cheent, la tusse est forte, l'appetit est fieble e l'aleine est estreite. En ceste manere put hom saver queldour le empic seit ptisic ou noun: si il est ptisic, la fevre est continue, mes la chalor descorde poy de naturele chalor, tut le cors enmegrist, les un[f.123r]gles sont elevés e courvés, la selive put e ceo esproverét sicum nus avum avant dit el chapitre de empimate. E sachét ke il y a difference entre ptisike e etike, pur ceo ke en ethike le pomon n'est pas blescé e le patient ne tusse mie, mes en ptisike

le pomon est blescé e le patient n'est pas sanz tusse. E sachét si la selive seit pulente e medlé de quiture e si les chevus cheent e ke ceo seit flux de ventre, signifie mort. E sachét si ceste passion aviegne a un fleumatic e moiste, ke ele put estre estendue dekes a .xxx. anz ou .xx. Mes si ptisike avyegne a coleric e a sec, donc est incurable.

[106] La cure de ptisike est double. L'une est verraye, l'autre est blandisante. La verraye cure est, quant la maladie est curable, de mundifier l'aposteme del pomon e de enseccher le e pur defendre la reume e pur deboter la materie del pomon. Por mundifier l'aposteme donét cest gargarime ové le jus de la decoction de jus de licoriz ou l'eawe de la decoction d'orge ové la decoction de la racine de licoriz. Ausi commun esperiment est solum touz les au[f.123v]tors: pernét cancres de fluvie e quissét desouz les cendres e pus trehét hors la char e quissét en eawe d'orge escorché e fetes le humer de cele decoction. Cure blandisante [est], quant la maladie n'est pas curable, de doner choses ke soudent e ensecchent. E donét cest sirup pur mundifier l'aposteme: r[ecevet] capilli veneris manipulos .iii., pimpinelle, consolide maioris et minoris et medie, ysopi recentis, ceterac, politricum, adianthos, scariole, radicis ungule caballine aquatice ana manipulum unum, viole unces .ii., florum nenufarum, quatuor seminum frigidorum mundatorum, liquiricie mundificate ana unce une, candii, penidii, medulle seminis bombacis, seminis citoniorum, boli armenici, seminis lactuce, portulace, papaveris albi, mirtillorum, succi liquiricie ana unciam semis, dragaganti, gummi arabici, amidi, rosarum, spodii, sanguinis draconis ana dragmes .iii., seminis malve, seminis altee, uve passe ab arillis mundificate, caricarum, pistacearum ana dragmes .ii., ordei mundificati libram semis, zucare libras .iii. E fetes sirup ovekes eawe de pluuie e clarifiét e do[f.124r]nét matin e seir. Ausi donét checun jor let de chevre el quel treis peres de fluvie ardantes seyent esteintes.

[107] E sachét ke Avicenne dit en ptisike 'Jeo ay', fet il, 'sovent esprové en divers cors ke le ptisik serra garri si il use zucre rosette par l'espace de un an checun jor quanke il put e oveke pain, me[s] ke mult seit'. Nestpurquant si l'aleyne deviegne estreite pur les roses, donét a boyvre sirup de blanc popy aprés sucre rosette. E ne lessét mie ceste cure, kar ele ne faut mye, par ont Avicenne dit: 'Si jeo ne dotasse estre tenu mentour, jeo vus cunteraye coment une femme eschapa ke tant aveit esté ptisik ke ele fu a la mort. E donc leva sus son frere e la garist par ceste cure long tens e ele revist e devint grasse'. E a ceste maladie de checune manere de let vaut plus let de femme soucché de la ma[f.124v]mele, e pus aprés, let de asne e de chevre. Nestpurquant let de chevre piz vaut a user. Nestpurquant si la fevre seit forte, ne seit pas usé. E si il ad flux de ventre, metét el let la poudre de sanc dragon ou bol armenic. Veét ci piles desouz la lange ke valent encontre aspresce de la gorge e la tusse e defendent reume e font dormir, e ceo font sanz dolor: r[ecevét] tiriace magne dragmes .iii., succi liquiricie, seminis papaveris albi, dragaganti, gummi arabici dragme une, opii scrupulum unum. Confisét piles ové jus de blanc popi e deus seyent tenues desouz la lange dekes seyent defiés. Bayn a meme ceo esprové: pernét chaels esvoeglés e trehét hors lor entrayles e trenchét en veye lor extremités e pus les quissét en eawe e en cele eawe seit le patient baygné aprés manger par .iiii. houres. A meme ceo autre bayn esprové: quissét limaçons dé boys, ceo est a dire turtouses, e quant comencent a boyllir trehét hors lour meules e lor chars e lor extremités e quissét en la secunde eawe e de cele eawe [f.125r] baynét le patient. Si vus ne ayét mye turtouses, fetes bain de cancres de fluvie.

[108] La diete est ke il use freide choses e moistes glumouses sicum pés de porc, gelines, poucins de geline e char de joefne aynel e net payn e vin blanc e sotil e le patient eschue chose salee e acetouse e manjue pessons de fluvie, figes e dates.

6.

[f.125v][109] *Peripleumonie* est chaud aposteme el pomon ke vus conoistrét par ces signes; fevre continue, destresce de aleyne, grant roujor en les jowes e dolor par devant e par deriere entre les espaules e grevance del piz sanz puynture e sanz dolor e sanz chalor. En pleuresie e en peripleumonie est commune reule ke le patient seit seyné. Autre reule: le patient ne use nule chose acetouse par la bouche.

[110] Por assuager e pur enmeurer l'aposteme fetes cest emplastre: pernét les racines de wimauve e fenugrec e semence de lin e figes secs e ferine d'orge e quissét e confisét oveke vielle gresse de porc ou bure e surmetét. A meme ceo surmetét cyroyne. Si il eyt fevre ague, donét ly a boyvre eawe de la decoction de citruli, melons, cucumbre e cucurbite.

[111] La diete est ke il eschue choses salees, acetouses, pontics e stiptics e grasse choses e agues. E use blites, arage, spinache condiz oveke let de alemandes. E eschue freid ayr [f.126r] e chaud pain sanz leveine e beyve vin blanc aromatic bien medlé ovekes eawe chaude. E se garde de ire e de estudie.

7.

[112] *Pleuresi* est aposteme en les pels dé costes ke vus conoistrét par ces signes: fevre continue, tusse al comencement de la maladie, anguisse d'aleyne, dolor de cele coste ou l'aposteme est. E sachét ke quatre tens sont de pleuresie, ceo est asaver comencement, anoytement, estat,[21] declineson. Al comencement la selive est liquide e sotile [f.126v] e petite e rouje ou citrine e grevement ist hors. En l'anoytement devient grasse. En l'estat est blanche e viscouse medlé ové naturele selive. En declination, ceo est a dire la departye de la maladie, est blanche e mult viscouse e legerement ist sanz grevance.

[113] La cure de pleuresie est de acomencer oveke choses ke eschaufent. Pernét de camomille, d'anis e de roses ana unces .ii. e metét en deus sachels e tut chaud metét al lu dolent. Autre: pernét libram semis de milio e broyllét sur une chaude tuyle ou en une paele sanz liqor, pus metét en un sachel e chaud surmetét. Ceo fetes el premer jor. El secund jor ou le ters fetes le seyner de la veine cardiake de la destre part. Pus fetes le user cest sirup: r[ecevét] radicem feniculi, petroselini, anisi ana manipulum unum, capilli veneris manipulos .ii., endivie, scariole, scolopendrie, ceterac, politrichi ana manipulum unum, viole unces .ii., quatuor seminum frigidorum mundatorum, candi, seminis papaveris albi ana unce une, seminis lactuce, portulace, dragaganti,

---

21 i.e. paroxysm cf. G. Lafeuille (ed.), *Les Amphorismes Ypocras de Martin de Saint-Gille 1362–1365* (Genève, 1954), p.61 no.29 'quant les accidens sont tres fors et la matiere est esmeue contre nature'.

gummi arabici ana unciam semis, mirabolanarum, sebasten ana numero .x., ordei mundati libram unam, zucare libras .ii. Fetes sirup e fetes le user matin e seir [f.127r] ovekes eawe chaude ou eawe d'orge e donét ly al matin de zucre violette ovekes eawe d'orge. E devant le sirup al vespre donét ces electuaries: r[ecevét] diadragaganti frigidi, diapenidion sanz comin ana libram semis, medlét ensemble e donét ovekes ewe d'orge.

[114] Ausi solonc les quatre divers tens devez diversifier vos emplastres, car premerement devét user repercussifs. Pernét de foilz de mauve manipulos .ii., quissét en eawe e pus triblét oveke gresse de porc e ajostét unce une de la poudre de semence de lin, e fetes emplastre e metez sur les costes. En l'anoytement fetes emplastre, partye repercussif, partye dissolutif: pernét de foilz de mauve, de la racine de wimauve ana manipulum unum, quissét en eawe e pus colét e pus triblét en un morter e medlét ovekes libram unam de novele gresse de porc. Pus ajostét de semence de lin, de fenugrec e la poudre de acori ana unciam semis e fetes emplastre e surmetét si chaud cum il le put soffrir al lu dolent. En l'estat fetes emplastre maturatif: r[ecevét] radicem altee, radicem lilii, brance ursine ana manipulum unum. [f.127v] Quissét en eawe e colez e triblét les herbes ovekes libram unam de bure fresche e .x. figes blancs e fetes emplastre. Ausi en declination de la maladie usét mundificatifs sicum ptisane d'orge quite oveke licoriz mundé. Ausi fetes cest oynement mundificatif: r[ecevét] de bure, de novele gresse de porc ana unces .iii., de gresse d'owe, de gresse de madlard, de gresse de geline tutes fresches ana unces .ii., dragaganti, gummi arabici ana unce une, de cyre blanche unce une e fetes oynement e eschauf[ét] e enoynét le pis e le coste. E donét les electuaries avantdiz.

[115] La diete seit potage de ferine e son beivre seit ptisana. Si le patient seit costivé, donét ly laxatif de tamarindes e de cassiafistula e de violes.

8.

[f.128r][116] *Dolor del piz* a la foiz est de chaud encheson, a la foiz de freid. De chaud a la foiz oveke materie, a la foiz sanz materie. Si sanz materie, enoynét le pis checun jor matin e seir ovekes oyle violette e oyle nenufari. Pus pernét d'oyle violette libram unam e eschaufét sur le fu. E pus pernét libram unam de novel cotoun e moyllét leynz e surmetét, car il oste la dolor del piz.

[117] Dolor del piz de chaud encheson est curé par sirup, par medicine, par seiné, par bayn, par oynement, par electuaries e par fumigations. Fetes le user cest sirup premerement: r[ecevét] capilli veneris manipulos .ii.,[f.128v] endivie, scariole, rostri porcini, herbe viole, radicis ungule caballini aquatice ana manipulum unum, violarum, florum nenufarum ana unces .ii., quatuor seminum frigidorum mundatorum, seminis lactuce, portulace, seminis papaveris albi ana unce une, berberis dragmes .ii., jujube, sebasten ana numero .x., zucre libras .ii. Fetes sirup e le fetes user matin e seir ovekes eawe chaude. Pus quant la materie est defié, voidét la ové ceste decoction: r[ecevét] violarum unces .iii., florum nenufarum unces .ii., quatuor seminum frigidorum mundatum ana unce une, cassiefistule, manne ana unce une. Fetes une decoction dekes a demy livre e donét al matin. Le ters jor après la medicine, entre en un bayn de chaud eawe e sue, e quant il ist, se garde de freid ayr. Le ters jor après le bain seit seyné de la

veine cardiake. Pus use checun jor a matin zucre violette e al seir triasandali oveke diadragant freit. Pus enoynét le piz e l'estomac ovekes oyle e oyle de alemandes medlés ensemble. Pus pernét leine carpie, ceo est a dire 'floccles', e moyllét en oyle violette e metét sur le piz.

[118] Encuntre dolor del piz de freid encheson fetes le patient user premerement ceste decoction: r[ecevét] capilli [f.129r] veneris, ysopi recentis, marrubii albi, teneritatum feniculi, radicis lilii ana manipulos .ii., liquiricie mundate unces .ii. Quissét en eawe e donét matin e seir. E de nutant donét diadragant infusum, diapenidion sanz canele medlez ensemble. Ausi enoynét le piz oveke cest oynement: r[ecevét] olei amigdalarum dulcarum, olei de lilio ana quartoun un, adipis anseris et anatis omnium recentium ana unces .ii. Medlét tut ensemble en manere d'oyle e l'eschaufet e enoynét le piz par .viii. jors.

[119] Encuntre dolor del piz ke avient de l'esplen ou de l'estumac. Donét premerement cest sirup: r[ecevét] radicis yreos, thimi recentis, radicis lilii, marrubii albi, ysopi recentis, camedreos, camepiteos, gentiane, germandree, scolopendrie ana manipulum unum, capilli veneris manipulos .ii., florum boraginis, florum camomille, florum melliloti et maratri ana unce une, radicis capparis, liquiricie mundate ana unces .ii., zucure libram unam et semis, mellis libram unam e fetes sirup pur user matin e seir pur defier la materie. Pus voydét la materie ové ces piles: r[ecevét] paulini dragme une, yerapigre dragmes .ii., agarici repressi cum succo liquiricie scrupolos .ii. Fetes piles e donét al seir ové vin de la decoction de ysope e cerflange e de licoriz mundé ana unces .ii. [f.129v] Ausi checun jor aprés manger e a nuyt use cest electuarie: r[ecevét] diacitoniton sanz peivre, diapenidion ana libram semis. Medlét e devant manger use ceste poudre esprové. Pernét de gingivre trié quartroun un, de semence de fenoil e de licoriz mundé ana unces .iiii. e fetes sotile poudre e use ceste poudre ke vin chaud bien medlé d'eawe. E pus enoynét ovekes oyle de lilie e de camomille.

9.

[f.130r][120] Encuntre *asma*, ceo est a dire destresce d'aleyne. Si ceo seit de sanc, ke vus conoistrét par les veines emflees e par roujor de la face, fetes le patient seyner. Si autre humor seit en encheson, pernét la poudre d'orpiment e temprét ovekes un oef e moyllét oveke ceo un drap e pus ensecchét le e ardét le sur les charbons. E le patient receive la fumé par sa bouche. Merveilousement prophite. Si ceo seit de seccheté, donét diadragantum freit e la decoction de figes secs e dragagant e yris illirica e jus de licoriz. A un pouvre issi aydét: fetes cauterie desouz la fourcele del piz e fetes le user matin e seir l'eawe de la decoction de ysope e de lovache e la racine de wimauve. E matin e seir enoynét le del menton dekes al piz ové bure par tut e le coverét de un cordewan e se garde de freide eawe kanke il put.

10.

[f.130v][121] *Paumeson* est defaute del movement de quer, si est apelé en latin de acuns *sincopis*. Des autres est apelé *lippotamia*, des autres *malfactio*, d'autres *exsolucio*. A la foiz avient des accidens de l'alme sicum ire, joye e poour. En checune paumeson jetét eawe freide sur le patient ou fetes le esternier e metét a ses narilz de bon odor sicum roses. Si la paumeson seit de joye, contét de triste choses, si de tristour, contét de joye.

[122] Paumeson ke avient des accidens del cors ou ele est de male complexion ou de inanition, ceo est a dire ke le cors est void, ou ele est de repletion ou de [f.131r] suor ou d'opilation dé veines ou de suffocation. Si ele seit de male complexion ou est de chalor ou de freidure: si de chalor, donc covient refreider le patient e remuer ceus ke sont entor luy; si de freidure, eschaufét le. Si de inanicion sicum de flux dé flurs, donc les estanchét sicum nus dirrum el chapitre de flux dé flurs. Si de flux de sanc dé narilz ou ayllors, estanchét le. Si de flux de ventre, estanchét le. Si de repletion, voidet le humor ke est en encheson. Si le sanc seit en encheson, fetes le seiner. Si autre humor, purgét le par medicine, ceo est asaver aprés l'accés. Si de suour, estanchét le sicum nus dirrum el chapitre de cardiake. Si d'opilation dé veines, ke vus conoistrét par ceo ke le patient paume sovent e par defaute del pouz, donét oximel oveke l'eawe de la decoction des racines d'ache, persil e fenoil e radich. De ceste paumeson plusors muront sovent sodeinement. Si de suffocation dé spiritualités, sicum suffocation del mariz, donc curét le sicum nus dirrum el [f.131v] chapitre de suffocation del mariz. Ausi pur paumeson ke avient del quer arosét la face sodenement ovekes eawe rose e lavét les plansons des [pés] e les mayns ovekes eawe rose. Ausi pernét une penne de geline e moyllét mult bien en vin egre e enoynét les narilz dedenz e meintenant serra garri. E cest esperiment est esprové. Si paumeson seit de dolor de l'estomac, fetes la cure sicum nus dirrum en son lu. Si ele seit de verms – ke vus saverét en ceste manere: donét a boyvre sirup violet e si la dolor acrest, donc ert por verms, si non, donc est de autre encheson – pernét jus de basilicon ou jus de rue e medlét oveke let de chevre e donét a boyvre. Si la paumeson seit de verms oveke fevre e as enfans, pernét de ferine d'orge libram unam, del jus de tetesoriz libram unam e fetes emplastre sur le umbril. Ceo est esprové. Si paumeson aviegne aprés seigné ou devant, pernét une lesche de pain e moillét en jus de poume ou de peyre e donét e ceo avant gardera de paumeson. A ceus ke ont paumeson de privé encheson mult vaut user electuaries ke receivent muscum, lignum aloes, or[piment?] par les [f.132r] os de quer de cerf e autre choses confortatives.

[123] Ces sont les choses ke nomément valent pur paumeson: borage, roses, ambre, ozimum, cardamome, cassialigne, cubebes, canele, saffran, epithime, thime, gelofré, galingale, mirte, minte, mirabolans, melisse, rosmarin, spicam, sené, satureye, calamus aromaticus, squinant, baume, blacca, bisantia, pulleole, rue, berberis, cuscute, touz les sandles, storax calamite, gingivre, carvi, amomum, noys mugette, carpobalsamum, xilobalsamum, vin, iacincte, emeraude.

11.

[f.132v][124] *Cardiake* est une passion ke fet tut le cors suer continuement. D'acuns est apelé *diaforetica*. A la foiz avient del quer, a la foiz de l'estomac, a la foiz de la foye, a la foiz de repletion dé veines, a la foiz oveke fevre, a la foiz sanz fevre, a la foiz de privé encheson, a la foiz de lumbriz ke sont en la bouche de l'estomac, a la foiz de ventosité. E donc est commune reule solom touz les autors de doner dianisum, diaciminum ou diaspermaton, e si vus ne les ayét mie, moyllét leine ou une esponge en l'eawe de la decoction de anis e surmetét al lu de la passion.

[125] Ausi a la foiz est de privé encheson, e donkes si vus metét ta mayn sur la region del quer, vus ne troverét mye le movement del quer ordiné, mes tremblant. Donkes est commune reule ke le patient seit espurgé en ceste manere: pernét ysope, lovache e satureye e la racine de licoriz e le jus de la racine de yreos, calamente e maroil e quissét ové mulsa e donét al matin e seir. E pus seit purgé ové yerapigra enagusé ové la poudre de la racine de licoriz.

[126] La cardiake ke est apelé *diaforetica* avient de forte chalor ke desoude le humor dé spiritualtés. De ceste [f.133r] parlent les autors sovent. Signifiance de ceste est ke tut le cors sue continuement e en les extremités est froid a la foyz, a la foiz tut le cors devient tenve. Le patient en dormant resemble mort. A la foiz avient aprés continue, a la foiz de lunge quarteyne, a la foyz de colere. Donc fetes le patient seiner e donkes mundifiét le cors oveke colagoge, ceo est a dire medicine ke espurge colre. Ausi solonc touz les autors en checune cardiake continue frotez les mains e les pés. Ausi moillét un linge drap en eawe rose e metét a[s] narilz. Ausi le patient seit en freid lu. Ausi enoynét le front e les temples oveke freides choses. Ausi donét electuaries ke confortent e repareillent l'espiris, sicum diamargariton, triasandali, rosate novele.

[BOOK VIII: THE STOMACH]

1.

[f.133v][127] *Bolismus* est trop grant appetit a manger ke de Alisandre est apelé *cinorodoxa*, ceo est a dire joye a chien, car il ne se delite en nule rien for soulement de vomir e de returner a manger. Ausi ces tutdis gettent e desirent de manger aprés. Ceste maladie avient a la foyz de fleume e de melancolie ke sont en la bouche de l'estomac sicum dit Constantin, e Alisandre dit ke a la foiz avient de chalor e de secchété. E jeo dis ke a la foiz est de lumbriz. Si ceste maladie seit de chalor e de secchété, donc fetes la cure ke vaut a ethike e ptisike. Si de lumbriz, fetes la cure de lumbriz. Si de freis humors, defiét la materie ovekes electuaries ke desoudent sicum diacalamentum, diaprassium. Pus espurgét le oveke yeralogodion checune semayne. Pus donét la grande tiriake, ceo est asaver aprés la purgation ové vin de la decoction de galingale. Ausi solonc les autors vus dorrez grasse choses al comencement del manger pur abatre l'appetit. E jeo le grant bien si melancolie seit en encheson, mes si fleume seit en encheson, jeo nel granteray mye.

[128] Ausi il y a un autre [f.134r] bolisme particuler ke n'est pas fort cum est *cinorodoxa*, mes avient en houres. E sodeinement survient grant appetit e nestpurquant de petite viande est assuagé. E si le patient ne ad mie a manger quant talent le prent, paume, e en tel bolisme est mon cunseil ke si tost cum le patient sent le premer appetit, ke hom ly doune acune diete ou acun electuarie confortatif.

[129] La diete seit grosse sicum char de boef, pain demayne, chasteins, feves, chiche, prunes blanches, jujubes, pastinakes, poumes gernettes, char de poon, char de bouk, owes, columbeus, viel furmage.

2.

[f.134v][130] *Seif* a la foiz avient de trop grant destemperance en chalor del quer e del pomon. E donc vaut plus l'ayr freid e moiste ke medicine reçue dedenz. E donc deit le patient meindre entour funtaynes e fluvies. Ausi a la foiz seif est de l'estomac e donc est de chalor sanz moisture e donc vaut freide diete sicum letuse, purcelane e freis electuaries sicum rosata, triasandali. A la foiz est de sausefleume e donc vaut purgation ke espurge fleume. A la foiz est de colre rouge e donc espurgét le patient oveke trifera ou diaprunis.

[131] Veét ci esperiment pur seif ke vient de colre. Pernét la semence de psillium e temprét en eawe tedve par une nuyt e al matin le pressét hors parmy un linge drap fortment. E ceo ke curra hors serra muscillage, ceo est a dire ke il serra espés ou viscous ausi cum glette. Cele muscillage metét en un poket de linge drap e metét desouz ta lange. Ceste muscillage vaut a maladies de colre sicum fevre terceine e a eschaufure de la foye e remollit le ventre e les entrayles e espurge de colre. Si est usé [f.135r] en confections e en decoctions. Ausi est doné par sey ou ovekes eawe freide ou tedve ou vin. Ausi ces trocisces seyent tenuz desouz la lange: r[ecevét] portulace, seminis cucumeris, dragaganti ana dragmes .iii., seminis melonis, cucurbite, lactuce, viole, sandali, gummi arabici, an[isi], psillii ana unces .ii. Fetes poudre e temprét en eawe rose ou muscillage de psillium e formét sicum une feve e metét desouz la lange.

[132] Ausi seif avient a la foyz de glotonie de manger e de beyvre. E cele est estanché par dormir e par abstinence. Seif avient a la foyz de destemperance dé reins en chalor. De cele dirrum la cure el chapitre de cele maladie.

3.

[f.135v][133] *Fastidium* est apelé de Galien *anorexia*, si est dit de *a*, ke est a dire 'sanz', e *orexis*, ke est a dire 'appetit', sicum 'sanz appetit'. Une reule est ke si ceste passion aviegne a un coleric, a peine ou jammés ert garri; si a un fleumatic, legerement. Ceste passion a la foiz est de chaud encheson e donkes oveke vice de humor ou sanz vice. Si oveét vice de humor, donc sent le patient grevance en l'estomac, punctions, arsures, si ad la bouche amere e seif. Si ceo seit de soule destemperance, donc n'i a poynt grevance, mes les autre signes remaynent.

[134] Si ceo seit de freid encheson, donc est oveke vice de humor ou sanz vice. Si oveke vice de humor, donc y a grevance e freidure el parfond de l'estomac, la bouche

dessavoré e acetouse eructuation. Si ceo seit de soule destemperance, donc n'y a mye grevance, mes les autres signes remaynent. Si ceo seit de chaud encheson ou freid, dementers ke le humor seit en encheson est une reule ke eawe chaude vaut pur fere vomir. Ausi si ceo seit de destemperance, [f.136r] donc vaut freide eawe bue. Ausi lavét la bouche de l'estomac oveke vin egre tedve. Ausi vin egre seit usé en sauses e en sirups. Ausi vaut electuarie de jus de roses pur espurger. Ausi vaut de user electuaries confortatifs freis sicum triasandali. Ausi vaut d'estre seyné de la veine epatike.

[135] Si ceo seit de freid encheson oveke vice de humor, la materie seit defié. Pus seit espurgé oveke benedicta. Ausi une reule est ke checune semaine seit tiriake doné. Ausi Alisandre cumant ke l'estomac seit enoynt oveke marciaton ke vaut en freis enchesons. Ausi ceste passion avient a la foiz de feblesce de l'estomac. E donc donét fors electuaries e en viandes donét la poudre de gelofré, noiz mugette e minte. Ausi fetes emplastre e surmetét a l'estomac, ceo est asaver a la bouche de l'estomac. Poudrét minte e payn tosté e roses e confisét oveke vin aromatic. Ausi donét al patient coinz quiz desouz les breses e moyllez en vin. Ausi le jus de poumes gernettes acetouses reparaylle appe[f.136v]tit. Meme ceo fet vert jus de verte grape. Ausi veét ci bone poudre pur feblesce de l'estomac de freid: r[ecevét] an[isi] unces .ii., zinziberis, origani, pulegii, samsuci, mente sicce, salvie, satureie, calamenti, thimi ana unce une, piperis longi, galange, cinnamomi, gariofile, folii, spice nardi, maratri, macis, nucis muscate, xilobalsami, carpobalsami, calami aromatici, cassieligni ana unciam semis, eufrasie, sileris montani, seminis rute, camedreos, meu, sinoni, ameos, seminis coriandri, sandali albi, salis ar[moniaci], squinanti ana dragmes .iii., omnium mirabolanorum, ana dragme une, panis zucare dragmes .iii. Fetes poudre e donét checun jor une cuylleré devant manger oveke vin blanc ou bru el comencement del manger.

4.

[f.137r][136] *Aposteme* avient a la foiz en la bouche de l'estomac, a la foiz de chaud humor, a la foiz de freid humor. Signes d'aposteme chaud sont grant chalor entor l'estomac, seif, fevre continue e dolor poygnant. Signes d'aposteme freid sont feble appetit e pou de seif e de dolor e sanz fevre e sanz chalor.

[137] La cure d'aposteme chaud est ke le patient seit seiné de la veine ke est apelé *basilica*, pus use cest sirup: r[ecevét] endivie, scariole, scolopendrie, rostri porcini, epatice, herbe viole, capilli veneris, ceterac, politrichi ana manipulum unum, radicis feniculi recentis, radicis petroselini recentis, ana manipulum semis, viole unces .ii., prunorum damascenorum .xx., florum nenufarum, quatuor seminum frigidorum ana unce une, seminis lactuce, seminis portulace ana unciam semis, jujube, sebasten ana numero .x., ordei mundati libram semis, uve passe unciam semis, zucure libras .ii. Fetes sirup e clarifiét e fetes le patient user le matin e seir ové la decoction d'endive. E il covient ke al comencement facét cest emplastre: r[ecevét] omnium sandalorum ana unce une, farine libram semis, radicis herbe viole manipulum unum. Fetes emplastre ovekes eawe de morele e d'endive. [f.137v] Quant l'aposteme est encressant, fetes cest emplastre: r[ecevét] omnium sandalorum ana unciam semis, abscinthii, melliloti ana manipulum unum. Quissét les herbes en eawe e medlét ové la poudre de sandles e fetes

emplastre ovekes oyle viole. E ajostét de ferine d'orge libram semis e bien chaud metét sur l'estomac. Si l'aposteme seit en estat, fetes cest emplastre: r[ecevét] radicis altee, radicis lilii, camomille, melliloti, abscinthii ana manipulum unum, omnium sandalorum ana dragmes .iii., ficuum alborum .v., farine frumenti libram semis. Fetes emplastre ovekes oyle de camomille e oyle de lils.

[138] Si l'aposteme seit de freid humor, defiét la materie oveke cest sirup: r[ecevét] radicis feniculi, petroselini, ysopi recentis, radicis apii, radicis lilii, capilli veneris, ceterac, politrichi, adianthos, radicis buglosse ana manipulum unum, violarum unces .ii., liquiricie mundate, maratri, florum camomille, florum melliloti, seminis brusci, seminis sparagi, florum boraginis ana unce une, zucre libras .ii. Fetes sirup ke le patient usera matin e seir oveke l'eawe de la decoction dé racines de fenoil e d'ache. Pus si mester seit, voidét la ové ceste decoction: r[ecevét] radicis buglosse, radicis yreos, radicis liquiricie mundate, radicum feniculi, radicum apii ana unce une, florum bo[f.138r]raginis, cassiefistule mundate ana unce une. Quissét les herbes en eawe e ové la decoction destemprét cassiafistule munde e donét par matin al patient. A meme ceo fetes cest oynement: r[ecevét] olei de lilio, olei camomille, masticeleon ana quartroun .i., adipis anseris, anatis, galline, medulle cervine, storacis liquide ana unciam semis, cere albe et rubee, ana unce une. E ovekes cest oynement enoynét l'estomac en l'estat de l'aposteme. Emplastre a meme ceo: r[ecevét] ficuum alborum .x., storacis liquide ana unciam semis, radicum lilii unces .ii., mastici, armoniaci unciam semis, farine fenugreci libram unam, vini albi quartroun semis. Boyllét le vin e ajostét la ferine al vin boyllant. Pus ajostét les gummes e les racines e fe[tes] emplastre.

5.

[f.138v][139] Encuntre *duresce de l'estomac* defiét la materie ovekes oximel e pus la voidét oveke decoction de yreos. E pus enoynét l'estomac ové la meule des os de cerf e la meule de l'os de quisse de vache. Veét ci bon emplastre a duresce de l'estomac: r[ecevét] melliloti, camomille, fenugrecum, baccarum lauri, radicum altee, abscinthii ana unce une, amoniaci, thuris albi ana unciam unam et semis. Resolét ces gummes oveke vin e mel e pus ajostét les meules e fetes merveylous emplastre. Autre emplastre: r[ecevét] masticis, thuris, abscinthii ana unce une, amoniaci, croci ana unces .iii. Fetes cyroyne e surmetét. E le patient seit payé de molle viandes sicum arage, spinache e bletes e viandes ke legerement defient sicum poucins, perdriz, faisans e se garde de freid eawe e de chaude, mes beive eawe de zucre. Ausi a duresce de l'estomac triblét la char de dates oveke gresse de porc e surmetét. Merveilousement vaudra.

6.

[f.139r][140] De acetouse eructation .i. *soure balkinges* sont pres de iloeke touz mires deceu ke quident ke ceo seit tutdis de freid encheson. Mes a la foiz est de chalor ke overe la bouche de l'estomac par ont les fumosités montent sus e l'esperiz hors de l'estomac par ont il y a indigestion e acetouse eructation. En cest cas chaudes choses

nusent par ont serra gari par freis oynemens e freis electuaries. Ausi la diete seit freide
e grosse.

[141] De amerté de la bouche touz mires sont[22] pres de iloeke deceu ke quident ke
ceo seit tutdis de chalor e de colre. Mes a la foiz avient de freid humor resolé en fumé
e ke espessit en amere viscosité entor la lange e le palet sicum vus veét verte busche
ke n'est pas amere est resolé en fumé e espessit e devient amere fulige .i. *sot.* [f.139v]
Ausi amerté vient de freid e par chaudes choses deyt estre garrie.

7.

[142] *Emflure del ventre* est conue de ydropisie par ceo ke le patient est bien coloré
e si n'est pas le ydropic. Encontre cest mal le patient se garde de checune chose inflative
sicum novele cerveise e si deit user diaciminum, diacalamentum, diaspermaton. Ausi
use la poudre de comin, peyvre, cardamome, gingivre, fenoil. Ausi surmetét emplastre,
cyroyne ou diatarascos. Ou fetes emplastre de aloyne e de minte e de comin.

8.

[f.140r][143] *Dolor de l'estomac* a la foiz est de freid humor oveke ventosité, a la foiz
de chaud. Si de freid, ke vus conoistrét par freidure d'extremités e par pallor de la face,
purgét le premerement oveke yerapigra ague ovekes agarik ou piles orees ou piles de
elacterie ou benedicta. Pus use ces electuaries: diatrion pipereon, diaciminum, diaspermaton. A meme ceo vaut aurea alexandrina e tiriake. Si la dolor seit de ventosité
soulement, tutes chaudes choses prophitent. Ausi donét al matin la decoction de
comin e de la semence d'ache. Ausi moillét un linge drap en vin e eschaufét mult bien
al fu e metét desure e quant est refreidé eschaufét autre foiz. Meime ceo purrét fere de
leyne ou de une esponge.

[144] Si la dolor seit de chaud humor, ke vus conoistrét par citrinité de la face,
espurgét le oveke trifera sarracenica ou psillitico ou diaprunis ou donét la decoction
de tamarindes, cassiafistre, mirabolans citrins ou piles de elacterio. Ausi donét freis
electuaries sicum rosata, triasandali.

9.

[f.140v][145] *Vomit* a la foiz est de freid, a la foiz de chalor, a la foiz de habundance
des humors. Si de freidure, ke vus conoistré[t] par la urine descoloré e par habundance
de selive, donét diacitoniton chaud. Ausi fetes le user anis, mastic, minte confiz oveke
mel. Ausi surmetét emplastre a l'estomac d'encens e de mastic e de jus de minte ou
de rue. Si ceo seit de chalor, ke vus conoistrét par le urine bien coloré e par la selive
salee ou amere, espurgét le oveke psillitico ou diaprunis. Pus fetes le user cest

---

[22] MS *sont sont.*

electuarie: r[ecevét] rosarum, sumac, spodii, berberis, acatie, masticis ana unces .iii. Confisét oveke sirup roset e si vus ne eyét mie le sirup, donét la poudre. Ausi metét emplastre sur l'estomac ke seit fet de roses e d'encens e de ferine d'orge [f.141r] destempré oveke blanc de l'oef e vin egre. Si ceo seit de repletion, espurgét le humor ke est en encheson. Pus surmetét les avantdit emplastres.

[BOOK IX: INTESTINES]

1.

[146] *Flux de ventre* solunc Avicenne ou il est de mangers ou de l'ayr ou dé menbres. Si il seit dé menbres, ou il est de l'estomac ou dé veines meseraics ou de la foye ou de l'esplen ou de la teste ou des entrayles ou de tut le cors. E sachét ke il y a treis manere [de] flux de ventre. Flux ke est de vice de l'estomac est apellé *diarria*. Mes si le flux seit ovekes excoriation ou sanc ou quiture, donc est apelé *dissinteria*. E si il seit sanz change de viande, est apelé *lienteria*. Acuns l'apelent meneson sanglant.

2.

[147]Signe de *diar*[f.141v]*rie* est flux sanz sanc e quiture e il ne vient pas par certeine houre pur acrestre e amenuser. Flux del cervel vient aprés lung dormir e si vient par houres e ad signe de reume. Signe de flux ke vient de la foye est la fente semblable a l'eawe en la quele fresche char fu lavé e il y a dolor en la foye e la face ad color citrine. E ausi de flux ke est dé veines. Signe de flux splenetic est neire fiente e melancoliene e dolor de l'esplen. De flux ke est des entrailes, seit il oveke sanc ou sanz sanc, est dolor ou pointure des entrayles. Signe de flux de tut le cors est sanc pur e mult e sanz dolor e vient par houre e ad ses accés. La cure de flux de ventre est oveke choses diuretikes ke font suer sicum bain e medicines ke font vomir. E sachét ke mult dormir vaut encuntre flux e mult vaut de lyer les extremités oveke fortes bendes. E si le patient seit fort, fetes le suer en un bayn de l'eawe de la decoction de vielles roses libram semis, de balaustie unces .iii., de mirtilles, sumac ana unces .iii. E fetes le ser sur un quissin de vielles roses en meme [f.142r] le bayn ou desur un sachel plein de bren. E tiegne sa teste dehors e tiegne roses a ses narilz. Ausi pernét un lincel trebble e metét en eawe boyllante e pressét e metét sur le umbril e le penil e eschaufét le sovent. E quant il ad bien sué, donét ly a boyvre choses constrictives sicum sirup roset tempré ovekes eawe rose medlé oveke zucre rosette, oveke dragmes .ii. de sanc dragon. E fetes emplastre sur l'estomac tut chaud oveke jus de peyres vertes e jus de coinz e jus de minte ana libram semis e d'eawe rose unces .iii., de blanc vin egre unces .ii. E frotét bien l[es] extremités ke i seient eschaufez. Ausi une ventouse mise sur le ventre sanz fu, sicum Avicenne dit, estanche flux de ventre dedenz quatre houres, e nus l'avom esprové. Ausi enoynét l'estomac e les entrayles oveke ces oyles medlés ensemble: r[ecevét] olei citoniorum, olei mirtini, masticeleon, anitileon ana unces .iii. E le patient eschue freid ayr e chaud ausi.

[148] E seit nurri oveke choses stiptikes e freides sicum char de turtre quit ou rostie en vert jus [f.142v] e vin egre, car bien estanche flux oveke vin egre. Ou pernét novels coinz ou peres e trenchét a peces e metét en vin egre ou eawe rose e metét el ventre de turtre e rostét. E pus donét les peces a manger un poy e pus la char. Ausi pernét turtres ou perdriz e fetes pastes e esparpilét desure la poudre de canele e de gelofré e donét a manger. E pernét une vielle geline e appareylés oveke peyres sicum nus avom avant dit e quissét ovekes eawe de pluvie. E de cele donét al patient a manger. Nestpurquant al comencement donét les peires. E sachét ke vomit estanche flux. Fetes le vomir ovekes eawe chaude.

[149] E si ceo ne suffit point, donét plus fortes medicines sicum beivres, clisteres, poudres e electuaries. Par boyvres defiét la materie par deus jors oveke cest sirup: r[ecevét] rosarum veterum unces .iiii., violarum unce une, mirtillorum, balaustie ana unce une, zucure libram semis. Fetes sirup ovekes eawe de pluvie. Le ters jor aprés donét ly ceste decoction: r[ecevét] omnium mirabolanorum [f.143r] ana unce une. Poudrét e metét en libram semis d'eawe rose e lessét estre dehors desouz le ayr par une nuyt. E al matin colét e donét la colature. Pus fetes le user cest sirup constrictif: r[ecevét] succi plantaginis libram unam, virge pastoris, memithe, cameleonte, quin-quenervie, pentafilon ana manipulum unum, foliorum rosarum ru[?bearum] veterum unces .iiii., omnium sandalorum, mirtillorum, sumac, balaustie, ypoquistidos, acacie, berberis ana unce une, dragaganti, gummi arabici, spodii ana dragmes .ii., zucre libras .iii., seminis citoniorum unciam semis. Fetes sirup ovekes eawe de pluvie e clarifiét mult bien. E aprés le sirup donét checun jor matin ceste poudre: r[ecevét] boli armenici, gummi arabici, dragaganti ana unce une, spodii, sanguinis draconis ana dragmes .ii. Triblét e poudrét e donét de ceste poudre unciam semis oveke ptisane.

[150] Si le flux seit oveke chalor, donét ces electuaries: r[ecevét] zucure rosate alexandrine, triasandali ana libram semis, diacodion e medlét tut ensemble. Si le flux seit sanz chalor, donét ceste poudre: r[ecevét] gariofilorum unciam semis, cinnamomi, galange, mente sicce, masticis, mirre, thuris ana unce une. Fetes poudre e donét al comencement [f.143v] del manger.

[151] Si flux aviegne a enfans sanz fevre, pernét une esponge e moyllét mult bien en vin egre chaud e pus esparpilét desure ceste poudre.: r[ecevét] boli armenici, masticis, thuris albi ana unce une, spodii, sanguinis draconis ana dragmes .ii. E tut chaud metét sur l'estomac e les entrayles. Si il seit oveke fevre, r[ecevét] farine ordei libram unam, succi crassule minoris, succi plantaginis ana libram unam, aque rosate libram semis, aceti albi unces .ii. Fetes emplastre sur le umbril.

[152] Si le flux seit oveke tusse chaude, donét al matin cest sirup: r[ecevét] capilli veneris manipulos .ii., virge pastoris, arnoglosse, mirte ana manipulum [unum], rosarum, quatuor seminum frigidorum mundatorum, seminis papaveris albi, seminis portulace, omnium assatorum ana unce une, mirtillorum, sandali albi et rute, seminis coriandri ana unciam semis, dragaganti, gummi arabici, omnium assatorum ana dragmes .iii., zucure libras .ii., ordei excorticati assi libram semis. Fetes sirup ovekes eawe de pluvie. E il covient ke le pis seit enoynt checun matin de cest oynement: r[ecevét] adipis anseris, anatis, galline omnium recentorum ana unce une, butyri sine sale, [f.144r] olei violacei ana unces .iii., cere albe unce une. Fetes oynement e oveke cest oynement chaud enoynét al seir le pis soulement.

[153] Ausi si le flux seit simple flux, donét constrictifs ke estanchent flux de ventre

sicum coins, medles, poumes, mirtilles, chous, peyres nient meures, cancre de mer .i. *se-crabbe*, l[es] escales des oystres, coagle de levre, let quit, let de asne, furmage, amidun, ris, feves, la semence de neir popi, minte, roses, boli terre, asele, mastic, sumac, berberis, sanc dragon, ypoquistide, acacia, balaustie, spodium, planteyne, cincfoil.

3.

[f.144v][154] *Dissinterie* est meneson sanglant ke vus conoistrét par ceo ke la fiente est sanglante e par tortion del ventre e par dolor poygnant. E sachét ke dissinterie a la foiz acomence en bien e termine en mal e le contrere. Pur ceo est commune reule ke tel flux ne seit pas estanché avant ke la materie seit bien voidé la grenore partye, fors si il ne seit issi ke le patient est trop fieble e le flux seit trop violent. Autre reule: si le patient seit fort, fetes le seiner. Ausi premerement donét mundificatifs e pus constrictifs. Autre reule: ne donét pas grosse diete. Autre reule: donét divers mes, ke le patient eyt talent a manger. Fetes legere purgation en ceste manere: quissét violes e prunes, colét, e a la colature medlét cassiafistula e tamarindes. E autrefoiz colét e donke medlét la poudre de reubarbe ou de mirabolans citrins e donc l'endemain donét. Le ters jor fetes un bayn ové l'eawe de la decoction de roses e de plantayne. Aprés le bain donét requies oveke owele medlé de athanasie ou miclete. Mundificatifs sont mege de chevre e l'eawe de la decoction d'orge non pas [f.145r] escorcé oveke mel rouge descumé ou zucre, ke mielz vaut. Constrictifs sont: emplét une turtre ou un perdriz de cyre virgine, quissét e donét. A meme ceo fetes chous de plantayne e de su de bouk. Ausi quissét les moels des oefs e donét. Autre: pernét un oef e ostét hors de l'escale quanke il y a hors pris le moel e esparpilét desure la poudre de peivre mult bien e ardét tut a poudre e donét la al patient checun jor oveke ses viandes, si garra. La poudre de omfacii (?) vaut a meme ceo.

[155] La diete seit ke le patient se garde de vin par les treis premers jors e beive freide eawe, sicum dit Avicenne, car ele estanche le ventre. E le patient use payn demayne e al comencement del manger use peires, coyns quiz en eawe e eschue pain chaud e de superflue manger e boyvre e use viandes ke sont de tarde digestion.

4.

[f.145v][156] *Lienterie* est flux de ventre sanz change de la viande, ceo est asaver quant la viande vient hors a la chambre foreine tant e tel qu'el est reçu en l'estomac. A la foiz avient de aposteme de l'estomac, ke vus conoistrét par grant e par fevres agues. E donc fetes la cure avantdite de aposteme de l'estomac. A la foiz avient aprés dissinterie ke vus saverét par le patient par ardor de l'estomac e des entrayles. E donc est incurable. A la foiz avient de fleume e donke y a flux reumatic e l'estomac est pesant. Donc espurgét le oveke diacitoniton chaud oveke dragmes .iii. de mirabolans keblis. E fetes un bayn ovekes herbes constric[f.146r]tives sicum mattefelon, moleine, rose canine, minte. Pus aprés le bain donét miclete ou athanasie oveke l'eawe de la decoction de minte. Si lienterie seit de chaud encheson, espurgét le oveke unciam semis de diadragant freid oveke dragmes .iii. de mirabolans citrins. Le ters jor aprés fetes un bayn de roses e plantayne. Aprés le bayn doné[t] requiem e miclete en owel peis. Ausi en l'un e l'autre encheson vaut tiriake doné ové le jus de minte. La diete seit tele cum en dissinterie. Sachét ke la poudre de turtre arse vaut pur checun flux de ventre.

5.

[f.146v][157] Ore dirrum de *lumbriz*. Sachét ke ceus ke ont lumbriz a la foiz resemblent frenetics, a la foiz maniacs, a la foiz melancoliens, a la foiz colics ou yliacs, a la foiz epilemptics. Ces sont communes signes. Mes propres signes sont prurit de[s] levres e de[s] narilz, puor de la bouche, grele voyz, dolor de l'estomac e tortion des entrayles. Pur ceo est commune reule ke le patient manjue checun jor matin. Autre reule est ke vus dorrez ameres choses oveke douce choses, mes ke plusors esperimenz seyent ke occient lumbris. Nestpurquant veét issi les plus especials. Destemprét la poudre de corn de cerf ars ové mel e donét. A meme ceo vaut le jus de persicarie ové let de chevre. A meme ceo vaut aloyne, ysope. A meme ceo veét ci bon electuarie: r[ecevét] centonice libram unam, seminis canabi unces .iiii., zucare dragmes .iii., cardamomi unces .ii., cornu cervini unciam unam et semis, mellis quod sufficit. A meme ceo vaut electuarie de centonike soulement e de mel. Pus pur fere les venir hors pernét l'escorce de la racine de poume gernette e l'escorce de [f.147r] fresne e triblét o vin e quissét e donét matin e seir. Ceo est esprové. A meme ceo vaut la poudre de corn de cerf oveke vin egre, e ceo est esprové. Par dehors enoynét le ventre oveke fel de tor e jus de centorie. Le patient se garde ke il ne manjue nul frut.

GLOSSARY

Given the length of the text the glossary is more selective than for the shorter works and excludes botanical names and the names of simples already included in the other glossaries, for which instead I provide a simple listing. All medical terminology, including the names of compound medicines, is fully recorded. References are to paragraph numbers. AN = **Antidotarium Nicolai** ed. W.S. van den Berg.

Abstinence s. 132   abstinence
Accés s. 37,40,47,49,122,147   bout, attack, onset
Accident s. 121,122   symptom
Acharistum s. 102   a kind of antidote (AN 3)
Alener v.n. 59,103   to breathe
Als s.pl. 53   garlic
Amerté s. 141   bitterness
Analemptic a./s. 43   (one) suffering from analepsy
Analemptie s. 37   analepsy, gastric epilepsy
Anitileon s. 147   'anethelaeon', oil of dill
Anorexia s. 133   lack of appetite
Anoytement s. 112,114   increase
Antimonii s. 67   stibnite, sulphide of antimony
Aperitif a. 11   aperient, opening
Apoplexie s. 54,58–62   apoplexy
Aposteme s. 18,20,21,25,34,62,80,91,98,103,106,109,110,112,136,137,138,156
impostume, boil, ulcer
Aromatic a./s. 30,83,111,135   aromatic
Arsure s. 133   burning sensation
Arterie s. 85   artery
Artetique s. 43   gout affecting the joints **freide a.** 43
Asma s. 120   asthma
Aspresce s. 103,107   roughness
Athanasia, athanasie s. 102,154   a medicament (AN 4)
Aurea(m alexandrina(m s. 62,143   a medicament (AN 1)
Autor s. 24,42,62,64,81,82,83,84,97,99,106,124,126,127   author, authority
Aventurousement adv. 48,90   accidently
Basilica s. 86,137   basilic vein
Benedicta s. 62,134,143   a medicament (AN 9)
Blandisant a. 106   soothing, palliative
Blite s. 111   beet see **Plant Names** sub **blitis**
Bolisme s. 128   bulimy, excessive appetite
Bolismus s. 127   bulimy, excessive appetite
Bru s. 29,36,47   broth
Brusure s. 10,17,101   fracture. rupture
Canin a. 27,28   see **manie**
Cantarides s.pl. 49   blister beetles (Cantharis vesicatoria)
Cardiake s. 71,122,124,126   heart ailment marked by pain and palpitation
Cathalemptie s. 37,38,49   catalepsy
Cendal s. 94   a silken fabric, cendal
Cephalargia s.1   type of headache

Cephalea s. 1   type of headache
Chacie s. 68   rheum, matter in eyes
Chael s. 29   whelp, pup
Chapitre s. 105,122,132   chapter
Chiche s. 99   chickpea (as a measure); 129   chickpea
Cince s. 87,94   strip, bandage
Cinorodoxa s. 127,128   bulimy, excessive appetite
Citrin a. 147   yellow
Citrinité s. 144   yellow colour
Clistere, clystere s. 18,24,25,35,62,98,149   clyster, enema
Clisterizer v.a. 24,25,35   to administer clyster to
Coagle de levre s. 42,153   rennet of the hare
Coilz, coylz s.pl. 38,49,56,86   testicles
Colagoge s. 126   cholagogue (for drawing off bile)
Colature s. 24,98,99,149,154   strained, sieved matter
Coleric a./s. 55,85,105,133   choleric, (one) suffering from bile
Colic s. 157   one suffering from colic
Collirie s. 67,70,72,74,77,78,81   collyrium, eye salve
Colre s. 1,34,39,98,130,131,141   choler, bile
Complexion s. 1,31,54,55,122   complexion (med.); 62   facial complexion
Concave a. 84   hollowed out
Concaver v.a. 91   to hollow out
Confection s. 131   medical preparation
Confortatif a. 33,47,98,122,128,134   soothing
Constrictif a. 147,149,153,154,156   constringent
Coriza, corize s. 89   flow of humours to nostrils
Costivé a. 35,115   constipated
Costiveson s. 22   constipation
Courvé a. 105   bent
Crampe s. 22   cramp
Cyroyne s. 110,139,142   wax plaster (AN 46)
Cyrurgie s. 29   surgery
Cyrurgien s. 88   surgeon
Darz s. 46   dace
Declination s. 112,114   decline, recession
Declineson s. 112   decline, recession
Decyrer v.a. 21   to tear
Demoniac a./s. 37,45   insane
Dessavoré a. 133   unsavoury, distasteful
Destemperance s. 130,132,133   excessive exposure (to)
Diacalamentum s. 127,142   medicament containing calamint (AN 29)
Diacelidonion s. 98   medicament containing celandine
Diaciminum s. 124,142,143   medicament containing cumin (AN 24)
Diacitoniton s. 52,119,145,156   medicament containing quince (AN 34)
Diacodion s. 102,150   medicament containing poppy (AN 31)
Diadragant(um s. 104,113,117,118,120,156   medicament made with gum tragacanth (AN 27)
Diaforetica a. 124,126   sudorific, name for 'cardiake'
Diagalanga, diagalange s. 47,52   medicament containing galingale (AN 38)
Diamargariton s. 126   medicament containing pearls (AN 14)
Diamoron s. 9   medicament containing mulberries (AN 16)
Dianisum s. 124   medicament containing aniseed
Diaolibanum s. 68   medicament containing frankincense (AN 21)
Diapenidion s. 104,113,118,119   medicament containing barley sugar (AN 23)

Diaprassium s. 127   medicament containing white horehound (Marrubium vulgare L.) (AN 20)

Diaprunis s. 130,144,145   medicament containing plums (AN 19)

Diarria, diarrie s. 146,147   diarrhoea

Diasené s. 33,52   medicament containing senna (AN 33)

Diaspermaton s. 124,142,143   medicament containing whale sperm

Diatarascos s. 142   a kind of wax plaster

Diatrion pipereon s 143   a medicament containing three types of pepper (AN p.37)

Digestif s. 49   digestive, aid to digestion

Dissinteria, dissinterie s. 146,154,156   dysentery

Dissolutif a. 114   solvent, having the property of dissolving or dissipating a condition

Diuretik a. 147   diuretic

Drasche de vin s. 72   lees of wine

Ebullissement s. 75   inflammation

Electuaire, electuarie s. 41,52,102,104,113,114,117,119,122,127,128,130,134,135,140,143, 144,145,149,150,157   electuary

Emathides s. 102   haematite, native iron oxide

Embruer v.a. 86   to soak, steep

Emigranea s. 1   severe headache

Emoptoicus s. 101   one suffering from haemoptysis, spitting blood

Emoptois s. 103   haemoptysis, spitting blood

Emorroides s.pl. 27,31   haemorrhoids

Empic s. 105   one suffering from empyema

Empicus s. 103   one suffering from empyema

Empima, empimate s. 103,105   empyema, collection of pus resulting from pleurisy

Enaguser v.a. 30,33,125   to sharpen, render tart or pungent

Enbruer v.a. 3,23   to steep, soak

Enmeurer v.a. 98,110   to ripen

Enmoister v.a. 32   to humidify

Entempré p.p. 32,52   mild, temperate

Epilemptic a./s. 37,38,42,157   (one) suffering from epilepsy

Epilemptie s. 37,41,42   epilepsy

Eruct(u)ation s. 133,140   belching, retching

Escoper v.n. 101,103   to spit

Esdra s. 62   a medicament (AN 39)

Esperiment s. 29,45,48,52,64,72,74,83,106,122,131,131,157   experiment, proof, test

Esplen s. 119   spleen

Estapir v.n. 88   to lodge, lie hidden

Estat s. 112,114,137   paroxysm

Esternier v.n. 44,62,83,89,121   to sneeze

Estront s. 86,98   excrement, dung

Estumac, estomac s. 119,124   stomach

Et(h)ike s. 105,127   hectic fever (accompanying pulmonary tuberculosis)

Excoriation s. 146   loss or removal of skin (epidermis or membrane of internal organ)

Exsolucio s. 121   syncope, faint

Fastidium s. 133   lack of appetite, distaste for food

Fecche s. 44   ? vessel, measure

Festue s. 35   blade of straw

Fievre s. fever **f. cotidiane continue** 36   continuous quotidian fever (i.e. with daily paroxysms)

Fleumatic s. 55,105,133   one who is phlegmatic

Fleume s. 1,4,34,62,65,97,98,127,130,156   phlegm

Flurs s.pl. 31,85,90,122   menses

Flux de ventre s. 38,107,122,146,147,153,156   diarrhoea

Foutre vbl.n. 42   sexual intercourse

Frenesie s. 20,22,23,26   madness, delirium, frenzy
Frenetic a./s. 8,34,157   (one) suffering from frenesis, madness
Fulige s. 141   soot
Fumigation s. 11,41,42,76,79,89,90,91,117   treatment with aromatic fumes
Fumosité s. 4,6,8,29,49,140   hot gas within the body, vapour, exhalation, fume
Funtaynele, fontaynele s. 63,88,91   hollow (at back of neck), fontanelle
Gargari(s)me s. 62,91,98,106   gargle
Garse s. 29   scarification
Garser v.a. 95   to scarify
Gingive s. 93,95,96,97   gum
Glette s. 131   mucus, phlegm
Glumous a. 79   sticky
Goute s. **g. cheve** 37   epilepsy
Gruel s. 36   gruel
Gule s. 101   throat
Haterel s. 95   nape of neck
Humable a. 49   swallowable
Humor s. 38,50,52,54,58,62,79,88,89,91,120,122,126,127,133,134,144,145   humour
Inanition s. 122   morbid depletion of bodily humours
Inflatif a. 142   promoting swelling or wind
Inversion s. 66   inversion
Juliani s. 82   a medicament
Juner v.n. 42   to fast
Laveure s. 11   lotion
Laxatif a./s. 62,115   laxative
Lenitif a. 24   lenitive, soothing, softening
Lentille s. 90   freckle
Lesche (de pain) s. 122   slice (of bread)
Lienteria, lienterie s. 146,156   a type of diarrhoea, 'meneson sanglant'
Limure s. 94   filings
Lippotamia s. 121   syncope, faint
Litargic a./s. 35   (one) suffering from lethargy
Lithargie s. 34   disease of the brain from an aposteme in the rear ventricle causing lethargy
and forgetfulness
Lumbriz (de terre) s. 15,86,124,127,157   earthworm
Lune s. 39,47,84   moon
Lupin a. 27,28   see **manie**
Lunatic s. 37   lunatic
Lus s. 46   pike
Malascher v.a. 3,17,52,64   to knead
Malfactio s. 121   syncope, faint
Malicious a. 38   malignant
Maniac a. 51,157   suffering from mania
Manie s. 27–29   mania **m. lupine** 27,28 **m. canine** 27,28
Marciaton s. 135   marciaton, a green ointment (AN 130)
Mariz s. 85,86,122   womb
Masticacion s. 41   masticatory, medical substance designed to be chewed
Masticeleon s. 138,147   oil of mastic
Maturatif a. 80,98,114   ripening
Mayle s. 69   leucoma
Melancolie s. 1,3,4,27,31,32,65,71,127   back bile **m. sanguiniene** 31 black bile mixed with
blood **m. naturele** 37
Melancolien a./s. 29,33,55,157   (one) suffering from melancholia (black bile); mixed with
black bile
Meneson s. 146,154   diarrhoea

Meule del cervel s. 20   brain marrow
Miclete s. 154,156   an electuary (AN 58)
Mitigatif a. 80   pain-reducing
Mordificatif a. 24,35,62,98   caustic, corrosive
Mundificatif a. 98,114,154   cleansing
Muscillage s. 131   mucilage
Nature s. 38   semen
Nectilopa s. 71   nyctalopia, dimness of vision after sunset (often misunderstood as hemeralopia, dimness of day vision)
Niwele s. 29   cake
Obtalmia s. 63   aposteme in the eye, inflammation (of the conjunctiva)
Opiate s. 62   opiate
Opilation s. 11,67,122   blockage, obstruction, stopping up
Opopira(m s. 62   a medicament (AN 69)
Orexis s. 133   appetite
Oximel s. oxymel, preparation of vinegar, herbs and honey (AN 72) **o. squillitic** 47   made with squills
Palet s. 141   palate
Pan s. 90   blotching or discoloration of the skin, esp. the face
Pareye s. 21   wall
Parlesie s. 43,54,60   paralysis, palsy
Paulini s. 119   a medicament, 'Paulinum antidotum' (AN 74)
Paumeson s. 121,122,123   syncope, faint
Pel s. 112   costal pleura
Perche s. 46   perch (fish)
Peripleumonie s. 109   aposteme in the lungs, pmeumonia
Pica s. 71   nuthatch
Pile s. 47,62,97,99,107   pill **p. diacastorum** 62 (AN 80) **piles orees** 143 (AN 79) **piles de elacterie/elacterio** 143,144   pills made with sediment or precipitate of wild / squirting cucumber (AN 88)
Pillule s. 62   small pill **pillulis fetidis** 62 (AN 90)
Planson s. 23,122   sole (of foot)
Pleuresi(e s. 20,109,112,113   pleurisy
Pliris s. 47,52   an electuary, 'pliris arcoticon' (AN 41)
Plume s. 25   lead
Pointure s. 147   pricking or stinging sensation
Poket s. 91,131   little bag
Polipus s. 86   polyp
Pontike, pontic a./s. 98,111   (something) tart, astringent
Por s. 88   pore
Pres de iloec adv. 37   almost
Prurit s. 68,74,157   itching, pruritus
Psillitico s. 144   'emplastrum psilliticum' (AN 45) made from fleawort
Ptisane, ptisana s. 98,104,114,115,145,150   infusion, tisane
Ptisic a. 105   consumptive
Ptisik(e a./s. 57,103,104,105,106,107,127   consumptive, (one) suffering from phthisis; phthisis
Pulent a. 105   foul, filthy
Punction s. 133   pricking sensation
Purgation s. 84,130,154   purging
Quarteyne s. 126   quartan fever
Quartroun s. 4,33,56   quarter (measure)
Queldour conj. 37,41,105   whether
Quiture s. 75,80,82,83,103,105,146,147   pus, discharge
Remedie s. 52,62,90   remedy

Repercussif a. 25,35,63,80,98,114   designed to reduce swelling, expelling harmful matter
Repletion s. 43,89,122,145   morbid excess of humours; excessive intake of, indulgence in
(e.g. eating and drinking); fullness
Requies, requiem s. 154,156   a medicament (AN 95)
Retention s. 90   retention
Reule s. 9,24,29,35,38,41,42,62,63,64,71,78,80,88,89,90,91,98,109,124,125,133,135,154,
157   rule, practice
Reumatic a. **flux r.** 156   flow of rheum
Reume s.76,88,89,91,99,106,107,147   rheum, matter in the eye; nasal mucus; cold in the
head
Rosata s. 130,144,150   electuary containing essence of roses (AN 42)
Rosate novelle s. 52   a medicament made with roses (AN 93)
Ruptorie s. 49   ruptory
Sachel s. 113,147   little bag
Salvatelle s. 86   the vein known as salvatella
Sanguinien a./s. 31,85   see **melancolie**; 55 one who is sanguine
Sargiotides s.pl. 42   veins beneath the tongue
Sausefleume s. 62,130   sauceflegm, 'salt phlegm'
Savo(u)n s. 62   soap **s. de France** 90 soda-ash soap
Scotomie s. 51   scotoma, dizziness accompanied by dimness of vision
Secundime s. 44   afterbirth, placenta
Seif s. 130,131,132   thirst
Sei(g)né s. 117,122   bleeding
Selive, salive s. 103,105,112,145   saliva
Sincopia s. 121   syncope, faint
Sirup s. 41,56,102,106,113,117,119,134,137,138,149,152   syrup **s. roset** 145,147   syrup of
roses
Soda s. 1   type of severe headache
Soniz s. 11,81   buzzing noise (in ears)
Sourdesce s. 84   deafness
Spasme s. 22,43   cramp, convulsive seizure
Spiritual a. 59   pertaining to bodily fluids esp. the vital spirit; respiratory
Spiritual(i)té s. 61,122,126   vital spirit, bodily fluid
Splenetic a. 147   emanating from the spleen
Squinantie s. 98   quinsy
Stiptic, stiptik a./s. 46,111,148   styptic
Suffocation s. 122   suffocation
Suffumer v.a. 86   to suffumigate
Suffumigation s. 99   suffumigation, treatment with aromatic fumes
Suppositorie s. 25,35,62,98   suppository
Tente s. 86   tent, pledget, seton
Tercein a. 131   tertian (of fever)
Teye s. 69,74   web or cataract in eyes
Theodericon euperiston s. 62   a medicament (AN 117)
Tiriake s. 42,62,90,135,143,156   theriac, medicine effective against poison **t. mitridatum**
62   a medicament (AN 56) **la grande t.** 'Tyriaca magna Galieni' (AN 111)
Tortion del ventre s. 154   colic, stomach cramp **t. des entrayles** 157
Tran(s)glo(u)ter v.a. 31,99   to swallow
Triasandali s. 126,135,144,150   medicament containing three kinds of sandalwood (AN
116)
Trifera s. 130   soothing medical preparation (AN 113,114) **t. sarracenica** 144 (AN 113)
Trocisce s. 131   trocisk
Tusse s. 99,103,105,107,112,152   cough
Tusser v.n. 105   to cough
Tutie s. 66,72   tutty, oxide of zinc

Ungle s. 69   'nail', 'haw' (growth in the eye)
Veine s. vein **v. capitale** 2,18,23,29,35,50,52,63,64,71,91,95,98   cephalic vein **v. cardiake** 113,117   cardiac vein **v. epatike** 134   hepatic vein **la mene v.** 17   median vein **v. meseraic** 146   mesaraic vein
Ventoser v.a. 29   to bleed (with cupping glass)
Ventosité s. 4,19,79,124,143   morbid wind in body, flatulence
Ventouse s. 2,29,63,88,91,98,99,147   cupping glass
Verm s. 91,122   worm
Vertin s. 37,51   giddiness, vertigo
Vescie s. 22   blister
Veye de l'urine s. 38   urinary tract
Viscosité s. 141   viscosity
Viscous a. 112   viscous
Vit s. 86   penis
Vomit s. 27,42,148   vomitory; 101,145   vomit
Ydropic s. 142   one suffering from dropsy
Ydropisie s. 85,142   dropsy
Yera fortis s. 62   a medicament (AN 146 'Yera fortissima Galieni')
Yeralogodion s. 33,47,62,71,91,127   a bitter medicine containing aloes (cf. AN 141)
Yerapigre s. 47,119,126,143   a bitter, purgative medicine containing aloes (cf. AN 143)
Yliac s. 157   one suffering from disease of the kidneys
Yris illirica s. 120   Iris, prob. Yellow Flag (Iris pseudacorus L.)
Yveresce s. 54–6   inebriation

Middle English Words

Floccle 118   (leine carpie) lint
Flocke s. 17,52   'courte leyne' lint
Hnotehech s. 71   nuthatch
Kousleppe s. 91   cowslip
Maddocke s. 87   earthworm
Meriswermode s. 15   'sea wormwood' (Artemisia maritima L.)
Popy s. 99,107   poppy
Se-crabbe s. 153   sea crab ('cancre de mer')
Sot 141   'fulige', soot
Soure balkinges 139   'acetouse eructation'
Turtouse s. 107   'limaçon dé boys'
Wanhede s. 90   discoloration (**livor**)
Wodecrabbe s. 81   crab apple
Yecche s. 68,74   itching

Arabic Words

Karabicus s. 20   frenzy, madness, delirium
Sirsen s. 20 =   'karabicus'

Proper Names

Alisandre 8,37,48,98,127,135   Alexander (of Tralles)
Almasor 20   title (Liber ad Almansorem) of a compendium by Rhazes
Amphorimes, Amforimes 44,85   Aphorisms (of Hippocrates)

REPERTOIRE OF SIMPLES[1]

Vegetabilia

abscinthium
acacia
ache (racine de, jus de, semence de)
acorus (poudre de)
adianthos
agaricus
agarik
alemande (amere)(oyle de, let de)
allia
aloe
aloen cicotrin
aloes
alosne
aloyne
altea (semen, radix)
aluine
amidoun
amidum
amigdala dulcis
amilum
amomum
anet
anetum
anis
anthos
antophali
apium (radix)
arage
armoniac
arnoglossa
asa
aveyne
averoyne
ayl
balaustie
basilicon (jus de)
baume
berberis
betonica
betoyne
bisantia
blacca
blete (jus de)
blite
bombax (medulla seminis)
borage (jus de)
borago (flores)
brance ursine (foilz de)
bren (de furment)
bruscus (semen)
buglossa (radix)
buglosse (jus de)
bux (foylz de)
calamente
calamentum
calamus aromaticus
camedreos
cameleonta
camepiteos
camomilla (flores)
camomille (jus de)
canabum (semen)
candi
canele
canv(r)e (tendrons de)
capilli veneris
capparis
cardamome
cardamomum
carica
carpobalsamum
carui
cassiafistula
cassiefistre
cassialigna
caulis (albus) (succus)
celidonia
celidonium

---

[1] Latin names are asterisked. Specified parts of the plants are indicated in brackets. For compound medicines see Glossary.

centonica
centonike (jus de)
centorie
centrum galli (greins de)
ceraser (gumme de)
ceterac
chastein
chenilé (racine de)
chiche
cholet (jus de)
chou
cicoree
cinamomum
cincfoil
cinnamon
citonia
citruli
coin
columbine
comin
consolida major
consolida media
consolida minor
coriandrum (semen)
coudre
coyn
crassula (succus)
crassula minor (succus)
crocus
cubebe(s)
cucumbre (savage) (racine de)
cucurbita
cuscuta
cynoglossa
date (char)
daucus
diptayne (poudre de)
egremoyne (foilz de)
ellebre (poudre de)
encens (blanc)
endive
endivia
enula
epatica
epithime
epithimus
euforbe (poudre de)
euforbium
eufrasia
eupatorium

everoyne
faba
feniculus (teneritates, radix)
fenoil (racine de, jus de, foilz de, jus e la
    racine de, semence de)
fenugrec
fenugrecum
ferine (potage de)
festue
feve (ferine de)
fige (blanc, sec)
figer
filipendula
folia lauri
folium
foylz de bux
frasere (jus de)
fumeterre (jus de)
furment (greins de)
gaia muscata
galanga
galingale
galle
gariofilum
gelofré (poudre de)
gentiana
germandrea
gingivre (poudre de)
grape (verte) (jus de)
gumme arabic
gummi arabici
heyre terrestre (jus de)
jubarbe (jus de)
jumente (let de)
junevre
jusquiame (summés de)
kousleppe
lactuca (semen)
ladanum
lancelé
lange de chien
laureole
laurus (bacca)
letuse (jus de)
leveine
licium
licoriz (racine de, jus de, poudre de la racine
    de)
lignum aloes
lilie (racine de)

lilium (radix)
lin (semence de)
linum (semen)
liquiricia (succus)
lorer (bays de)
lovache
macis
malva (semen)
maratrum
maroil
marrubium album
mastic
mastix
mattefelon
mauve (foilz de)
medle
melisse
mellilote (jus de)
mellilotum
melo (semen)
melon
memitha
menta (sicca)
meos
merculiale
meu
milium
minte (jus de)
mirabolan (citrin, keble)
mirabolanum
mirta
mirte (foilz de)
mirtille
mirtilli
mirtus
moleine
morele (jus de)
mustarde
nenufar (flor de)
noys mugette
nux muscata
olibanum
opie
opium
opopanac
ordeum
orge (farine d', payle d', eawe d')
origanum
orobi
oynon (jus de)

ozimum
papaver albus (semen)
parele (rouge) (racine de)
paritarie (jus de)
pastinake
peivre (lung)
pelestre (poudre de)
pentafilon
peoyne
persicarie (jus de)
persil
petrosilium (radix)
peucedanum
peyre (jus de)
pimpinella
piper (longus)
piretrum
pistacea
plantago (succus)
plantayne (jus de)
policarie
politricum
pome (grenette, savage, aromatike) (escorce
       de, escorce de la racine de, jus de, vin de)
popi (neir) (semence de)
popy (blanc)
poret (jus de)
portulaca (semen)
prassium
primerole savage (jus de)
prune (blanche)
pruner (gumme de)
prunus damascenus
psillium (semence de)
pulegium
pulleole
pulpa colloquintide
purcelane
quinquenervia
radich (racine de)
rapistre
ris
rose (foilz de, poudre de)
rose canine
rosmarin
rostrum porcinum
rue (jus de; fumigation)
ruta
saffran
salvia

sambuc
sanc (de) dragon
sanguis draconis
sandalus albus
sandles
sanigle
sarcocolla
satureia
satureye
sauge
saus (foilz de)
scamonee
scariola
scolopendria
scordeon
sebasten
sena
sené
senecion
serpillum
siegle (pain de)
sinonum
sisimbrium
sparage
sparagus (semen)
spica nardi
spigornele
spike
spinache
squinant
squinantum
staphizagre (poudre de)
sticados

storax liquida/calamite
sumac
tamarinde
terebentine
tetesoriz (jus de)
thime
thimus
thus (albus)
titimal (let de)
tormentille
ungula caballina aquatica (radix)
uve passe
valeriana
verveine (foilz de, racine de)
vervena
vin blanc, pur, v. egre blanc
vine (blanche)
viola
viole
violette (flur de, foilz de, jus de)
virga pastoris
wimauve (racine de)
wodecrabbe
xilobalsamum
ypoquistidos
yreos (racine de)
yris illirica
ysope
ysopus
zinziber
zucre (rosette)
zucura

Animalia

aignel (joefne) (char de a. de un an)
ambre
anas (adeps)
angille/angulle (gresse de, sanc de, fel de)
anser (adeps)
arunde
asne (estront de, let de)
boef (char de, fel de)
bouc (sanc de, su de)
bure (fresche)
butyrum (sine sale)
cancre de fluvie/de fluvie
cantarides
castor (poudre de)

castoreum
cerf (quer de, la meule des os de, corn de)
chael (blanc)
chapon
cheveril (char de)
chevre (char de, foye de, let de, mege de, urine de)
chien (estront de)
coc (sanc de)
columb (sanc de, sanc dé pijuns de)
columba (sanguis)
columbel
corn de cerf (rasure de, limure de)
cornu cervinum

darz
faisan (char de)
geline (gresse de, char de)
heyron (gresse de)
let de femme
levre (coagle de, char de, fel de, peils de)
limaçon dé boys
limasoun (rouge) (gresse de, poudre de)
lumbriz de terre
lus
maddock
madlard (gresse de)
medulla cervina
mel
moton (char de, coilz de, pel de, pomon de)
mulsa
musc
oef (blanc de l', moele d')
owe (gresse de)
oyseus ke vivent en riveres/de rivere/de
  ravine (les fels de)
oystre

perche
perdriz
pesson (de fluvie)
pica (hnotehech)
poon (char de)
porc (char de, grasse char de lard de, vielle
  gresse de, novele gresse de, char de jeune
  porc non pas gras, pés de)
poucin
samsucus
sancsue
savon (de France)
se-crabbe
sengler (coilz de)
spodium
tor (fel de)
tortouse
turtre
vache (char de, la meule e l'os de quisse de)
yreine (teile de)

Mineralia

alum de plume
ambre
amoniac
antimonium
arnement
camphora
camphre
ebor (limatura)
emathides
emeraude
iacincta
lapis armenicus

lapis lazuli
lithargire
nitre
orpiment
piz
pomiz
salgemme
salisgemme
sel
tutie (poudre de)
vitreole

Oils

oleum mirtinum, oyle de anet, oyle de
  camomille, oyle laurin, oyle de lils, oyle
  muscellin, oyle nardin, oyle de pulleole,
  oyle roset, oyle viole, oyle violette

Miscellaneous

courte leine   leyne carpie
cyre blanche   rouge cyre cyre virgine cera
  nigra

cyroyne
blanc vin (aromatique)
merum

payn (net, demayne)(cruste de)
oximel (squillitic)
furmage
let
encens (blanc) (poudre de)
penides
bolus (armenicus)
bol (armenic)
candii
penidii

sucre rosette
jujube
manna
ozimum
pain demayne
furmage (viel)
acetum album
mel rouge

CHAPTER FOUR

The Trinity 'Practica'

The present work is by far the most extensive medical compendium to include vernacular material which has survived in England. With only a few fragments of English, the work essentially mixes Latin and Anglo-Norman. The design of the work is that of a 'Practica Medicinae' in which material is arranged topically, *a capite ad calcem*. This structure is disturbed by the incorporation of lengthy sections on phlebotomy, prognostications, and urines. The section on the stomach appears to have been fragmented and misplaced. For ease of consultation I have divided the work into books and paragraphs.

Contents

The compendium begins with conditions of the head, distinguishing 'apoplexia' (3–4), 'epilencia' (5) and 'cephalia' (6), the latter subdivided into 'mania' (7), 'frenesis', 'litargia' (8–9) and 'melancolia' (6). Complaints from internal causes are completed with 'cephalia' (10) and 'scotomia' (11). Complaints with external causes (12) are listed as 'favus' (13), 'acora' (14), 'tinea' (15,20*,27*,28*,31*)[1] and 'canicies' (16). The appearance of 'vertigo capitis' (17,14*,24*,26*) marks a return to internally caused conditions like 'emigranea' (19,20*). Several sections (18,21–23,25) are composed of remedies for a variety of conditions involving headache. It is noteworthy that detailed consideration is given to infestations of the head (see 'tinea' above) and hair conditions (28*,29*,30*). There then follow sections on the throat (32*) and facial complexion (33*,34*,35*,37,38).

Book Two deals with eye conditions, distinguishing the terms 'strabo', 'paetus', 'luscus' and 'lippus' (39). Again there is a distinction drawn between internally and externally caused complaints (40*). Conditions arising from external causes are listed as 'tela', 'macula', 'ungula', 'pannus', 'albugo', 'ulcera', 'sanguis' (41). The sections of remedies contain a high proportion of vernacular entries (42*,43*,44,45*,46*,47*, 48*,49*, 50*,51*) and the use of charms (52*). The use of charms appears to have been the motivation for three sections on sleep (53*,54*,55*).

Complaints of the ear constitute the material of Book Three. Again the distinction is made between internal (56) and external causation (57), the latter including infestation by fleas and invasion by dust particles or grit. Conditions dealt with include tinnitus (58*), deafness (59*) and auricular infestation (60*). Not surprisingly this is one of the shortest books in the treatise.

---

[1] An asterisk denotes the use of Anglo-Norman, whether in whole or in part, in a given section.

Book Four (61*,62*) is devoted to the nose and is even shorter than Book Three.

Book Five deals with the mouth including halitosis (63*), ulceration (65), complaints affecting the ysophagus ('squinantia') which include 'peritunia' and 'suffocatio' (66), scalding, excessive saliva production etc.(67*).

The teeth are the subject of Book Six which covers dental decay and discoloration and gum disease (68*,69,70*71*,72*) and includes the use of charms (73*). This Book is interrupted on f.13 by a passage on the stomach which is insititious and has been relocated in the text printed below as Book Ten (91–95). There is a short section on chapped lips (74). There follow in the MS a number of misplaced passages (75 and see note 286).

The subject of the next section, which draws on Bede's *De minutione sanguinis*,[2] is phlebotomy, its virtues (76*), recommended days and 'Egyptian days' (77*).[3] As in Book Six (68*), the Anglo-Norman remedies are in verse (78*,79*) drawn from the 'Physique Rimee'. The Book ends with a number of charms (79*). Phlebotomy was an important subject which has been shown to have an interesting theoretical basis in the Middle Ages.[4] A large number of short treatises '(Epistola) de phlebotomia' were produced, along with a number of Salernitan works which were published as a series of German doctoral dissertations.[5]

Book Seven deals with the hands and feet, particularly rheumatic conditions and types of gout and skin eruptions (80*,81*,82*,83*,84*).

Book Eight deals with the penis and once more versified Anglo-Norman receipts are given (85*). There is one item of Middle English (86*).

The bladder attracts more extended treatment as Book Nine and covers the usual conditions like vessicular calculus or bladder stone (88*) and strangury (89*). Nephritis is also included, as is swelling of the testicles (89*).

Book Ten is the relocated passage on the stomach (91–5) which contains no vernacular material. It is likely that the passage on 'lienteria' (95) should be followed

---

2   See *PL* 90, cols.959C–962C.

3   See J. Loiseleur, "Les jours égyptiens. Leurs variations dans les calendriers du moyen âge", *Mémoires de la société des antiquaires de France* 33 (1872), 198–253; R.S. Steele, "Dies Aegyptiaci", *Proceedings of the Royal Society of Medicine* 12 (suppl.) (1918–19), 108–21; W.R. Dawson, "Some Observations on the Egyptian Calendars of Lucky and Unlucky Days", *Journal of Egyptian Archaeology* 12 (1926), 260–4; M. Förster, "Die altenglischen Verzeichnisse von Glücks – und Unglückstagen" in K. Malone and M.B. Ruud (eds.), *Studies in English Philology. A Miscellany in Honor of Frederick Klaeber* (Minneapolis, 1929) [pp.258–77] pp.261–5, 270–7; O. Södergård, "Notes sur les jours périlleux de l'année", *Neuphilologische Mitteilungen* 55 (1954), 267–71. See also Ps.-Bede, PL 90, 960D–61C.

4   As an introduction to the subject see P. Brain, *Galen on Bloodletting* (Cambridge, 1986); P. Gil-Sotres, '*Scripta minora' de flebotomia en la tradición médica del siglo XIII*, Cuadernos de historia de la medicina 1 (Santander / Pamplona, 1986); id., "Derivation and Revulsion in the Theory and Practice of Medieval Phlebotomy" in L. García-Ballester *et al.* (eds.), *Practical Medicine from Salerno to the Black Death* (Cambridge, 1994), pp.110–55; L.E. Voigts and M.R. McVaugh, *A Latin Technical Phlebotomy and its Middle English Translation*, Trans. Am. Philos. Soc. 74, ii (1984), pp.1–69; J. Baier, *Geschichte der Aderlässe* 2nd ed. (München, 1966).

5   For example, A. Morgenstern, 'Das Aderlassgedicht des Johannes von Aquila' diss. Leipzig, 1917 and H. Erchenbrecher, 'Der Salernitaner Arzt Archimatthaeus und ein bis heute unbekannter Aderlasstraktat unter seinem Namen', diss. Leipzig, 1919. See also the *Flos medicinae* Pt.8, c.x in Renzi, *Coll. Sal.* 5, pp.78–82.

by that on 'dissinteria' which concludes the compendium on f.29. I have repositioned the latter accordingly.

Book Eleven treats the intestines (96,97*) and Book Twelve the kidneys (98,99*). Book Thirteen deals with the anus (100*,101*).

The knees,legs and feet form the subject of Book Fourteen, covering gout, swellings and skin eruptions in a somewhat random manner (102*, 103,104,105,106*,107*).

This is where the 'Practica' comes to a natural end.

There now follows a treatise on prognostications which is something of a jumble, the Latin section (108–111) being based on the first two books of Hippocrates' *Prognostics* with section 112 drawing on the *Aphorisms*. Section 113 is a compilation of Anglo-Norman prognostic receipts whilst 114–116 represent an Anglo-Norman translation of the pseudo-Hippocratic prognostic treatise known as *Capsula eburnea*.[6] The Anglo-Norman sections are accurate enough, but the Latin sections suffer from frequently garbled statements and omissions which leave the context and significance of many symptoms and signs unclear. For example, the highly pessimistic Latin original is concerned almost exclusively with acute febrile diseases, though this fact is scarcely apparent from the excerpts offered in the present work which appear in almost random order despite being derived predominantly from the first book of the *Prognostics*. I therefore give a detailed account of this section of the Trinity 'Practica'. In addition an interesting elucidation of the pseudo-Hippocratic text will be found in the commentary composed by the twelfth-century Salernitan master, Maurus, whose most important work was a commentary on the *Aphorisms*, followed, probably late in his career, by that on the *Prognostics*.[7] However, a tradition of pseudo-Hippocratic prognostic texts, including versions of the *Capsula eburnea*, had arisen much earlier in the monasteries, as Paxton has shown.[8] The Trinity text proceeds as follows.

The text begins with consideration of the patient's posture in bed (M4–5; Prog.3).[9] It is a good sign if the patient is able to lie on one side or the other and if his limbs are relaxed (but not too flaccid) and his whole body in a flexible position, in fact if the patient's position resembles as closely as possible that adopted in normal health. Ominous signs are the patient's lying with his neck thrown back, his mouth open, or his feet twisted. Equally undesirable is to lie on the abdomen (if this is not customary in the healthy patient) which indicates delirium or pain. A further dangerous sign is

---

6   See K. Sudhoff, "Die pseudohippokratische Krankheitsprognostik nach dem Auftreten von Hautausschlägen, 'Secreta Hippocratis' oder 'Capsula eburnea' benannt", *Archiv für Geschichte der Medizin* 9 (1916), 79–116 (repr. 1964) and P. Kibre, *Hippocrates latinus* (New York, 1985), pp.110–23.

7   See M.H. Saffron (ed. and tr.), *Maurus of Salerno, twelfth-century 'optimus physicus', with his commentary on the Prognostics of Hippocrates*, TAPA n.s. 62,i (Philadelphia, 1972).

8   F.S. Paxton, "*Signa mortifera*: Death and Prognostication in Early Medieval Monastic Medicine", *Bulletin of the History of Medicine* 67 (1993), 631–50. On the early MSS Cass. 69 and 97 see S. Adacher, "La Trasmissione della cultura medica a Montecassino tra la fine del ix sec. e l'inizio del x sec." in F. Avagliano (ed.), *Montecassino dalla prima alla seconda distruzione: momenti e aspetti di storia casinese (Secc. VI–IX)* (Montecassino, 1987), pp.385–400.

9   The references are to Saffron's edition of Maurus and his indications of the passages in the *Prognostica*.

if the patient, in distress, attempts to pull himself suddenly upright and if he moves violently from the head of the bed to the foot.

If an ulcer occurs in the body (M7; Prog.3), it should be noted whether it developed before or during the illness. A dried ulcer indicates different things according to whether it is blackish, greenish or yellow. Cold sweat (M10; Prog.6) implies a more serious illness, warm sweat a lesser one. Cold sweat in the region of the neck and head is a dangerous sign. A favourable event is when sweating occurs on the critical day appointed by nature for the task and uniformly throughout the body. A good and laudable sweat is one which appears on the critical day in all acute illnesses, for it relieves the patient and renders him more comfortable.

An important diagnostic procedure is to examine the patient's facial appearance (M3; Prog.1). If the temples are sunken, or the forehead is parched and red, or the skin drawn tight, these are unfavourable signs. If the eyes shun light, are sunken or seem restless and tremulous, discharge freely, or if one eye appears smaller than the other, if the eyes lachrymate involuntarily, or protrude on account of breathing difficulties or if the whites of the eyes are tinged with blood, these are negative signs. If in sleep only the white of the eyes can be seen through half-closed eyelids, this is a bad sign. So is insomnia. If the ears are cold or contracted, with the fleshy part inverted, a poor prognosis is indicated. If the nostrils appear sharp and constricted or the tip of the nose is white, these also are bad signs.

There follows a lacuna where we must supply the information that we are dealing with the situation where only the white of the eyes can be seen through half-closed eye-lids. In this case (M3; Prog.1) if it is not the result of diarrhoea or of the operation of a cathartic and if the patient does not normally behave [the context indicates sleep] this way, then it is a highly dangerous symptom. By these signs, alone or in association with those mentioned, death can be confidently predicted.

We now come to cases where the gathering of pus forms a tumour (M11; Prog.7). Often there is a useful flow of blood from the nostrils within a period of seven days. If cold air is exhaled through the nose and mouth (M9; Prog.5), a fatal outcome can be expected [similarly, if food or drink is spewed out through the nostrils]. If the lips / eyelids (M3; Prog.1) are blueish, or white, or drooping, this is a bad sign. Another inauspicious sign is if the tongue is weak and shrinks (not in Prog.).

On the symptom of the grinding of teeth in fevers (M6; Prog.1) we learn that it is bad if this takes place more than is habitual or characteristic in children, for it portends death or madness.

An abscess in the throat (M38; Prog.23) accompanied by acute fever is bad and if other unfavourable signs develop amongst those already mentioned, the patient will die. Sneezing with catarrh (M29; Prog.14) in all diseases of the lungs and chest is serious. There follows an acknowledgement that these signs of life and death are extracted from the 'Liber prognosticorum' of Hippocrates.

The compiler now draws on the *Aphorisms* for the significance of the discharge of gall or blackish blood.

The return to the *Prognostica* (M27; Prog.13) is marked by the argument that vomiting is useful. If vomitus resembles the juice of leeks, is greenish or lead-coloured or blackish, this is a bad sign. Sputum (M28; Prog.14) which is globular (indicating, according to Maurus, cold producing mortification) is useful, but if frothy, it is a bad sign and black sputum indicates a fatal outcome. Further ominous signs concern breathing (M9; Prog.5): if breathing is hurried and there is sign of pain and excessive heat in the organs which lie above the diaphragm, if breathing is deep and with interruption and alienation of the spirit results. A good sign is when breathing is easy and follows a regular rhythm during acute illnesses accompanied by fever.

So far as sweating is concerned (M10; Prog.6), a cold sweat is harmful and when confined to the head and neck is dangerous.

Owing to an elision the next argument is out of context, but concerns the case where an ulcer appears on the patient's body and the importance of noting whether it developed before or during the illness. A dried, greenish ulcer or a yellowish or blackish one is a bad sign. Similarly, a context has to be supplied for the next observation. The context is the preliminary examination in all acute diseases of the patient's face and posture (M3; Prog.1). After attention to a list of symptoms (duly listed in the *Prognostica*) it is important to inquire from the outset whether the patient has long been sleepless or has experienced persistent diarrhoea or has suffered from lack of sustenance. If it is found that any of these symptoms occurred before the illness, there will be less cause to fear them. If they continued through the preceding day and night, they will not be considered very dangerous, but if none of these circumstances is confirmed, then death is to be expected. If the disease continues for three days, the preceding symptoms must be investigated no less thoroughly and attention must be paid not only to the body's appearance, but also to the eyes.

A bad sign is if the arms are rigid, and a good sign if the hands are not tense as in a spasm (M4; Prog.3). Concerning the mobility of the hands (M8; Prog.4), it is noted that in acute fevers, such as in pneumonia and a false phrenitis and severe pain in the head, the patient's hand may be raised to the head or he may move his hands here and there as if collecting or searching for something, or he may pick something of his clothes or may be seen to pick at the walls. These are all bad signs.

In the case of greenish discoloraton of the nails (M16; Prog.9), death may confidently be expected.

There follows the Anglo-Norman translation of the *Capsula eburnea* (114–116). After this comes another Anglo-Norman translation of a prognostic text, corresponding to the Latin found in MS Bodl. Libr. e mus. 219 f.83v under the title 'Pronostica .G. dierum timendorum in incepcione omnium egritudinarum' (117), to which is appended in our compendium a short text of prognostications according to the movements of the moon (118)[10] and a brief list of 'perilous days' (119).[11] The most important of the prognostic texts is the full Anglo-Norman translation of Hippocrates'

---

[10] See P. Saintyves, "De l'influence de la lune sur les maladies d'après les médecins astrologues des origines au XVe siècle", *Hippocrate* 2 (1934), 289–313, 405–33, 492–524 and see next note.

[11] See L. Thorndike, *A History of Magic and Experimental Science* 1 (New York / London, 1923), pp.685–91 and 695–6; G. Keil, "Die verworfenen Tage", *Sudhoffs Archiv* 41 (1957), 27–58. For a survey of such prognostic texts, especially lunaries, see I. Taavitsainen, *Middle English Lunaries: A Study of the Genre* (Helsinki, 1988) and C. Weisser, "Das Krankheitslunar aus medizinhistorischer Sicht", *Sudhoffs Archiv* 65 (1981), 390–400 and *id.*, *Studien zum mittelalterlichen Krankheitslunar. Ein Beitrag zur Geschichte laienastrologischer Fachprosa*, Würzburger medizinhistorische Forschungen 21 (Pattensen / Hannover, 1982). For early MSS see Beccaria, *I Codici di Medicina*, Index sub *Lunari*.

De urinis (120–133) which follows accurately the Latin text in MS e mus. 219 ff.127r–129r, except for where the latter is defective. It is preceded and followed by excerpts from the section on urines in the 'Lettre d'Hippocrate'.

The rest of the MS is made up of a miscellany of treatments which cover panaceas (134), a variety of conditions which include quinsy and treatment of the humours (135), complaints of the stomach (136), of the chest (137), cough and phthisis (138), hoarseness and vocal difficulties (139), complaints of the heart (140), of the spleen (141), of the lungs and lateral areas of the body (142), of the stomach (143), intestinal worms (144), tumours (145), dropsy (146) and diarrhoea (148). The concluding, incomplete Latin passage on dysentery is probably misplaced and should follow the other passage already displaced on f.13 (91–5).

The Manuscript

MS Cambridge, Trinity College 0.5.32 (1313) is made up of two volumes, the first being principally concerned with divinatory texts. The second volume is occupied by the medical compendium printed below. James's collation is 1^{12}, 2^{16} (16 canc.), 3^4. Folio 13 is insititious (see catchword *guta* on f.12v and the beginning of the text on f.14). At the bottom of f.15 is written 'Wigornia'. The top of the first folio bears the name Thomas Richards 'Thys is Thomas Richards [booke]'), an inscription found elsewhere (vol.1, ff.8v, 20v; vol.2, f.31v). Richards owned both volumes in the late 15th – early 16th centuries. At the top of f.11v is written 'Anno regni regis Ricardi 11 vto' i.e. 1382.

On f.29v there is a text beginning 'Domine T. hispaniarum regine Johannes hispaniensis salutem. Cum de utilitate corporis olim tractaremus . . .' This is a brief medical extract from the Pseudo-Aristotelian *Secretum secretorum*, namely 188 lines of Suchier's text preceded by a letter to a queen of Spain (perhaps Tharasia who died in 1130), possibly (though the matter is still disputed) the work of John of Seville.[12] This is then followed (f.30v) by a text on the seasons beginning 'Veris inicium est in cathedra sancti Petri[13] . . .' and (f.31r) by a set of receipts for medicinal powders. Folio 31v is badly stained and the text illegible in many places. The final entry, following a Latin receipt for oximel, is in French:

> Aliter oximel: pernez racines de persil, de ache e de raiz e de glehul e herbe seint Johan de chescun .i. poiné, pernez cerelanghe, cicoré, violette, copere de chescune .i. poiné, e triblez bien en un morter e quisez en treis galons d'ewe deske a la tierce partie, pus le colez parmi un drap e mettez del mel e quise[z], medlez ensemble e pus le reboilez desque seit espés. De ce degutez une goute sur vostre ungle e si elle se tent e pas ne decourt, donke est assez quit. Cest seit usé matin chaud de ceus qui ount mestier.

The rest of the page is occupied by lines in English beginning,

---

12 See L. Thorndike, "John of Seville", *Speculum* 34 (1959), 20–38. Cf. M.A. Mazaloui, *Secreta secretorum: Nine English Versions* 1, EETS 276 (London, 1977), pp.xiv–xv.
13 I.e. 22 February, the Feast of St Peter's Chair.

Ipocras þis bouk herknyth to me and I ȝew wole telle lente do also þis bouk hit bit hit techiþ goud for everech manere yvel . . . .iiii. umurys þat susteyniþ manys body that is thulke whyche they beth. Þe furste is hete, the oþer is colde, the prydde drowþe, þe ferþe is moist. By þes .iiii. humours beth ysusteynyd all thynge were throw we liveth. Oure bonys beth drye that ȝyviþ strenthe to suffry travayl. Oure innewarde is cold war þorw we breþiþ, and þe bloud is moyist which norschip þe lyf and by þe ynewarde comyth þe veynis whiche receyviþ the bloud. Þe bloud þe lyif sus[t]eyniþ. Now loke hen. . .[14]

The name of Thomas Richards reappears at the bottom of the page.

Sources

As indicated above, parts of the Trinity 'Practica' are translations of identified Latin treatises. References to authorities are rare, much rarer than in the *Euperiston*, and occur as follows: Galen [21,22,23,92,98 ('in Organon'), 108]; Hippocrates (Aphorisms) [3,40,93,98] and [51] 'esperment Ypocras'), [77] ('Ypocras iubet'), [110] ('de libro pronosticorum Ypocratis'); 'ut testatur auctor' [40]; Trota [68]; Constantine the African [91]; Master Bartholomew (of Salerno?) [94][98] ('magister Bartolomeus in Practica sua'); Master Andrew (of Salerno?) [94]. Use is made of charms in sections 28,48,52,53,54,61,67,73,79,107,113 and 134. Latin verses are cited in sections 39,40,90,95,108. Vernacular sources include the 'Lettre d'Hippocrate' (see notes) and the 'Physique rimee' (also see notes). The materia medica included covers a wide range of compound medicines as illustrated in the *Antidotarium Nicolai*. There are first-person anecdotes in sections 8,56,64,66 and 98.

Language and Lexis

The predominant languages of the treatise are Latin and French. Short passages of English are found in sections 27, 28, 54, 86 and 135. In general the languages are kept apart, but there are certain consistent exceptions. The first is glossing, of which the following cases are found:

[14]   acora . . . a vulgo appellatur *teine, skale*
[28]   la escorce / .i. suber /
[30]   sicute / .i. *homlok* /
[30]   *chavçoris* / .i. vespertilionis /
[35]   viticelle / *wild nepe* /
[35]   bombace / .i. *coton* /
[36]   ombre de fosse / *feltrid* /
[57]   auricularis / *erewike* /
[66]   corpusculum quod in arabica lingua appellatur 'nern' et in greca 'isophagus'
[68]   andre / .s. *bischopiswort* /
[70]   flaunbe / .s. *gladeine* /
[95]   liz / .s. *lilie* /
[114]   *brenetes* / alias burbices /
[129]   *routet* / .i. ructat /

[135]   tussis et dicitur anglice 'chinke' vel 'chekhost'
[135]   singultus est anglice 'yiskinge'
[137]   *seel* / .i. sal /
[141]   coopere / .i. *livrewort* /

A relatively common form of code-switching occurs in receipts where the indication is in one language and the directions in another, as in the following examples:

[26]   *Ad felon del chief:* + Latin
[28]   Item ne cadant: + French
[28]   Item si cadant: + French
[28]   *Ad espescer ch[everel]:* + Latin
[31]   *Pur puces:* + Latin
[32]   Item *ad enflure de goitrun et de maschel:* + Latin
[33]   *Face techelé:* + Latin
[34]   *Contre lepre:* + Latin
[38]   Item ad faciem dealbandam: + French
[42]   Item aqua: + French
[42]   *Autre:* + Latin
[43]   Aliud quod et visum prius turbat sed postea clariorem reddit: + French
[44]   *Autre:* + Latin
[45]   Ad ruborem oculorum: + French
[46]   *Autre:* + Latin
[47]   Ad albuginem oculi: + French
[49]   Ad caliginem oculorum: + French
[52]   *Cherem:* + Latin
[52]   Item *pur le mail:* + Latin
[52]   Item *ad oilez:* + Latin
[52]   *Autre:* + Latin
[55]   *Pur faies:* + Latin
[58]   Item ad surditatem: + French
[59]   Item ad surd[itatem] auris: + French
[61]   *Nes estoupé:* + Latin
[62]   *Ad poriture de naril:* + Latin
[63]   *Puor de la bouche:* + Latin
[70]   *Ad dent dolour:* + Latin
[73]   *Charme ad dentz:* + Latin
[73]   Item *cherme:* + Latin
[79]   *Autre, e s'il doult,* faba cocta in vino
[79]   *Cherem:* + Latin
[81]   Item ad scabiem manum et brachiorum aut aliorum menbrorum: + French
[81]   *Autre:* + Latin
[82]   *Autre:* + Latin
[82]   *Autre e ad goutte e ad parlesie:* + Latin
[82]   *Et pur roin[e]:* + Latin
[83]   *Autre:* + Latin
[83]   Item *cirons:* + Latin

[84]   Item *si ungle commeste sont kancré*

[84]   *Ad blauncher les meins e col*: + Latin

[86]   *Vit que seine*: + Latin

[88]   Ad petram que impedit urinam: + French

[88]   *Autre*: + Latin

[89]   *Estale*: + Latin

[90]   Item castrare homines: + French

[100]   *Fundement*: + Latin

[106]   Item *podagre*: + Latin

[116]   Item de eodem: + French

[134]   *Ke maladie ne vous touche*: + Latin

[134]   *Ad touz medicines que vous donez e charmez que vous ditez, dites cest*: + Latin

[134]   Item *ad toz mals del cors*: + Latin

[136]   Item *[pur] purger le stomak*: + Latin

[136]   *Ki vomit e ne puet maunger*: + Latin

[137]   Item *ad dolour*: + Latin

[137]   *[Pur] purger le piz*: + Latin

[138]   Item *ad touse e ad le piz*: + Latin

[138]   Item *ad purger le piz*: + Latin

[144]   *Verms denz le ventre*: + Latin

[144]   Item ad tineam: + French

[147]   Item *charme ad flux de sanc*: + Latin

A related phenomenon is code-mixing which is also well illustrated by our treatise:

[24]   *pur tot dolour* capitis

[24]   *de pel de gras chat covrez*, ut supra, *e des herbes* et cetera

[27]   *feltrey* genus herbe est

[28]   sicuti scabiosis et *teinus* et cetera

[28]   *si metez* vel *oinez la cheverel*

[30]   succo rafani et edere unge .iii. dies, *poi lez ostez*

[33]   vel *de oil fet de nogagk* vel *de sanc de levre*

[34]   scrupulus *peisit* .iii. *quadrantz*

[42]   Preterea *ad cest avantdit euye*

[45]   *Ad la chace des oils* distemperetur *mel*

[47]   *boilez od cerfoil* et post cole

[51]   *pere que est appellé* celidonius

[52]   per anulum illum in oculum, *ce est la medecine*

[52]   Item *en noun del Pere e del Filz e del Seint Esprit*, Teda, Nicea et Aquilina.
         Teda dixit 'stamus', Nicea dixit 'sic faciamus', Aquilina dixit 'maculam
         de oculo deficiamus' . . .

[52]   herbam que dicitur *wakerwort*

[53]   *sa giouye* et cetera ut supra

[53]   *Cherme* ut infirmus dormiat

[55]   *Pur faies*: Conjuro vos, *elves*, per Patrem et Filium

[60]   fac jus feniculi *ke si il ad plaie dedenz* . . .

[61]   Ad sanguinem restringendum ubi volueris *cherme*

[68]   e ut supra *recevez*
[71]   e *recevez la fumé* ut supra
[71]   e *tenez* ut supra *en la bouche*
[71]   *boilez en estale cervoise semence de chanilé* ut supra
[71]   *tenez* ut supra *en bouche*
[71]   et tresura aut *bevez le od vin* . . .
[72]   *te[nez] en la bouche* et cetera ut supra
[72]   vel *mult masch[ez] le herbe*
[74]   *Levers*, ad rimas labiorum
[80]   viltrit *vous prendrez en ewe*
[80]   *viltrit* genus est herbe
[81]   *de ce oinez ad feu*. Probatum est.
[83]   surmitte
[84]   *si ungle* commeste *sont kancré*
[88]   sicut *testmoinent parfiz mires*
[90]   *herbe r[ecevez] ke est appellé* regina
[106]   une herbe que est appellé *sourethestil* et *watercresces*
[106]   *en mati[n] trois* 'sponful'
[116]   *ce est* signum de morte
[134]   vel tecum habeas vel *portez sur vous la racine*
[135]   *une grasse ouye* et cetera ut supra
[138]   *Tussick*, ad tisicos
[142]   *Pomoun*, ad pulmonis vicium
[142]   *Coste*, ad dolorem lateris
[147]   Item *flux de sang* res probata

To these may be added those lists of ingredients which mix Latin and vernacular forms, sometimes producing such hybrids as *flur de paniwort* [36], *jus de mogwed* [60], *racine de gletoun e foxesglove* [81], *la racine de rouge doke* [81], *la souredoc* [86], and *la wedrof e cel bois* [89].

Since the size of the treatise renders a complete glossary impractical and largely unnecessary, on account of duplication with the other glossaries in *Anglo-Norman Medicine*, it is sufficient to draw attention to some less familiar plant names, whilst referring the reader to T. Hunt, *Plant Names of Medieval England* (Cambridge, 1989), W.F. Daems, *Nomina simplicium medicinarum ex synonymariis medii aevi collecta: semantische Untersuchungen zum Fachwortschatz hoch – und spätmittelalterlicher Drogenkunde* (Leiden etc., 1993) and *Anglo-Norman Dictionary* (London, 1992). Of note are *amblette* [83][145],*bilre* [36], *feltrey* [27], *feltrid* [36], *garre* [27], *gaudine* [27], *oculesconce* [27], *ombre de fosse* [36], *paniwort* [36], *verge ad pastor* [27], *viltret*, *viltrit* [36], *wakerwort* [52], *yerre arbrine* [27].

More general lexical items which deserve to be recorded are: *arcisons* [28], *arsepan* [48], *artisons* [31], *blast* [41], *borsize* [71], *brenete* [114], *causon* [125], *cerne* [123], *chaudepisce* [89], *date* [43], *emigranie* [20], *esrakeure* [115], *fundriaile* [115], *fundril* [124], *gist* [125], *goisterin* [114], *gulinz* [113], *maschel* [32], *nue* [124,127], *orpree* [68], *pleureisin* [124], *roventele* [35], *sinoce* [125], *tribleid* [20], *vanité* [20], *winderor* [27], *wndour* [60], *[y]postas(i)e* [127].

Problematic Latin words are *frellata* [67], *gabrio* [28], *lenderta* [40], *martali* [64], *orola* [84], *poka* [48], *reverencia* [5].

The Edition

There is no denying the interest of the medical compendium, but unfortunately the evidence is that it is an inaccurate copy with many scribal blunders which pose serious problems to an editor. The Latin is often incorrect, particularly in respect of flexions (often through assimilation to adjacent case-endings), and there are frequent signs of unintentional omissions which interfere with the sense of what is left. Emendation is often necessary and yet without clear evidence of the scribe's model, and given the heterogenous nature of his material, the form of the required emendation is all too often incalculable. Nevertheless, the compilation is too important to be ignored and accordingly an attempt has been made to provide a comprehensible, though not 'correct', text. Rather than obliterate unsatisfactory readings, which might nevertheless suggest possible emendations, I have in cases of doubt retained such readings and marked them with (?). Where correction may confidently be made, I have relegated the MS reading to a footnote. In order to keep footnotes to a manageable number I have permitted myself silent correction where little more than a single letter was at stake and where the error was a sign of inadvertence.

The Trinity 'Practica'

[BOOK 1: THE HEAD]

[f.1r]¹[1] Quoniam omnia vicia a capite procedunt ex quibus oculi et aures et dentes paciuntur, oportet congruo tempore gargariss(i)mis et aliis medicamentis facere purgacionem capitis et tunc aures, oculi et dentes nullam sustinebunt pascionem. Cerebrum continetur in capite et caput est quasi lucerna corporis et dignior pars. Ideo a morbis capitis incipiamus.

[2] Capitis pasciones sunt varie et plurime. Sed tamen generaliter quelibet capitis pascio **cephalia** dicitur /.i. appellatur / quasi capitis lesio, a cephas quod est caput. Et fere omnis morbus capitis inicium habet a cerebro. Igitur de morbis cerebri dicemus.

[3] Inter omnes **apopl[ex]ia** periculosior est. Apopl[ex]ie ergo difinicionem dicemus et divisionem atque signa. Apopl[ex]ia est exuberacio humorum ventriculos cerebri implens, animales virtutes perdens. Item apopl[ex]ia alia maior alia minor alia media. Minor est in qua corpus caret sensu, in .vii. diebus interficit, et est vero quando omnes nervi cerebri nec ex toto opilantur. Media est quando caret motu et sensu, cum difficultate tertia die interficit, et fit quando omnes² nervi cerebri opilantur, sed non ex toto. Maior est quando caret motu³ [et] sensu et anelitu, sine dificultate in prima vel in secunda die interficit, et fit quando omnes nervi cerebri opilantur ex toto. Maior et media incurabiles sunt et minor vix curatur. Unde Ypocras in **Aforismis**: maiorem apopl[ex]iam curare inpossibile est, minorem non facile.⁴

[4] Cura, si curabile est: caput primo radetur, deinde attrahatur sanguis de utroque brachio, unguatur capud unguentis calidis atque oleis calidis, ut oleo petroleo, oleo

---

1 The righthand margin of f.1r contains the following entries which essentially represent headings under which the material in the main text is treated: 'Partes capitis sunt prora .i. anterior, puppis .i. posterior, sinistra, dextera'; 'Pasciones capitis sunt apopl[ex]ia triplex – maior, minor, et media – epilencia, emigrania, epigrania. Mania genus est descipiencie et est duplex: canina et demoniaca. Malina frenesisque, et letargicio [que] dicitur litargia, cephalia, vertigo, skotomia, acora, tinea, ulcus, fa[v]us, dolor, fractio, unisacio(?), monopagia, sigraropha, inflacio, feloun, formicaciones, plaçons, fer peil crestre, oster peil, canicies, colerer peil, crisper peil, oster lentes et vermin, ne concalescat sole, [ne] intumescat'; 'Cerebrum dicitur esse frigidum et humidum, cor calidum et siccum, stomacus frigidus et siccus, epar calidus et humidus'; 'Apolixia [sic] est quando humores ascendentes privant homines quinque sensibus que est mors subdita. Epilencia quando descendens strenuit [sic] hominem sed non interficiunt que est gutta caduca; an[a]lenpcia eiusdem est nature, paralisis per totum, catalenpcia est tertia species. Descipientia idem est quod mania et dicitur duplex, canina et demoniaca. Canina fit de enela adusta ex sanguine habens talem descipienciam superridet et talis est curabilis.'

2 MS *omnis*.

3 MS *notti*.

4 See *Aphorism*. Bk 2 ch.42 'Apoplexiam soluere fortem, impossibile est. Debilem vero non facile'. (Articella, Venice 1523 f.38va). Cf. also *De egritudinum curatione* in *Coll. Sal.* 2, p.111 'Unde Ypokrate: solvere apoplexiam fortem quidem impossibile, debilem vero non facile'. Martin de Saint Gille translates '[Forte] apoplexie est impossible ou de fort curable, et la foible n'est pas de legier curable', see G. Lafeuille (ed.), *Les Amphorismes Ypocras de Martin de Saint-Gille 1362–1365* (Genève, 1954), p.63.

laureo, olio mucillino; unguentis calidis, marciaton, Agrippa, benedicto aureo. Dieta sit calida et sicca sicut in paralisi quia species paralisis est. Nulla evacuacio debet in hiis fieri. Preter fleobotoma[m] detur ei opopira ad modum castanie cum vino calido, tyriacam sub lingua teneat.

[5] **Epilencia,** que est gutta caduca, fit de humori apopl[ex]ie, sed hic ad presens de ea omitto quia postea de ipsa in isto libro suo loco dicetur.

[6] Nota quod antiqua pascio proprie appellatur **cephalia**. Sicut caput in quatuor partes dividitur, sic humor humori quamlibet partem sibi occupat. Caput in proram et puppem dividitur et in monopagiam[5] et in emigraneam. Prora antereor pars capitis est in qua parte calidus humor principalis habundat .s. sanguis.[6] In dextra parte capitis calidi humores habundant, in sinistra frigidi. In anteriori parte capitis est quedam cellula que fantastica appellatur in qua parte maxime dominatur sanguis et quandoque purus, inde nascitur quedam species decipiencie que **mania** dicitur. Est et alia celula media que rationalis cellula dicitur in qua parte maxime dominatur colera rubea et in illa parte nascitur quedam species descipiencie que **frenesis** dicitur. In parte posteriori habundat fleuma in cella que memorialis dicitur. Ibi generatur quedam species discipiencie que **litargia** dicitur. Melancolia totum cerebrum occupat quasi [c]operculum tocius et inde generatur quedam species decipiencie que **melancolia** dicitur et fit ex colera nigra que melancolia dicitur.

[7] **Mania** quandoque in mulieribus, quandoque in viris fit. In mulieribus fit ex retencione menstruorum cuius sunt singna hillaritas, luxuria,[7] in tota ventura predicit. Cura est precipue menstrua provocare hoc modo: primo purgetur cum theodoricon yperiston. Deinde fiat ei talis subfumigatio: recipe archiemesiam, urticam maiorem, marubium, calamentum, mentastrum et decoquantur in vino fortiter in una olla et ita preparetur ut fumus non possit intrare in vulvam nisi per embotum[8]. Deinde post subfumigationem utetur trifera magna cum decoctione arthimesie, calamenti, origani. Fiat ei pessarium tale: accipe electarium et farina[m] cum melle ad quantitatem degiti et supponat sibi. Tunc cum folio debet ligari. Et ne liquefactum ibi ex mora ledat accipe radicem rubie maioris et subponat sibi recentem. Et si ista non subveniunt, flebotoma de venis saphenis[9] vel de varice in fronte. Dieta[10] sit [. . .].. In viris fere signa manie sunt hec: yllaritas frigida et humida, [f.1v] predictio venture. Curentur per fleobotomam factam de varice in fronte. Deinde raso capite per localia adiutoria prius dicta .s. popilion, de olio violaceo, olio roseo, purgetur cum decoctione[11] cassiefistule, tamarindorum, reubarbari, mirobolanorum. Utetur dieta[12] frigida et humida ut pane et aqua, seminibus melonis,[13] lactuca, portulacis, piris coctis. De **frenesei** alias dicetur post suo loco in libris et in primis[14] maioribus.

[8] **Litargia** est egritudo quasi universalis que a cerebro procedit, unde dicitur litargia oblivio mentis sine recordacione preteritorum cum sompnietatis opressione.

5 MS *nonopagiam*.
6 MS *s. et colera*.
7 The intrusive 'de purgacione menstrue deberet poni' which occurs in the MS between 'luxuria' and 'in tota ventura' makes no sense.
8 MS *ombotum*.

9 MS *sophenis*.
10 MS *dicta*.
11 MS *decoctacione*.
12 MS *ditta*.
13 MS *servibus melonibus*.
14 MS *i p"nis*.

Unde litargia quasi lephargia a fluvio infernali, quoniam secuti anime transvecte tradunt oblivioni quicquid dediciti apud suos superos .i. apud imaginacionem racionis memorie. Fit autem ex fleumate in memoriali cellula collecto huius hec sunt signa: stupor mentis, insensibilitas, sompnus continuus et quandoque ore aperto, quandoque oculis apertis. Cura est dicta talis: ponetur in loco lucido et claro ubi fient confabulaciones hominum coram eo, exitetur a sompno vocando proprio nomine et attrahendo eum per barbam, per capillos, per aures. Radetur capud et ungetur unguentis calidis et oleis calidis ut petroleo, olio sinapis. Fiat emplastrum tale circa caput: recipe piretrum, castorium, euforbium, adarcis .i. caro marina. Fiat pulvis de omnibus hiis et conficietur cum petroleon vel cum marciacio[n][15] et raso capite apponatur. Castorium teneat semper ad nares. Excitetur a sompno per adiectionem sinapis per nares. Purgetur cum diacastorio. Dieta[16] sit calida et sicca ut caro animalis, angni, galline, perdices. Abluciones pedum fient et in aqua in qua coctum sit sulphur vivum et calamentum, artemesia, origanum, pulegium, urtica maior, mentastrum. Hoc modo curavi comitem nevensem. Cum vidi eum desperatum aperui dentes . . .[17] Dedi ei medicina[m] nominatam et transacto spacio trium horarum cepit ructare et eructare. Quibus[18] factis quidem incepit vomere et facto vometo convaluit et locu[tu]s est. Et postea paulatim dietavi eum et suavi dieta et leni et iunxi ei quietem et naturaliter dormivit[19] et convaluit.

[9] Item ad litargiam speciale emplaustrum: recipe pulverem piperis, peretri, castorie, euforbii, sinapis, et distempera cum melle et modico aceto et raso capite superponatur calidum. Et de illis fiat unguentum cum olio.

[10] Illa passio que appellatur **cephalia** quandoque habet originem a capite et tunc continue infestat, quandoque a stomaco et tunc interpolate. Et dividitur in diversas species: in emigrania, epigrania, monopagia. Cephalia quandoque est ex calido humore, quandoque ex frigido. Ex calido secuti ex sanguine vel ex colera, hec sunt signa: dolor in fronte et in temporibus, saltus eiusdem vel pulsus, rubor oculorum, sompnia ignea ut combustiones domorum vel sanguinea ut carnes crudas et sanguinem videre, cuius cura cum dieta[20] talis fiat: fleubotoma de vena cephali[c]a vel de vena in fronte, purgetur cum decoctione cassiefistule, tamarindorum ut supra[21] dictum est. Unctiones fient eis de unguentis frigidis et oleis frigidis. Abluciones pedum fient eis de frigidis herbis ut de jusquiano, barba jovis, ut superius dictum est.[22] Dieta[23] sit frigida et humida, ut panis et aqua et extremitates porcium, pisces fluviales squamosi duras carnes habentes ut pertice, luces, et cum aqua vinum aquaticum vel mulsum,[24] fructus ut pira. Post cibaria omnia ligumina et omnia olera nociva [sunt] nisi fuerit de lactucis et frigidis herbis ad sompnum provocandum. Eadem est cura de cephalia ex colera. Item cephalia ex fleumate quandoque et aliquando ex malancolia. Eius signa familiaria sunt et continua nisi quia fleuma in posteriori parte capitis [f.2r] magis infestat et melencolia in sinistra parte. Signa hec sunt: gravitas capitis, dolor lentus in respectu

---

15 The abbreviation for final '-on' has been incorrectly resolved as '-io'.
16 MS *dicca*.
17 Illegible superscript insertion.
18 MS *comunibus*, probably arising from a misunderstanding of initial *q* as 9.

19 MS *dormium*.
20 MS *dicta*.
21 MS *sepe*. See [7] above.
22 See [8] above.
23 MS *dicta*.
24 MS *mullum*.

aliar[um] et si vicio erit capitis et continu[u]s dolor et ex fleumate sequitur stuporum [. . .], ex malancolia[25] quasi quedam species descipiencie. Dieta sit cruda et sicca ut pulli, perdices, caro animalis agni, pisces carnes crudas habentes squamosi fluviales. Vinum sit album et subtile. Utetur oximelle diuretico vel paulino simplici. Purgetur cum pillulis aureis vel 'pillulis sine quibus esse nolo'.[26] Purgata materia utetur aurea alexandrina ter in septimana cum ibit ad mansionem cum [vino] calido. Eadem cura valet ad cephaliam que fit ex stomaco ex frigida materia nisi quia vomitus sic precipue valet.

[11] **Scotomia** est quedam capitis passio que a vulgo 'vertigo' appellatur quia paciens verti se in giro credit. Quandoque [fit] a capite, quandoque a stomacho. Quando[27] est a capite, tunc continue infestat cum tenebrositate oculorum, quando a stomaco .i. a vicio stomachi, cum nausia et voluntate vomendi et paciens ex stomaco per vomitum aleviatur. Sed quia ex fleumate grosso cum ventositate inclusa fit vertigo secuti ex fleumate, eadem est cura et dieta.[28] Cum si fuerit vicio capitis, in fronte epicranei cauterium valde utile est; si vicio stomachi, in orificio stomachi superiori. Cavendum est a leguminibus indigestibilibus, a ventositate digentibus, a coitu, a nimia potacione, a tarda cena.

[12] Sunt autem capitis passiones extrinsece quibus localia adiutoria necessaria sunt, sicud favus, acora, tinea, canicies.

[13] **Favus** est morbus postulosus in capite et dicitur ad similitudinem favi mellis. Sicud mel liquedum [de] favo exit, ita sanies exit de posticulis istis. Eius cura talis est: purgetur universaliter cum yera vel cum pillulis aureis vel cum pillulis diacastorie vel per nares in balneo raso capite, et attractis mortuis pilis scarificetur caput. Et deinde recipe testes avelanarum et fac comburi et sparge pulverem super caput et in tertia die lavetur caput cum urina propria vel urina vaccinia vel bovina et coque usque ad spissitudinem liqui[di] mellis et cum ea unge frequenter caput. Vel aliter accipe nasturcium aquaticum et attrahe succum et accipe fuliginem et confice quasi unguentum cum succo et unge caput.

[14] **Acora** est morbus capitis qui a vulgo appellatur *teine*, *skale* et dicitur acora quasi sine corio, quia totum caput exulceratum est. Eadem est dicta cura. Cura[29] facta, tamen, pulvis de plumbo combusto hiis est necessarius. Comburitur plumbum hoc modo: pone illud in vase terreo et cum inceperit liquifieri, appone sal movendo[30] semper spatula et cum liquefactum fuerit, sale admixto, et combustum erit, cepera[31] sal a plumbo et fac pulverem et supersparge capud. Vel accipe allium et fac pulverem et distempera cum melle ut fiat quasi unguentum et frequenter inunge caput. Et frequenter ungetur capud cum propria urina vel cum urina vaccina vel cum bovina ut superius diximus.[32] Item accipe stercus caballinum, cum melle combure, commisce ad modum unguenti et unge caput. Probatum est.

[15] **Tinea** est adhuc passio capitis et est quasi squame et capilli inde commeduntur. Cura est: accipe buxum et fac cinerem combustione et lexivam et cum lessiva illa

[25] MS *malancta*.

[26] See *Antidotarium Nicolai* ed. W.S. van den Berg, p.117, no.78 (hereafter AN followed by the number of the Latin receipt).

[27] MS *quandoque*.

[28] MS *dicta*.

[29] MS *cum cura*.

[30] MS *et movendo*.

[31] i.e. 'separa'.

[32] See [13] above.

lava caput frequenter. Vel accipe corticem fabarum et paleas avene et fac cinerem, deinde lessivam, et lava caput.

[16] **Canicies** capillorum est vicium capitis quandoque naturalis, quandoque accidentalis; naturaliter in senio quia proprium est hominis in senectute canescere. Illa ergo canicies removeri non potest quia est naturalis. Accidentalis fit ex frigida complexione cerebri vel ex labore vel ex dolore. Unde illud est remedium. Per talem curam hoc modo retinetur. Si capilli primo [f.2v] fuerunt nigri, accipe vitreolum .i. alcanum et gallam, in aqua calida distempera, et cum aqua lava caput. Vel eciam sola galla perforata et pulverizata cum aqua calida distemperata et inde caput lava. Si capelli prius fuerunt croci, accipe lupinos et corticem fabarum et fac pulverem et in aqua distempera et lava capud. Item ad idem: accipe fecem aceti et amurcam .i. fex olei et combure omnia et in aqua calida pone et lava caput eodem modo quo prius.

[17] Vertigo capitis: ita fit .s. ex vicio stomaci .i. ex indegestione. Indigestio autem fit ex nimia frigiditate sicut stomacus quandoque est nimis frigidus et non potest facere bonam degestionem, unde surgit ventositas et ascendit [ad] cerebrum et inficit illud et obscurat opticum nervum per quem fertur visibilis spiritus ad oculos et de hac causa[33] fit vertigo et scotomia. Cura est talis: accipere debet pigram[34] ad evacuandam stomaci frigiditatem et ventositatem et hoc ante prandium. Si autem hoc modo curari non potest propter ventositatem fleumatis, comedat escas spongeas .s. cepas, casium, piscem siccum. Et post cibum per unam horam vomitum provocamus penna oleo intincta vel etiam digitis, sed et prius ad provocacionem aquam calidam bibat. Item sinapismum calidum capiti apponere debes vel calamentum bene coctum in saculo positum vel origanum. Dieta sit[35] calida et sicca. Item ex nimio calore quandoque stomacus nimium calidus est et adurit cibum et ex tali adustione iterum fit indigestio et cerebrum infectum et impedit opticum nervum qui inde induratur. [Si] vertigo est ex colera, curacio talis [est]: debes curare stomacum de colera que est in ore ipsius et per frigidum vomit[um], ut dictum [. . .] aceto et melle et rafano vel trifera cum utraque coleram purgat.

[18] Ad dolorem capitis: absinthii radices et edere terrestris tere et adde simul albumen ovorum, induc in lintheamine et capiti appone. Item: succum crissonis misce cum olio et aceto et unge caput. Item: herbam rute cum vino potaberis et post hoc cum oleo rosaceo et aceto caput perunges et sic mirifice sanaberis. Ne caput a sole concalescat herbam pullegium tecum porta aut super aurum aut super argentum. Hoc est estivo tempore nec gravedinem senties neque perfricacionem. Item ad dolorem capitis: herbe plantaginis radix in collo suspensa capitis dolorem mirifice tollit. Item: quinquefolium circumscriptum ter digito medio et pollice sublatum et capiti illinitum efficaciter sanat. Vel radix eius capiti alligata mirifice sanat. Item: herbe verminacie corona facta et capiti imposita dolorem tollit. Item: accipiat alloes et teratur et postea succo caullis temperetur et deinde skamonea apponatur et detur pacienti, statim liberabitur. Item mixtura capitis: recipe betonice, viole albe, panis mundi, malage,[36]

---

33 MS *hac de causa.*
34 i.e. 'picram'.
35 MS *Ditta sunt.*
36 For *malache* 'mallow'? J. Jörimann, *Frühmittelalterliche Rezeptarien* (Zürich / Leipzig, 1925; repr. 1977), p.10 has *malagma.*

edere terrestris, piloselle, agrimonie, simph[on]ie, salvie.[37] Ne intumescat, tere betonicam – dolorem tollit et sanat; salvia aufert passionem, edera terrestris curat et
mundat, viola sanat, plantago soluit dolorem, et emendat agrimonia et pilossella sanat,
melagia[38] iuvat ut claudatur vulnus. Ad capitis fracturam: herbe gladioli segetalis
superior pars trita [et] sicca equis ponderibus mixta capitis ossa fracta trahit cum olio
rosacio aut si quit in corpore sopetum vel si pedibus calcata sunt ossa. Eadem contra
venenum efficax est.

[19]   Ad illam capitis passionem que **emigranea** dicitur: accipe lignum juniperi et
ex eo fac lessivatam crudam et ex inde lava caput .iii. diebus veneris. Probatum est.
Item ad idem: abrotanum et mel et acetum mixtum et appositum licet veteriores tollit
dolores. Item ad idem: oleum et acetum mixtum et super dolores positum mire facit.
Ad eos qui cerebrum habent inflatum: rutam, pulegium, cepam, satureiam, anetum,
oleum, butirum et mel calidum induc in lanam succidam et sic capiti inponis.

[20]   Si tinea fuerit in capite, ex felle vituli capud inunges et lindines exterminat.
Si les oreils tentisent ou sonnent o s'il se(i)nt une vanité [f.3r] *en la teste ou s'il sent les
humours courre par le chefe et puis se arestent as oils et il veit devant ses oils ensement come
neirs musches voler que sont unz noirs estencelsce*[39] [o] *neire ombre, ceo*[40] *signifie avuglement
des oilz ad vener et une manere de mal que hom tient oilz overtz et goute ne veit .i. tribleid.
Si la meité del chef li deut et les temples li sonnent, ce signefie emigranie, une goute que saisit
le meité del chefe.*

[21]   Item videamus si capitis dolor duobus modis potest considerari, vel ex se
proprie vel ex membris sicut stomaco. [Si] quasi modo presens modo recedens sit,
aliunde procul dubio venit, unde Galienus 'Si dolor est in capite nulla cura certa [est]
extrinsecus veniente'. Humores collecti pregnant stomacum et maxime acutus[41] dolor
inde est in summitate capitis quia ex regione est stomachi, qui si sine intermissione
fuerit, proprie ex capitis[42] venis et quolibet humori humorum fit. Si sit ex sanguine,
calorem patitur in capite, gravitatem in fronte et oculi[43] rubescunt, vene faciei sunt
plene, urina rubea et pi[n]guis, et corpus molle, pulsus mollis. Si ex colera rubea, infra
nares nimium habet calorem et lingue siccitatem, vigelie et scitis non desunt, et maior
in dextra parte est dolor. Si ex colera nigra, in sinistra parte erit dolor cum frigore,
vigiliis et gravitate. Si de fleugmate, sustinet gravidinem et spiritus gravem retrac-
tionem cum querela et dolore in occipitio. Universalis habundancia colere[44]: signa
erunt urina intensa tenuis cum clara et lucida substancia, aliquando pinguis. Si ex
colera vitelina fuerit vel ex illius degestione vel admixstione vel humorum pertur-
bacione, cum alba spuma /erit urina[45]/. Si vero epar compaciatur, [facies] citrina, pulsus
vero frequens et durus dolor in anteriori parte capitis et ad radices oculorum maxime
infestatur a tertia hora diei usque ad nonam eiusdem. Facies et alba oculorum apparent
citrina et totum corpus quandoque insompnietas aderit, sompnia in ignium fulguris et

---

37 The last four names are written in the
   lefthand margin and there is an insertion
   mark.
38 For 'melago', balm?
39 Cf. *Coll. Sal.* 4, p.470.
40 MS *et ceo*.

41 MS *acuti*.
42 MS *capm~*.
43 MS *oculorum*.
44 MS *colore*.
45 Superscript addition.

lampadastorum, avaricacio[46] et asperitas lingue et siccitas, nausia et vomitus, in plurimis colericisque[47] [. . .] citrinus .s. vel veridis, defectus appetitus cibi cum desiderio potus, egestiones citrine et verides, totius corporis desiccacio, extenuacio et calor acris. Sed totum corpus solet colere superhabundancia contingere calidis et siccis usis, calida et sicca dieta in simili regione in consuetis uti catharticis,[48] colagogis[49] et eis preter consuetudinem pretermissis. Ex genere quoque egritudinum determinamus ex causa[50] inde terciana yctericia et similibus coleram superhabundare discrivimus.

[22] Ergo capitis purgatio primo est ponenda quam Galienus et alii medici probaverunt que talis est: recipe ysoppi, satureie fasciculum unum, vini optimi eminam unam et coque in olla nova ad terciam et ex eo jejunus gargariza; corpus calefacit et caput purgat. Unde te cooperi donec omnis humor desiccetur. Tamen post aliquam moram potes lintheo caput tergere. Ordinamus igitur antidotum ad vicia capitis utile: antidotum Johannis Damasceni[51] vellet ventositati grosse, visus obscuritati, gravitati tocius corporis propter ventositatem ex flegmate et colera nigra: recipe aloe dragmas .xv., epitimi, costi ana .v., euforbii, croci, spice, camedreos ana .iii., gariofolii scripulum unum, acorii, calami aromatici et masticis ana .viii., cassielignee m. .viii., diagridii cocti m. .ii., mellis quod sufficit. Dabis pensum unius vel .iiii. denariorum cum aqua calida. Pillule Galieni ad flegma deponendum et ad omnem gravedinem capitis et ad fumum ascendentem oculos purgant et stomacum: recipe aloes epatici, diagridii, colloquintide interioris, absinthii, masticis ana m. .ii., tempera cum succo solatri[52] vel scariole .i. lactuce agrestis, fac in modum ciceris, dabis .vii. vel .ix. ante cibum. Pilule Johannis Damasceni[53] [que] valent ad mundificacionem [f.3v] capitis et stomachi accipiantur omni tempore: recipe aloes .m..vii., masticis et turbit et rose ana m. .iiii., fac pillulas in modum ciceris, da .ix. vel .xiii. ante sompnum cum aqua calida.

[23] Stomaticon Johannis Damasceni purgat coleram rubeam et nigram et flegma sine ulla molestacione: recipe yerapigre et mirobolani citrini ana manipulos .iii. et vitri [et] agarici ana manipulos .ii., turbet manipulos .vi., salis gemme, ephitim[i], ameos, anisi ana manipulos .ii., scamonee manipulum unum, tempera cum succo skariole et fac pillas quasi grani piperis cum aqua calida. Si dolor capitis ex sanguine vel colera rubea natus fuerit, incidamus venam cefalicam nisi etatis contrarietas vel temporis, consuetudinis et virtutis occurrat. Si igitur ad flebotomandum non sufficit, scarificemus pleno palmo ab utriusque pedis calcaneo. Fumum anisi Galienus confirmat prodesse capiti. Idem facit succus mente si nares et tempera ungamus. Item antidotum probatissimum ad capitis dolorem scotomianis et sanguini[i]s et oculorum

---

46 Probably an error for *amariscatio*. Compare the following passage from Gilbertus Anglicus, Bk 2 f.xc 'Signa colere . . . paucus somnus et somnia rubeorum corporum ut ignis et fulguris, alba oculorum citrina, et quandoque totius corporis et cutis, oris amariscatio, et quandoque sputum citrinum et asperitas lingue et siccitas, nausea et vomitus, quandoque co. citrine et viridis, defectus appetitus'.

47 MS *colericus que*.

48 MS *catericis*.

49 MS *calagogis*.

50 MS *causo*.

51 I.e. Johannes Serapion (Ibn Sarabi d. ca. 1074). There is a long list of antidotes in his *Practica, Jo. Serapionis Practica* . . . (Lugd. 1525).

52 MS *salatri*.

53 See *ed. cit.* f.lxxviii 'pilule de mastice et aloe mundificantes stomachum et conferentes ad sodam'.

dolorem [tollit], lacrimas potenter stringit et visum clarificat, humoresque malos in capite congestos desiccat, stomacum calefacit et confortat: recipe aristologie manipulos .xxviii. .s. binos,[54] spice, costi, croci, jusquiani, cinoglosse, omnium usque manipulos .ix. et semis, singulos melanopiperis manipulos .iiii., laseris manipulos duos, mellis quod[55] sufficit cum aqua.[56] Item gargarismus preciosus ad omne flegma totius capitis et corporis et ad dolorem eius auferendum: recipe peretri manipulos .iiii., sinapis totidem, pullegii regalis, calamenti, zinziber, staphisagrie, ysoppi, piperis, omnium sex manipulos duos[57] conficiatur, sic omnia simul tere et crebra et secundum quantitatem pulveris adde acetum et super lentum ingnem fac bullire. Parum postea mellis quatuor partes adhice et permitte ebuliendo sic inspissari ut[58] gutta super unguem posita adhereat. Item antidotum philonium[59] hoc operatur: caput purgat, pectus lenit, capillaturam fluentem confirmat, vocem clarificat, auditum reddit, stomacum confortat, vesicam purgat, calculos solvit[60], urinam provocat, vomitum restringit, malum anelitum tollit. Recipe hec: piper, ciminum, gingiber, peretrum, baccas lauri, semen feniculi, aneti, petrosilini, livestici, apii ana omnia ista tere in mortario, addatur eis mel coctum et bene despumatum et reponatur in pixide bene cerata et sumatur mane et sero ad modum avelane.

[24]   Vertigo, precipitium .i. revolutio. *Ad vertin del chef:*[61] *reez le chef e mettez enplastre fet de comyn e de mastic e de oint de cat et beve vetoine quit en estale cervise e facez ton chef laver de lessive fet de vetoine. Pur vertin:*[62] *pernez la rue e edre de la terre une [poiné], batez le ben, e pernez le jus tant com en purrez trahire. Puis*[63] *pernez mel e aboun de oef / e un drape linge veuz ou nef,*[64] */ ben le plastre[z], ne vous seit grief, / issi le mettez sur vostre chef. Item: averoune triblé o vin o od oximel bevez. [Item:]*[65] *frotez les temples de jus de neire bete. Item ad dolor del chief:*[66] *mettez as narils puliol quit en eisil ke ils sentent la odour e de cel puliol curonnez la teste. Item:*[67] *quisez en ewe rue e edre terestre e foiles de lorer, de chescune une poiné e .ix. baiez de lorer e de ce oignez ben le chef. [Item:] bevez sovement averoigne triblé od mel vel oignez les templez od rue triblé od oile. Item: oignez le front e les temples od fel de levre e mel ouelment trebien triblé ensemble que tout seit de rouge colour. Item: puliol*[68] *od sa fleure triblé od ewe beive june, pus june deke noun. Item: beive destemperez od ewe averoigne, sauge, trifoil e ere terestre. Item:*[69] *mettez enplaustre ad*[70] *le chef fet de rue e seel triblé od mel. Item:*[71] *si vous est avis que le chef la sus est enfundré*[72] *cum une fosse, les foils de egrimoine quesez od [f.4r] mel e mettez le enplastre sur, si garra. Item:*[73] *quesez celidoine*[74] *ben en bure, pus si la colez parmi un drap, si gardez en boistez.*

54 I.e. aristologia longa and rotunda.
55 MS *et*.
56 MS *cum te aqua*.
57 MS *duas*.
58 MS *si*.
59 See AN 49 (Filonium maius).
60 MS *solum*.
61 Most of the succeeding vernacular receipts are found in the 'Lettre d'Hippocrate' (hereafter *LH*), see Hunt, *Popular Medicine*, pp.100ff.
62 See *Physique rimee* (hereafter PR) in *Popular Medicine*, pp.142ff, ll. 97–100, 101–4.
63 MS *plus*.

64 MS *nez*.
65 See *LH* 13.
66 See *LH* 7.
67 See *LH* 8.
68 MS *piliol*.
69 See 'Novele cirurgerie' (hereafter *NC*), in C.B. Hieatt and R.F. Jones (eds.), *La Novele Cirurgerie* (London, 1990), ll.37ff.
70 MS *od*.
71 See *LH* 8a.
72 MS *enfleure*.
73 See *LH* 9a.
74 MS *en c*.

De ce ungez le chef e lavez le en la ewe en laquele le celedoine fut quitez. Item pur le feie eschaufé e a le chief s'il seit tout enflé:[75] *greise de cerf e mel e farine d'orge e ere terestre e mel triblez tot ensemble, reez le chef, si mettez icel enplastre eschaufé en une aumusce sur la teste dekez il seit garriz. Item pur touz les mals del chef:*[76] *triblez bien rue e mettez en fort eisel. De ce oignez bien le chief desus. Item:*[77] *rue e fenil quesez en ewe e de ce lavez la chief. Item:*[78] *la neire bete estanpez e del jus ungez le front e les temples. Item pur tot dolour capitis:*[79] *les moles foiles de ere triblez mult bien od eisel e od oile roset e ungez le front e les temples.*[80] *Item:*[81] *betoine, vervaine, aloine, celedoine, plantayne, rue, eble, sauge, de l'escorce de seu, vint greins de peivre neir*[82] *tot triblez bien ensemble, puis quesez en vin, si en bevez chescune jour jun e couchez desque seie[z] sain. Item:*[83] *puliol chaud of sa fleure bevez jun, si vous destenez de manger desque ad nonam*[84] *horam. Item ad le chief: quesez en stale cervoise fenuil e ere terestre, sauge, betoine,*[85] *sandre, rue e bevés par .ix. jours, ad matin freid, ad sere chaud e de cestez herbis covrez li le chife, si garra. Si escorez un chat*[86] *madle e de la pei[l] li coverez le chef .iii. jours e si ert gariz denz poi de houre. Item ad dolour del chief: fenuil, ere terestre, sauge, verveine (si), sander, rue, si liez triblé ad le chef, si le carsés. Aprés de pel de gras chat covrez, ut supra, e des herbes et cetera. Item:*[87] *puliol quit mettez ad*[88] *les nariles, si que ils sentent le odour e fettez une coroune de ce puliol quit e crounez le chief. Item piles arabiks ad la dolor de la teste provees*[89] *[s]on[t], [meme] si par cent anz la eut en,*[90] *e si purgent*[91] *tresbien touz humours e engendre[nt] le[e]sse*[92] *e acuic[ent] le penser e rend[ent] le vewe e gardent le memorie e si ne suffre[nt] chaniz avant [le] dit age e sane[n]t le stomak e le vertin e nomément del mal*[93] *q'est appellé emigranium. Si purgent denz e langke e oilz e tot le cors de maus humours*[94] *e le soun des oreiles e toutz complexions conservent.*[95] Pernez *.iiii. ouncez de aloen epatic, brionie, bacca, scamoiné, mirre ana .i. once, confiez od jus de fenuil e fetez piles .v. o .vii. o .ix. o .xi. et cetera.*

[25]   Item electuarium pro nimia sal[i]va [que] a capite descendit: zinzibra, juniperi ana .i., piperis .iii., mellis quod sufficit, accipe .ii. coclearia sive .iii. cotidie donec stringatur saliva. *Item pouder ad purger la teste: [pernez] de gilgano e de gingivre e de pelettre e de organe e de ysoppe e temperez od mel e eisel e gargari[s]és en la bouche. Item pur la teste pille:* recipe peritri, staf[i]sagrie, gingebri, piperis, seminis sinapis ana dragma una, omnia trita cum melle conficiantur et cum uti volueris, unam sub lingua tene et fleuma attrahet a capite disolu[tu]m et sic caput purgabit. Item pillule Galieni[96] ad delendam omne fleuma et omnem gravem fumum caput adscendentem et oculos atque

---

75 See *LH* 10 which has *morele* in place of *mel*.
76 See *LH* 12.
77 See *LH* 11.
78 See *LH* 13.
79 See *LH* 14.
80 The scribe here recopies a receipt and clears it by underlining: *Item ad touz les mals del chief: rue triblez bien e mettez en fort eisel e de ce oignez bien le chef desus.*
81 See *LH* 16.
82 MS *mei.*
83 See *LH* 21.
84 MS *unam.*
85 MS *botoine.*

86 MS *chaud.*
87 See *LH* 7.
88 MS *od.*
89 See *AN* 87: 'etsi per .c. annos duraverint ... generant leticiam et auferunt tristiciam, mentem acuunt, visum reddunt, auditum restaurant, memoriam tribuunt ...'
90 MS reading unsure. Cf. note above.
91 MS *purgez.*
92 MS *les l.*
93 MS *de la madle.*
94 MS *h. mundetur.*
95 MS *conservient.*
96 See *Antidotarium Nicolai* ed. van der Berg 89.

stomachum purgabit: recipe aloes, diagridii, colloquintidis, agarici, mastici, absinthii ana dragmas .iiii., temperabis cum succo solatri et fac pilas. Item ad purgandum caput et vocem clarificandum: absinthii fasciculum unum et marrubii et piperis grana cum farina[97] fabarum ben[e] cocta[98] coclearia .iii., mellis dispumati eminam et coque ad specitudinem[99] mellis et refrigerantur in ampulam et repone inde accipe cotidie coclear .i. et illis diebus caveat a lardo, [f.4v] butiro et oleo. Item: mirra et aloe aceto acerimo[100] distempera et [in] nares per .iii. dies infunde; caput et pectus ex flegma multum purgat. Item: radix peretri manducata et pituitam patefacto ore mirifice expellit et caput a flegma educit et purgat. Item: oleum rosaceum[101] tepide in nares infunde et caput purgat.

[26] *Ad vertin quele ke seit e [a] amender la vue: pernez une medicine, pillule castorie, en ewe tefe ou[102] seit destemperé le peis de une maile. Item ad vertin:[103] triblez rue od eisel e oinez sovent les temples. Item: sav(a)ine, averone e peivre triblez od vin e aukes de mel e bevez matin fraid, ad cocher chaud.* Item et ad pectus: bibe jus marubii et mel et butirum quam calidum potes quando vades dormire. Ad fracturam ossis capitis: lava caput cotidie cum aqua cocta cum betonica et de eadem herba bibe jejunus et cetera. Quere ubi de plagis agitur. Ad ulcus capitis: fove ulcera[104] urina tauri aut sepo aut modico sale; efficacissime sana[n]tur. Ad formicaciones capitis: frontem et timpora perunges oleo cum aneto cocto. *Ad felon del chief:* r[espice] ubi de fel[one] agitur. Frontis dolorem curat folia sambuci et radix urtice agrestis trita cum melle fortiter, et inde perunge frontem. Ad formicaciones et sirones ubicumque fuerint in homine maxime in fronte vel facie: frumentum distempera cum vino et pulverem olibani appone et in modum enplastri appone.

[27] *Teste teingnus: reez la, metez sur un drap piez[105] e rue boili ensemble, illucque seit deke le nefime jour, si garra pur veir. Item: ail triblé od mel mettez ad le chef. Item:[106] de jus de neire bete oinez le chef sovent. Item: reez le chef e boillez ensemble piz, rue e fevez [e] teve mettez et cetera ut supra. Item: boille tedcline one boutere ad suye, do it ye nrt of an finere, yer mide ofte. Item:[107] raez le chef, fel de tor od eisel garit mult ben de cel peril. Puis pernez seu de tor e la teste de ail pelé e medelez od sel ars e oile e oinez la teste.[108] Item oignement pur teine: 'Feltrey' genus herbe est. Ceo pernez e les racines de rouge doke e de rouge fenuil e de lovesche ouelment e mult secs seient tous, ke ewe ne mosture ne i seit e issi les triblez, pus les friez mult bien en sein de pork maydle e en bure de mai, tant de .i. cum d'autre, pus le colez parmi un drap. Donke pernez peivre tant cum entreit en .i. escale de .i. oef e bone partie de vif argent, si triblez mult menu et metez en le vant-dit jus e ben le movez que seit trebien medlé e mettez en boistez. Pus trahez de .i. winderer les maveis peiles que creisent en la teine. Aprés reez la teste, pus le lavez chescun jour. Avant que vous le oignez si se garde du soleil e dedenz meison seit la teste descoverte. Quant serra sein, si le faut peil, pernez rouge foille e pur mel, si medelez e de ce si le oignez. Item ad teine, roine, derte e chescun kancre: pernez moleine, avence, archangelie, blionie, ermoise, qui[n]quefoil, gaudine,*

---

97 MS *farinam.*
98 MS *b. si coctam.*
99 I.e. 'spissitudinem'.
100 MS *acerino.*
101 MS *oleo rutato.*
102 MS *ewe que tefe s..*
103 See *LH* 12.

104 MS *ipsa sed u.*
105 I.e. 'peiz', 'pitch'.
106 See *LH* 14.
107 See *PR* 1679–82.
108 See *PR* 1685–90. This and the previous receipt are combined in Sloane 146 (see *Popular Medicine,* p.272, no.37).

medwort, trifoil, osmunde, ausne, frasier, agrimoine, taneseie, maruil, cham[om]ille, burnette, ambrosie, comperon de ronce, comperon de seu, mauye, w[i]mauwe, oculesconce, chefrefoil, verge ad pastor, herbe s. Johan, ruge paril, sure parele, milfoil, al(i)oine, yerre arbrine, amerosche, rouge centurie, cerfoil, chanfe, warance, nepte, entrerus de freine, eglenter, garre, lauriol, restebuf, saneroile, de toz icés du poignez la meité, meins de moleine e autretant de kersons de fonteine e le bugle, sanigle ouelment, .ii. itant de pigle, atant de plainteyne e de lancelé, conferie, premerole, foilz de raiz, petite consoude, chenlange, jubarbe, violette, fenuil, brioine, maufe de cortil, gletoner, [f.5r] matefelon graund e petit, pionie, betoine, alisaunder, luvesche, liz, treis itaunt de herbe water,[109] autant de herbe, autant de orpin, morele, pimpernole, dragaunce, celidonie, navett, .ii. itant de peluete triblez od sein de motoun e bure de mai e fetez quere en eisel e en ewe deke le jus seit tot vert e le herbe jaune[110] e premez le, pus [l]e purez e i mettez oile de olive asez e cire e poudre de ensens e mastick e reseine blaunche. Quant ert boili e refreid[i], metez en boistez.

[28]   Item in prima quadragesime accipe sagmen carnis, in eodem die elixe, et ad gabrionem valet et ceteris aliis sicuti scabiosis et teinus et cetera. Item cherme[111] certeine e esprovee ad testes tenues: pernez en ta main cru lard de pork madle bone partie e le teinus sece devant vous, si mettez le lard sur la teste e dites 'cum as tu a noun crestien?' e il nomera sun noun. Sequitur 'In þe faders name and ine þe sones + and ye holi gost'. Quant ce dites, de la lard croisez la teste od ta mein destre e puis tenez le lard sur la teste e ditez 'Loverd yif it is yi wil, of yis evel hil his man .N. for þe love and for ye honour of sent Sompne, seint Chome, seint Dome and seint Damien'. Ditz .iii. foiz. Ad chescune fiez ditez oveke Pater Noster et Ave Maria e le bien quiez cum avant est dit. En cel manere ditez deke seiz aiez. Dit[es] .ix. feiz et se garde la teste trestout le an d'ewe e de chescune moist[u]re ne mye tant que ewe beneite i touche e checun jour un foiz oinez la teste de cel lard. Si le lard defaud, triblez autre od ce. Quant il se oigne, die 'que avez a noun crestien? Jeo ai a noun .N.'. Quant mester est, de cisur forcés le peil. Adprés le an, quant il est sein, la le peil faut esparpillez poudrez arses. Item:[112] ad lieus placous ou pil faut / ben vous dirrai que mult vaud: / moschez[113] e és, si mettez / en un nuef pot, si les ardez, / ad ceo metez jus de cerfoil / e noiz petites, de cel b[r]oil, / en poudre arsez mult sotilement / e mel e oile tot ensement e de ce oignez. Item pur fere chef [creistre]: mettez la ou faut [peil] foils de sauz, qui[s]etz od oile, si recrestra ben. Item: ardez le cheforele de femme, si medle[z] od mel e oinez ou volez que creisch. Item: limnatoras cornu caprini cum farina siliginis miscas et combustas cum oleo lauri, capiti appone, capillos confirmat et renasci facit. Item ad fer crestre: la escorce /.i. suber/ de houz e les racines de sauz e de ros triblez e quisez od oile e de ce oignez. Item ut pili nascantur:[114] agrimoniam tritam cum lacte caprino appone. Item: de cinere vitis et ossibus pecoris et verris[115] uncto fac unguentum et unge per .vii. dies. Probatum est. Item ad pilos percreandos: ladanum triticum in tegula ustum et stercora murium et vitella ovorum cocta,[116] hec pulverizata cum olio ad modum ungenti conficia[n]tur et locum ubi producturi sunt pili sic para: salnitrum in aceto tempera et ex illo aceto locum grosso panno laneo frica donec rubescat. Deinde medicinam induc, probatum

---

109 I.e. Herb Walter.
110 MS fauue.
111 MS cherene.
112 See PR 1691–8.
113 MS moltez.

114 See LH 74. A Latin version is found in the *Speculum medicorum* in MS Oxford, Merton College 324 (s.xv) f.17r.
115 Correct *veteri*?
116 MS *costa*.

est. *Item ad cheveril que chet: quisez les entrailes de levres medlé od oile de merte e mettez e cresteront. Item: ees od oile et cetera, ut supra.*[117] Item: agrimoniam cum lacte caprino, ut supra.[118] Item: bulli simul sal et vinum et inde lava et balnea simul cum croco dulci. Item ne cadant:[119] *ardez lin e medelez od oile e oignez le chef.* Item si cadant:[120] *oignez de meule de cerf.* Item ut pili nascantur ubicumque volueris:[121] panem ordeacum cum sale combure et tere cum adipe ircino et unge locum. *Ad espescer ch[everel]:* fac saginum de lardo porcino, inde sepe perunge. Item: agrimoniam, radicem ulmi, vervene, radix salicis, absintheum, abrotanum, semen lini combustum et in pulverem radicis canne adde, radantur radica. Hec omnia coque in lacte caprino vel in aqua ablue. *Item ad fer recrestre que est cheuye par arcisons:*[122] *poudre de neil molu medlez od mel cru e si mettez vel oinez la cheverel.* Ad faciendum longos capillos: radicem altee cum sagmine [f.5v] porci recentis vel veteri diu fac bullire in vino et post appone ciminum bene tritum et masticum et vitella ovorum bene cocta, hec omnia simul misce postquam bene cocta fuerint, per pa[nnum] cola,[123] que frigerate pinguedinem collige supernatantem et capite prius abluto inunge capud et elongabuntur nec in capite remanebunt pediculi. *Item:*[124] *moilez*[125] */.i. per capillos/ votre chef de la roucee de maii chescune jour .iii. foiz, prové est.*

[29] Si mulier voluerit habere lot[um] caput et nigros capillos:[126] acc[i]pe viridem lacertam et remotis capite et cauda coquatur in oleo communi, tali oleo caput inunctum reddit capillos longos et nigros. Item ad nigros capillos: preparentur capilli ut invenientur abiles ad tincturam[127] suscipiendos ut postea dicetur. Galle cum oleo in olla comburantur et pulvis cum aceto distemperetur et apponetur atrimentum, inde unge. Item ut pili nigri flavi fiant:[128] decoque celidoniam, agrimoniam, rasuram buxi et folia et infunde super stramen avene et sineres similiter et fac lixivam et inde caput lava. Item *ad [cheveus] espés e jaunes: rouge cerfoil e oint de pork medlé boilez en ewe e lavez le ch[everel]. Prové est.* Item experimentum [A]driani(?)[129] ad flavendos capillos: accipe radices mirte et rubee maioris et celedonie ana, tere diligenter cum olio in quo cuminum et rasura buxi et parum croci decoctum sit et capud inunge et maneat inunctio die ac nocte et lixivum[130] cineris cal(l)idum et pane ordei et multum valet. Item ad coloracionem[131] capillorum ut flavi fiant: accipe corticem exteriorem nucis maioris, illud .s. viride et amarum ipsius arboris et coque in aqua et cum hac distemperabis alumen et gallas et cum istis distemperatis caput illius bene illines folia subponendo et pilo ligando per .ii. dies. Pect(in)e caput et illud quod capillis adhesit tanquam superfluum recedat. Post appone tincturam que fit ex croco orientali et sanguine draco[nis] et [de] alecanna[132] cuius erit maior pars.[133] Ista distemperentur

---

117 Cf. entry at n.107.
118 See entry above at n.108.
119 See LH 72.
120 See LH 71.
121 See MS Merton Coll. 324 f.17r.
122 See LH 77.
123 MS *li cola.*
124 See LH, *Popular Medicine,* p.127. Also in Latin in MS Merton Coll. 324 f.19r.
125 MS *mouez.*

126 See MS Merton Coll. 324 f.19r.
127 MS *tuncturam.*
128 See MS Merton Coll. 324 f.18v.
129 The MS appears to read *driañ.*
130 MS *lixiva.*
131 MS *coleracionem.* The receipt is found in MS Merton Coll. 324 f.19r with variant readings as follows: 'viride et corticem illius a. . . . hoc locum ilines illud supponendo cum fascia ligando . . .'

cum decoctione brasilii et sic remaneat per .ii. dies vel per .iii. Post in tercia die lavetur cum aqua capud et [n]unquam[134] de facili removetur. *Ad ch[eveus] espisses: oignez les de jus de milfoil od oil[e].* Item ut per .ix. dies crispentur: sepius forti cervisia lavetur caput. Item: cornua arietis combusta cum olio tere et inde sepe unge. Item: radicem eliburi trita, caput inunge et cum oleo super caput liga. Si vis aliquem nunquam canescere agnum nigrum qui habet caput candidum, decoque et inde caput sepe unge.

[30] Ut fiat perpetua ablacio capillorum: accipe ova formicarum et gummi edere[135] et auripigmentum rubeum et cum vino conmisce in unum et quemlibet locum ubi vis confricabis. Item:[136] *la semence de sicute / .i.. homlok/ e le sank de chavso[r]ez e le jus de verveine medelez ensemble e aracez le peil de quil lieu que vous vuilliez et pus lavez le liu e aprés en oignez de cest e jammés ne recrestra peil.* Item: semen urtice in aceto tere et corpus calefactum inde line. Item sanguisugarum [pulvis cum][137] succo edere inmittus crescere non permittit. Item: *ostez le peil, pus lavez la lieu de leit de lesche. Item: oefs de formicez, gumme[138] de ere, orpiment ensemble medelez e touchez ou voillez que checent e cherount ne mes ne cresteront. Item: ardez cinc[139] de chavçoris / .i. vespertilionis/ e les cendres od afronito / .i. lapis calcedonio/ triblez et oignez.* Item:[140] succo rafani et edere unge per .iii. dies. *Poi lez ostez.* Sume aliquotiens serum cum acerimo aceto et liberabis nec nunquam postea renascantur.

[31] *Item: lavez vostre chef de jus de rue e boilez, lentz cherunt.* Item ad pediculos: oleum olive et pulverem cuiuslibet cineris de foco bene cribrato simul conmisce [f.6r] et ita tere ad spissitudinem mellis, deinde cum opus fuerit ex eo caput unge. Item: lava cum succo viridis bete. Item: cinis vitis cum oleo et melle mixtus lentes et pediculos spargit. Item ad [illos] qui in pectine vel in acella inhabitant: cineres in oleo distempera et inunge. Item ad illos qui circa oculos sunt, ad ruborem oculorum et ad mitigacionem eorundem unguentum: recipe aloes .iii., ceruse, olibani[141] unciam .i., lardi quod sufficit conficitur. Sic dum subtile terimus et cetera, pulverizata apponimus. *Pur puces:* semen coriandri pone vel herbam . . ..[142] *Poudre ad engeter artisons de drap o de pane o de forure: triblez soufre e seel e bren e esparpilez, frotant bien de vostre main.* Collum ad cuius malum atque scapularum: melle perunge et postea farinam fabarum et folia edere superpone cum melle. Item: artimesie succum, oleum, ceram ana conmisce et inde unge. Maxillarum dolori testa ovorum unde pulli excluduntur et ovorum coctorum vitelli et parum olei rosacei et cere quod sufficit. Item: cerotum in lintheo inductum appone.

[32] Item ad raucedinem et ad fauces: respice ubi de raucedine agitur. Gutturis dolor et faucium sic curatur: cimini[143] pugillum plenum coque bene in vino et bibe

---

132 MS Merton Coll. 324 f.19r confirms the reading ('de alcanna').
133 MS Merton Coll.324 f.19r has 'alecanna in maiori quantitate'.
134 MS Merton Coll. 324 has 'non'.
135 MS *g.et e.*
136 MS Merton Coll. 324 f.18v has a similar receipt in Latin.
137 Addition based on MS Merton Coll. 324 f.18v.
138 Corrected from MS *lerine* from the Latin version of this receipt at the beginning of the section.
139 For *sanc.*
140 Same receipt in MS Merton Coll. 324 f.18v.
141 MS *o. qñ.*
142 MS has *lto.* Expansion to *lectorica* (hazel) seems unlikely.
143 MS *ciminum.*

inde die ac nocte. *Item ad enflure de goitrun et de maschel*: accipe feniculum, apium, betonicam et coque eas in aqua. Postea tere illas et appone parum vini et farine siliginis et fac enplaustrum et appone per .iii. dies. Item: si intumuerunt cum dolore magno: radicem canis lingue cum cineribus assari facias et cum ausungia tere et subliga faucibus et sit ita per .iii. dies. Hec medicina prodest ubi tumor cum dolore fuerit. Item ad inflaturam gutturis que quin contra et pa[ciens] nec potest commedere: accipe malvam et archimesiam, cassilaginem et jusqueamum, absinthium, p[ar]ittariam, coque tritas cum melle et superpone calidas pacienti.

[33]   *Face techelé*: ciminum in aceto tunsum postea assatum si quis hoc commederet in omni cibo suo et facia(n)t inde salsam qua utatur .s. cotidie, faciem rubeam et postulas curat sine dubio. Item [*face te*]*chelé*: *oignez de la sanc de tor et la fra clere*, vel de *oil fet de nogagks* vel *de sanc de levre*. Item ruborem faciei aufert sagimen vetus tunsum et tritum cum foliis rampni et sulphure. *Item ad rouge teches en la face: triblez freis furmage od mel si que le furmage ne seit lavé de [. . .] ce enplaustre mettez sur la face. Item: triblés bien les peires que l'en trove en feies de buef e de tors e distemperés od oile, si oinez.*

[34]   *Item ad cele que ad emfle*[144] *de lepre o ad des boce[s]*: *pernez .ii. onces de soufre e veil oingt tant com i covent e triblez ensemble e oinez la face. Item ad face leprouse: oingt de ver e jus de creischon e jus de ortie, igalment de vif argent, triblez tot ensemble e oinez ad seir e matin, pus si le lavez. Ce fetes par .ii. feiz o .iii. o plus si mester est.* Contre *lepre*: accipe semen caniculate bene pulverizatum et da cotidie scrupulum .i. in cibo. Scrupulus peisit .iii. quadrantz. *Item ad lepre: pernez le fleurs titimali e triblez od reiseine e de ce oignez e ne crestra pas.*

[35]   Item ad ruborem faciei: accipe radicem viticelle / wild nepe / et pulveriza minutatim, desiccatum pulverem destempera cum aqua rosacea et cum bombace / .i. coton / pauco vel panno lineo subtili illinito induc faciei ruborem. Mulieri fiant albe naturaliter. Fac istum rubeum colorem si rubore careat illi que debet dealbari. Facimus colorem rubeum ut submentita et paliata specie albedinis color rubeus appelat quasi naturalis. *Ad palliour .s. oster: quisez ancusa od vin e usez ad hour terç*[145] *.ii. colerez. Autre ad femme pale:*[146] *lavez la viz o(d) de savun o d'ewe chaud, si leschiez sechir, pus mettez roventele od sa salive, .iii. jours durra.*[147]

[36]   Ad inflationem faciei sufficit sola fumigatio aque. Item ad inflationem oculorum: teratur ornecio(?) cum recenti ausungia porci et superponatur. *Deytre, roine e teine: ombre de fosse*[148] */ feltrid / triblés od gresse de pork et gise .xl. jours en pelotes [f.6v], aprés pernez meloine,*[149] *oculus sconse, femetere, feverfeue, aun(i)e, ameroske, rouge cheferfoil, peniwort, milfoil, surele, racine de rouge peril, rouge cholet, bilren, aloine, agrimoine, escorce de neir prunier, burjons de coudre triblés durement bien, de chescun herbe .ii. poinés, f[l]ur de paniwort e cholet une poiné, .iiii. de burjons de coudre, tot come le autre*

---

144   MS *emble*. The emendation is conjectural.
145   MS *tere*.
146   See *Pop. Med.*, p.272, no.40.
147   MS *dirra*.
148   Cf. *lumbre de fosse* glossed by 'ço est flectrit' in MS London, Wellcome Historical Medical Library 544 p.256 printed in Hunt, "Anglo-Norman Medical Receipts" in I. Short (ed.), *Anglo-Norman Anniversary Essays*, ANTS O.P. 2 (London, 1993), p.203 no.12 (cf. p.204 no.16).
149   I.e. 'moleine'.

triblez e issi en pel[otes] gisez .ix. jours, puis gisez en siu de motoun e bure de mai mult bien
e premez le jus e mettez en seire, encens, mastic, blanch ress[in]e, peiz liquide, soufre vif e
oripiment, vif argent, de chescun demi livre e fetes ent poudre e de ces que deivent estre triblés
la .iiii. partie de un livre, mes estreinez les bien od gresse de pork en une esquile en vostre
main e tot veis frotez od la greisse deke seit tot neire e mettez leinz do oignement, ostez del fu
e toteveis le movez deke soit refreid[é]. Pus me[ttez] en bo[istes]. Ad faciem rugosam: accipe
spatulam et gladiolam et extrahe succum et sero succo illo faciem inunge et in mane
erit cutus elevata et erumpetur quasi. Rupturam sanabis cum unguento in quo radix
lilii posita sit. Ad venas que apparent in facie: prius extrahendo pellem que prius
rupturam subtilis apparet [..]. Ad venas que apparent in facie vel in naso: tres partes
de sapone et quartam de pipere pulverizata apponimus loco et predicto modo sanamus.

[37] Ad ustionem solis super faciem: radix lilii domestici mundata et cocta cum
aqua pistretur, postea accipe pulverem masticis, olibani .i. s[crupulum], camphorie
uncias .ii., ausungie recentis porcine et cum aqua[150] conficiatur et cum aqua rosacea
similiter conficias et usui reserva. Conficiatur autem sic: mundamus ante lilii radicem
et bene lavamus et cum aqua decoquemus et decoctam fortiter terimus ausungiam et
ad ignem liquefactam et sale mundificatam et distemperatam infundimus. Postea [...?]
grossam in aqua rosacea tus solutam (?) ponimus. Deinde pulverizatam adiungimus.

[38] Ad faciem dealbandam et pilos tollendos: calcem vivam per mensem aqua
mutando et removendo ad solem pone agitando sepe. Primo per pannum subtile
coletur et desiccetur in modum seruse, tunc de altea vel butiro inungatur, oculos tamen
custodiat. Sed et cum unxerit, mane lava cum [aqua] tepida. Item ad faciem dealbandam: *neile triblé od fel de chefre e destemperez enb[l]aunche la face.* Ad ustionem faciei et
dealbandum: recentem porci adipem et ovorum semicoctam albuginem cum modico
farine simul contere, de baccis lauri unge. Item: bulli radicem levestici et ex aqua lava,
mirum est. Item [ad] hominis et mulieris faciem declarandum: accipe thus et cam-
phoram, masticem ana, cerusam mediam partem et os [s]epie, omnia pulverizentur
cum glarea, tamen exagitentur ut spuma elicitatur. Deinde in aqua bulliente ponatur
et paululum in ea moretur. Tandem extrahatur et in usui reservetur. Cum glarea
apponatur faciei. Item: fabas magnas vel alias frange inter duos lapides molendo et
ablue in aqua, bene inde sicca ad solem, postea fac molere et farinam bullire. Deinde
accipe albumen ovi et verbera fortiter usque[151] liquidum sit ut aqua et misce cum
fabarum farina et verbera. Sic fac per .iii. dies vel quatuor vel octo et misce sanguinem
galline vel auce aut columbe et iterum verbera ad solem. Quanto plus sic verberatur
ad solem tanto melior erit. Postea [mitte] in pixside et quando volueris uti, frica palmas
inde et cum palmis faciem et erit candida et nitida. Super omnes medicinas valet. Ad
totum corpus faciendum lucidum, clarum et purum lava totum in lia (?) fortissimi vini
vel servisie.

---

150 MS *cum aqua com̃ aqua.*
151 MS *usque dum l.*

[BOOK II: THE EYES]

1.

[39] Oculorum tria sunt vicia. Ipse qui habet oculos tortos, et dicitur a torqueo
-ques. Item strabo dicitur a sterno. Petus est ille qui sepe oculos claudit. Luscus est ipse
qui non potest bene videre, et dicitur de lux, lucis et careo, -es, quasi luce carens.
Cecus est qui omnino caret luce. Lippus est ille qui habet oculos aquaticos. Obliquum
visum gestans homo strabo vocatur.[f.7r] Cernit in obliquo strabo, lippus in altum.
Dicatur luscus qui videt id quod parum. Orbe carent orbi, sed sole lumine ceci. At
petus et illuc luscus proprie lippus acquescunt (?). 'Pulvis obest oculis, fletusque
fumusque famesque./ Allia, nux, nix, venus, vinum et vigilare'.[152] 'Allia vina venus
ignis fames fumus et estus, / ista nocent oculis, sed vigilare magis'.[153] 'Pulvis obest
oculis, vinum venus ac vigilare,/ allea, nix, nux, fumus lacrimare famesque'.[154]

[40] *Dolour des oils avent a la feiz de grand veiler e de grant eveilment, ad la fiez avent
od enfleure, a la fiez od perfusion de sanc, ad*[155] *la feiz od purlei*[156] *ad la feiz*[157] *od*[158] *chacie.*[159]
Encontre totes maners oez ici medicines. 'Feniculus, vervena, rosa, celidonia, ruta, / ex
istis fit aqua que lumina reddit acuta'.[160] Item: appone eufrasiam. Oculi sunt quasi
lucerna tocius corporis.[161] Colores et dolores oculorum quandoque veniunt ab intrensicis causis, ut a scotomia, que est vertigo, que tenebrositatem inducit oculorum;
quandoque accidit ex extrensicis causis. Ypocras in libro **Afforismorum** docet modum
curandi dolores oculorum acutos in flebotomia rubea; a causis intrensicis procedens
ut dicit 'meri pocio aut piria[162] aut lavali curavit flebotomia solvit'.[163] Si dolor
oculorum ex sanguine fuerit, hec esse signa: dolor oculorum acutus in flebotomia
rubea. Cura est flebotomia de cephali[c]a vena vel de vena in summitate narium vel
de venis intra nares. Deinde apponenda est aqua rosacea in oculo vel succus verbene
cum pastello eiusdem superposito.[164] Sillium in saculo positum in aqua infrigidata

---

152 See Walther, *Proverbia* 22890. See also Renzi, *Coll. Sal.*5, p.55 ll.1921ff (*Flos medicinae scholae
      Salerni*).
153 See Walther, *ibid.* 810,774,1915,1924.
154 See Walther, *ibid.* 22890 (cf.11399).
155 MS *de*.
156 Apparently an error for *od lermes*.
157 MS *face*.
158 MS *pur*.
159 See LH 26.
160 *Reg. San.* ed. Cummins ll.239–40. See also *Euperiston* above para. 73 and *Pop. Med.* p.232 no.79
      and p.289 no.197. See also *Liber de diversis medicinis* ed. M.S. Ogden p.11, ll.33–5.
161 Cf. the *Speculum medicorum* in MS London, B.L. Royal 12 E xxii f.24v '. . . cum sunt oculi lucerna
      tocius corporis'.
162 MS *tiria*.
163 See Lib.VI c.xxxi 'Dolores oculorum, mery potio, aut lavacrum, aut piria, aut flobothomia, aut
      pharmacia solvit' and Lib.VII, c.xlvi 'Oculorum dolores mery potio et lavacrum et flobothomia
      solvit'. (*Articella* 1523 f.133ra). Martin de Saint-Gille *ed. cit.*, p.93 'Pocion de vin, baing,
      fomentacion, saignee, medecine laxative, curent la douleur des yeux' (VI,xxxi).
164 MS *superposita*.

apponatur. Si ex colera rubea, hec sunt signa: dolor pungitivus cum facie[165] citrina. Cura ut autor testatur. Postea lavacio, balneum, aquee calide, per sudorem exiat materia tota. Singulariter fleobotoma confer[t] de cephali[c]a vena. Localia adiutoria apponenda sunt ut superius diximus. Si dolor ex fleumate fit, [hec] esse signa: dolor le[n]tus erit in flebotoma alba [et] copia lacrimarum. Cura ut testatur autor: (iiii.) potio interius sumpta in oculo posita. Item: rutam, celidoniam coque in vino albo et infunde in oculo. Item: thus, cerusam distempera cum succo feniculi et pauco mellis et conmisce insimul et cola. Instilla vel pone collirium album quod in vinacio(?)[166] reperitur. Recipe[167] amidum et cerusam et dragagantum, aloes, ana et de hiis fiat pulvis, cum succo rute distemperetur et in vase vitreo vel cupreo reservetur et utetur eo. Purgacio confert cum lenderta (?) et yerapigra. Si ex malencolia, hec esse signa: dolor extensitivus et gravans, color lividus vel subniger. Cura ut testatur auctor: purgacio cum melagoga, theodiricon vel yeralogodion vel pillulis de lapide lazuri vel pillulis aureis. Similiter localia adiutoria apponenda sunt ut in predictis.

[41] Sunt adhuc passiones oculorum extrensece ut est tela, macula, ungula, pannus, albugo, oculorum ulcera, sanguis ex coleracione[168] in oculo collectus. Contra telam: accipe papaveris rufi succum et frequenter in oculo distilla. Vel aliter: accipe radicem zinziber et pone in vino, deinde frica cum cote et pone in oculo. Ad idem: os [s]epie tritum cum lacte mulieris pone in oculo. Ad idem: limax rubea cum testa combusta et in oculo posita.[169] Item: thus tritum cum lacte mulieris in oculo positum constat. Ad idem: succus p[ar]it(r)arie similiter instillatus valet. Ad idem: succus celidonie cum melle valet. Ad idem: grana gallitrici .v. in oculo posita per totam noctem iuvant. Hec eadem remedia ad maculam valent. Etsi curabilis fuerit. Ungula macula indurata dicitur. Pannus qui operit totum oculum vel utrumque incurabilis est. Item propter turbitudinem hoc modo tingnatur: accipe corticem maligranati, attrahe succum et misce cum succo jusquiani et tinge per .iii. dies continue et ita tinctus erit. Vel accipe mirtillos et semina mirte[170] et tere et adde succum jusquiani et unge. Ad albuginem oculorum: accipe vitrum et tere cum melle et misce bene et unge et multum confert. Similiter: os sepie trita cum lacte mulieris et cum melle mixta, si apponatur, iuvat. Ad ulcera oculorum: accipe crocum et [misce] cum lacte mulieris et appone. Item ad idem: accipe crocum et gummi arabicum parum et conmisce cum lacte mulieris et appone. Ad sanguinem ex percussione in oculo: accipe pullum columbi [f.7v] et sub ala flebotoma et sanguinem calidum in oculo pone. Ad idem: accipe succum verbene et pone. Item: decoque ciminum in albo vino et pone vinum in oculo. Ad lacrimas oculorum: betonicam manduca et aciem oculorum clariorem reddit.[171] Ad pungciones oculorum: caprinum caseum recentem oculos impone, omnes dolores et puncciones tollit et capitis dolorem.

[42] Item: lé [grei]nes[172] de ere destemperez od urine e la[vez] le oil. Item aqua: rue, celidonie, verveine, eufrage, betonie, puliol, fennel, freses, sauge, fleurs de chefrefoil, flours de liz de ewe, fleurs de roses, de chescun festes par sei ewe cum hom fet ewe rose, pus mesurez

---

165 MS folio.
166 Corr. viatico?
167 MS quod r.
168 Corr. ex ulceracione or, perhaps preferably (see end of paragraph), ex percussione.

169 See LH 27.
170 MS mirre.
171 LH 35.
172 Conjectural emendation. MS leues.

chescun ouelment, pus les mettez ensemble. Preterea ad cest avandit euye: pernez .ii. onces de aloem epatic e .i. once de aloen citrin et fet[e]z mult menu poudre et quisez cest euye deske ad le premer boilon, pus en un basin sur charbons quisés le poudre des aloens e mult le movez bien, pus ad ce mettez jus de racine de fenuil triblé quant il seront refreidez, pus mult le movez, issi estoise .iii. jours e .iii. nutz. Chescun jur .i. fiz ben le movez. Aprés premez hors la clere e mettez en veire e sovent le mettez contre le soleil e le anmés que trop ne eschaufe e si vaudra plus. Collirie ad oilz: mettez un potel de blanc vin en .i. novel[173] pot, ad ceo mettez .ii. poinz de net forment e fennel, rue, trifoil, la rouge pimpernele e boilez bien deke ad la terce[174] partie, pus cole[z] parmi un drap, mettez en un veischel de latoun. La nuit mettez ad[175] oilz od une penne e garra. Prové est. Autre: piper, gingeber, salgemm[e], succus edere terristris et feniculi et rute, celedonie ana, bonum vinum, mel quod sufficit et repone in vase cupreo et unge ut supra.[176]

[43] Aliud quod et visum prius turbat sed postea clariorem reddit: emplez un novel pot de tere de date, ad se mettez fenuil, rue, aloine, consoude la petite, rouge cholez, ortie, planteyne, fente de veir e de bacinet d'escurie e sec oinez le fonz dedenz de mel e si le dentez(?) sur le pot .s. .iiii. jours. Le .v. jour coilez en un veisel le vert que troferez ad[177] le fonz de bacin, ce est bon coliri[e] ad[178] la chacie. Autre colirie:[179] colez le jus de bon partie de eufraisie ben triblé e colez seim fet meité de pork, la autre partie de owe o de geline, pus le eschaufez e i mettez cel jus e boilez oufeke, movant la fonz de la paeele de un pere rouge e quant est [refreidi] reserve[z] en bo[istes] e oinez et cetera. Autre: le jus de freses aprés que averont esté miz par .ix. jours souz terre e la meité taund de mel e demi colerié[180] de gingebra e de pevre, boilez un petit en cel jus, pus mettez en ve[ssel] de quivre e oinez ut supra.

[44] Autre ad omnia vicia presencia [et] futura et curat albuginem, pruritum, et omnem cecitatem, nam experto credas per .v. annos lumen oculorum amisisse, infra .xl. dies restituit. Collige[181] jus istarum herbarum: apii, feniculi, rute, verbene, betonice, benedicte, agrimonie, sanamandre, germandree, pimpernel, eufrasie, salvie, celedonie, equali mensura et .vii. grana piperis et cum .v. cocliaria mellis et urina pueri virginis, optime tere et cola per rudem pannum, hec pone in vase cupreo et unge ut supra. Cum siccaverit, auge urina pueri virginis.[182]

[45] Ad la chace des oils destemperetur (sic) mel, poudre triblé de aloen epatic e mettez i fel de livre e movez le un poi ke seit cler e mettez i [j]us de la [. . .] e oi[nez] ut supra. Item: jus de milfoil triblé e prent e poudre de qevre e de un keuz ad rasur mettez en cel jus, ad cocher

---

173 MS movel.
174 MS tercie.
175 MS od.
176 In the lefthand margin is the following remedy: A l'oil en que[i] crest la teye ou peyn par coup ou en autre manere: pernez les fleurs de solsecle, c'est assavoir les felurs rougez sanz nul autre chose de la dit fleur e medlés a ceo ouelment bure de mai fresch e la bruez ensemble e puis pressez cel (la) parmi un drapelet net e mettez un poi de ce en le un but de vostre oil quan vous irrez coucher e si deguttera en vostre oil e vous garra.
177 MS od.
178 MS od.
179 LH 31.
180 For coileré 'spoonful'.
181 MS collide.
182 This sentence is added in the lefthand margin with a insertion mark in the text.

mettez ad oil e garra. Item: mettez ent jus de lancelé, si garra. Item:[183] triblez ensemble arnement e aubun de oef e mel, ad cocher mettez sur les oilz, quiture e maufeis sanc tot engetera. Item: ensemble ouelment triblez la racine de fennoil e de planteine. Cest jus totes chaciez garrit. Item: metez rue od les racines de fenuil en un ves[sel] de areim [f.8r] od veil v(e)in, si seit en pes par .iii. jours. Pus de ce les oil lavez ad[184] cocher. Ad la manjue des oils: mettez ent jus de celidoine e rue et cetera ensemble. Oils enfl(u)ez: mettez sur creischon e veil oint ensemble triblé.[185] Autre: pernez la tendroun de la rounce e del rouge cholet e selfhelle e goute de mel e fleur de frument, batez ensemble e mettez sur.[186] Ad ruborem oculorum: poudre mult menu de commin mettez en une bourse .s. de ligne ad la gise de .i. o[r]iler e ad le mesure de l'oil e la bainez, que ben seit moilé en jus de morele. Ad cocher cochez sur le oil. Autre: ad home fel de buc e ad femme fel de chevre, le fendez parmi outre e ostez nettement la teie dedenz le escale de .i. oef. Cel liquor de fel mettez dedeinz od atant de eisel e le movez de un movor de coudre boilant sur cherbons, pus estoise .iii. jours en un veischel de latoun [o] de plombe. Mettez .ii. gouttes ad[187] oil et cetera.[188] Autre: destemperez aloen epatic od leit de femme que enfanta medle, [si] enferm es[t] [madle], si ce est femme,[189] [od] leit de cele que enfanta female, ce mettez ad[190] oil e garra. Autre: ardez .ix. feiz calamine, pus le destemperez od greisse de chapoun e vin blanc e mettez en veire o en plumbe e mettez od oil.

[46] Lipposis .i. aquaticis oculis caseum recentem in aqua coque et fac tortellos et oculis appone. Item ad lacrimas restringendas: accipe ciphum plenum fragorum et super asperge parum de salgema quo liquefacto cola per pannum et adde vitella ovorum in aqua coctorum et pulverem cimini et coque parum in vase eneo ad lentum ignem cum lacte mulieris et oculis inmitte. Item: conmisce rutam siccam cum melle, oculos unge, certum est. Item: une foile de cholet oinez en gleire e mettez la nuit sur les oiles. Item: quesez vetonke e la meyndre pulliol, de cel jus lavez les oils. Item: mangez sovent betonk. Aut[re]: degettez le jus en les oilz e esclariceront.[191] Ad oilz singlans:[192] jus de verveine e sank de columbe mettez denz les oils e beve pulioll. Autre: tolle pullum columbinum et sub ala incide et sanguinem qui exierit in oculo infunde. Oculis reversis: urticam grecam mitte in ollam rudem, postea[193] illine de to[to] totum fundum bacini spissa lacrima mellis et pone super ollam. Postquam aliquot diebus ibi moram fecerit si quid blavii

---

183 LH 28. See also Ogden, LDM p.9, ll.25–9.
184 MS od.
185 In the righthand margin is written Quando rubor oculorum accidit, quere ubi docet de cephalia et curacionem ibi invenies.
186 In the righthand margin is written the following remedy: Si oculus subtracto sanguine suderit, agrimoniam cum albumine ovi tere et superpone.
187 MS od.
188 In the righthand margin are written the following remedies: Ad sanguinem hauriendum ex oculis: coque albumen ovi et succum radicis feniculi et lac mulieris filium lactantis ana et conmisce et in oculum mitte. Ad oculos lacrimantes: succum tenuissimum betonice oculis infunde, clariores facit et lacrimas siccat. Ad lacrimas restringendos: jus rute cum modico melle destempera et per pannum exprime et inde oculos illine et in girum unge.
189 MS e. m. enfermes si ce est od oil de femme leit de cele.
190 MS od.
191 MS esclaricerent.
192 for 'sanglans' cf. cinc = 'sanc' in [30] n.139.
193 MS postea has i.

aut viridis pelvi adheserit, pone in pixide de cupro, postea aufer urticas illas et pone intus alias recentes. Sic fac .ix. diebus, inde unge et cetera.

[47] Ad eos qui appertis oculis non vident: serpillum campanum decoque in aqua et de ipsa oculos sepe fove. Ad albuginem oculi: *la fleur de milfoil triblez od leit de femme e mettez. Ad mal des oilz: lavez les oilz d'ewe, boilez od cerfoil* et post cole. Item: succus floris mente maculam oculi tollit efficaciter. Item: fimum humanum super laterem sicuti pulverem diligenter tritum in oculos pone, procul dubio tollit. Item: *leschez bainez e vin vermeil, si bevez leit de chevre blaunche attemprément. Ad comence[me]nt le sca[rifi]ez que vous aiez un poi de sank. Pus pernez le jus de ere terrestre e pimpernell et d'oil[e] d'olive [ouele] mesure, si oinez les oilz.* Item: *chescun jour de un mais degottez en lé oilz jus triblé de maufe, trebien prové est.* Item: tere fortiter in morterio ereo caprifiolium viride cum suo flore, succum per pannum lineum extorque et in ampula cuprea pone et unge et cetera. Item: succus jusquiani in .xii. diebus ita maculam delet ut nec vestigia appariatur. Item: imatithem[194] intinge in aceto vel in vino albo et frica et illud in oculis inmitte quod resolvitur. Item: zinziber humectatum in vino albo vel in aceto frica cum cote et quod resolvitur inmitte.

[48] *Teie des oilz: destemperez ouelment mel e fel de livre e oinez, esprové est. Item: jus de blanc cerfoil .iii. foiz. Autre ad teie cum espés quecumque seit: gingevre mult menu triblé batez parmi un boletel e le destemperez de mel que espés seit. Pus en une cince de lin le pendez en un hanape de vin mis en une paele sur le feu dekes le vin commence [f.8v] ad boiler, dunc tercez le jus ad le vin, issi fetes .iii. feiz, pus engettez la since, movez donc cel vin mult belement deke il espisse, pus le estuez en areim. De ce oinez ad coucher e toudra teie[195] e maile e totes enfer[tés].* Item: si in oculo poka sedeat, arsapan(?) et lac cerve conmisce et cola et purum in oculo mitte. Si in oculis sordicula ingressa fuerit, mulsam frequenter infunde et lac mulieris. Item: si arista vel quelibet sordicula oculum intraverit, claude sanum oculum et dolentem patefac, et duobus degitis, medio .s. et pollice, leniter pertracta et tribus vicibus dic hoc carmen et per singula expue: 'os gar bons basio'. Hec quoque sic ter vomes (?). Dicatur etiam de faucibus hominis vel jumenti (os) aut si quod aliud heserit potenter extrahit.

[49] *Oilz estoppez dedenz: pernez .i. chefroil de une colour, si pernez la curreie e quisez en feu de charbon, si donez ly ad manger e aprés pernez kanele, anys, fennel, percel e quesez en vin blanc e donez ly .iii. foiz ad bevre e garit. Ad caliginem oculorum: que si vous est avis que ombre les siue devant, quisez ben rue en blanc vin, de ce les lavez sovent.* Item: *jus de aloine medlé od mel e leit e totz passions des oilz sane.* Item ad pruriginem oculorum: aloen et mir[ram] tere subtiliter, confice cum vino et cum penna inmitte. *Item ad oilz: lavez les de ewe quite od racines de vetoine. Item ad dolour des oilz: triblez la racine de fennoil od vin, si le coverez ben en un bacin e le fouez issi en tere par .ix. jours, pus mettez ad oilz. Cest ostra le sanc et toute dolour. Prové [est]. Item ad oilz: triblez en un morter de areim o[196] de fer mult menu cum fleur .iii. onces de blanc calamine e une once de coperose, pus de vin blanc le destemperez molant que bien seit espisse, puis i mettez seim que il seit ausi tense cum caudel. Aprés fettes mult delié poudre de .ii. oncez de aloen epatic e atant de aloen citrin, ad ce mettez .iii. coiler[é]s de seim e boilez en une paele, pus purrez le parmi un drap e medelez as autres choses e ben les entremedelez movant, estuez en boistez, ad cocher mettez un petit*

---

194 I.e. 'emathites'.
195 MS *teie teie.*

196 MS *od.*

sur le cil aval de long en long, si ke ele entre en le oil. Pus dorme. Item: jus de fenuil e de rue
e le fel de perdriz e mel destemprez, de ce degottez en le oil ad coucher.

[50] Item ad caliginem: confice pulverem cinamomi cum succo radicum appii et rute et hec per pannum exprime et oculo appone. Preterea ipsum in aqua calida datur, mirifice lu[m]bricos expellit. Item ad clarificandum visum et oculos nebulosos: superpone calidum panem ordei et per medium cissum pulverem carvi vel cumini asperges et ante oculos pacientis tenebis. *Item ad esclarer les oilz: jus de eufrasie en cest [. . .] e la poudre en ivern mangez e averez bonz les oilez.* Item ad claritatem oculorum: fac pulverem de cumino et camphora et succum radicis apii et modicum albuginis ovi et parum mellis, omnia bene diu conmisce et cola per pannum et hec in oculis mitte, nebulam manducat et claritatem prestat. Item: succum rute et radicis feniculi et liastrai(?) folia equali pondere cum fortissimo aceto conde in vase enio et inde unge et cetera.

[51] *Item contre touz les mals des oilz vaut la greische de rouge limaçon*[197] *qit. Item: bevez chescun jur*[198] *aloine, si mangez, si esclaront les oilz, que ad le soleil lusant veras les estiles. Item tresbon esperment ad vewe: verveine rouge, turmentine, eufrasie, greines de ere ouelment pres fetz pouder e usez en toz voz mangers e voz bevres. Item ad anguisse des oilz e toteveis pur garder tres sein medicine: quisés en blanc vin ouel peis de verveine, eufrasie, tormentine e meins [. . .], aukes de rue ad vermeile [. . .], ben les quisez e mettez du vin, pus*[199] *cest usez chaud ad seir e matin freid. Si vous n'avez vin, pernez bon cervoise. Item: greines de blanc ensens, tanz cum vous plerra, mettez sur charbonz ardantz que gisent sur une tuile e les coverez de un bacin escuré que resceive tout le fumee e pus coilez del bacin ce que i est adhers par la fumee e ce destemprez od ewe rose, de ce lavez les oilez. Ce solt le rei Cesar fere. Item: la [f.9r] greische de touz pisschons de flums eschauf[é]s ad le soleil deke il i ert seim, ad se destemprez du mel e oniez e*[200] *il vous esclaront. Item ad oilz que ad la fiet dolent e [a] la fiez sont seinez: oinez de jus de centoire medlé od mel. Item: mangez vetoine jun e vous amendra la vewe. Item esperment Ypocras ad amender la vewe: feles de levre e de kokis e de anguilles destemperez od mel e od pur ewe e estuez en un vessel de areim e oinez et cetera.* Item contra dolorem oculorum: cum yrundinem primum in an[n]o audieris vel videris illico tacitus decurre ad fontem et inde fove oculos aqua et roga Deum ut in illo anno non censeas dolorem oculorum tuorum sed irundines illum auferant. Certum est. *Item la neire pere que est appellé celidonius que hom trove en ventres des aroundez, si les oilz vus doilent, triblez od ewe e inoignez les oilz e saneront.* Ad clarificandum visum: accipe fel anguille et leporis atque galli et misce cum aqua limphida .s. modica et adde modicum mellis et in vase eneo aliquantulum coque et cum ieris dormitum oculos perunge et infra .ix. dies stellas videbis in[201] meridie.

[52] Item ad maculam oculi: scribe in anulo aureo vel argenteo has litteras: + b h i a d a g d l s n a n + et fac(r) auferre (?) .iii. guttas de aqua benedicta per anulum illum in oculum, *ce est la medecine. Cherem:* prius limacium rubicundum combure super tegulam et fac inde pulverem et mitte in oculos. 'Adiuro te infirmitas per Patrem et Filium et Spiritum Sanctum ne hic tu remaneas. Absterge, domine, maculam ab oculo famuli tui .N. sicut abstercisti ab oculis famuli tui Tobie. Agyos Agyos Agyos, sanctus sanctus sanctus, Christus vincit, Christus regnat, Christus imperat.' Pater Noster .iii.,

---

197 MS *limacion.*
198 MS *jus.*
199 MS *plus.*

200 MS *e e.*
201 MS *in in.*

carmina ter.[202] Pone ante (?) hoc ligatum scriptum et si potes dic cotidie. *Item pur le mail: 'In nomine Patris et cetera conjur tei fete per Patrem et Filium, si tu es blaunchez, que tu t'en augez, si tu es rougez, que tu disrumpez, si tu es neire, que tu desçoivre. Tere e mere te susteine que te puent meuz sustiner de tei crestien'*, Pater Noster .iii. *Autre:* in nomine Patris et cetera glia nelia nec alia yrrippa de male. Si est macula super hunc famulum tuum .N. si est alba, Christus deleat, si est rubra, Deus destruet, si est nigra, Deus deficiet. Agyos Agyos Agios. Pater Noster .iii. Item si Teda,[203] Nicia et Aquilinia *se seeient sur le mere e dit si Teda,[204] Nicia et Aquilinia, quant pousu[n] nus la mei, tant puissent les mailes en les oilz cestem (?) Amen.[205]* Pater Noster .iii. *Item: en noun del Pere e del Filz e del Seint Esprit,* Teda, Nicea et Aquilina. Teda dixit 'stamus', Nicea dixit 'sic faciamus', Aquilina dixit 'maculam de oculo deficiamus'. Si fueris alba, Pater, te deleat et cetera ut supra. *Item:[206] ad vepres[207] e matin ditez .iii. feiz e[208] le oil malad [sanera]* + *'In nomine Patris et cetera', soflez .iii. feiz en croisant sur le oil, pus croisez disant 'In nomine Patris et cetera'. Aprés ditez* 'Inveniat te Pater, inveniat te Filius, inveniat te Spiritus Sanctus; circumcingat te Pater, circumcingat te Filius, circumcingat te Spiritus; destruat te Pater, destruat te Filius, destruat te Spiritus Sanctus'. *Si encloez le oil de voz ditz[209] e ditz la Pater Noster. Issi le charmez par dens (?) .iii. foiz e par .iii. jours.* Item: lutum fecit Dominus Deus Jhesus Cristus ex sputo unigenitus filius Dei et linivit oculos ceci nati et abiit et lavit et vidit et ipsum dominum verum Deum esse credidit Agios Agyos Agyos, sanctus Deus, sanctus fortis, sanctus et immortalis Deus, miserere huic peccatori .N. famulo tuo et libera eum de dolore oculi sui. Item + Agyos + Agios + Agios + sanctus Deus,[210] sanctus fortis, sanctus et immortalis . In nomine Patris et cetera, + Amen. Sanctus Nigasius minutam habuit variolam et oravit ad Deum ut quicunque nomen suum scriptum super se portaverit non haberet hoc malum. Sancte Nigasi, ora pro isto famulo Dei, Amen. Item: si tui oculi dolere inceperint, hoc modo illico ei subvenire poteris: accipe literas nominis eius et nominans totidem nodos in rudi ligno stringe et postea circa collum dolentis mitte.[211] Probatum est. Item *ad oilez:* Agne Dei qui tollis peccata [f.9v] mundi, miserere huic et depelle caliginem de oculis istius .N. Sanctus, sanctus, sanctus, Deus sabaoth, pleni sunt celi et cetera, gloria tua, osanna in excelsis, benedictus qui venit in nomine domini nostri Jhesu Cristi crucifixi, extollat dolorem de oculis .N. Lucas, Matheus, Marcus, Johannes illuminant oculos istos per Deum vivum, per dominum verum, per dominum sanctum, per eundem Deum qui in principio cuncta creavit ex nichilo, per thronum et majestatem eius, per lignum preciosum + sancte crucis .i. per merita eiusdem Dei genitricis sancte Marie et per .vii. candelabra aurea que in conspectu eiusdem Dei semper asistunt. 'Adiuro te, dolor, et omnis cura morbi mali ut hinc recedas et amplius in oculis istius .N. non noceas per .ix. ordines angelorum et per quatuor ewangelistas et per quatuor animalia plena (?) oculis ante et retro et per cxliiii milia innocentes martires et per omnes patriarchas et prophetas, apostulos, martires, confessores et virgines. Lutum fecit Dominus ex sputo

---

202 See NC p.10 IV.
203 MS *tera.*
204 MS *tera.*
205 The charm makes little sense as it stands. It looks as if, in addition to an obvious dittography, some material has fallen out.

206 Cf. NC p.56 VI.
207 MS *verpres.*
208 MS *el.*
209 I.e. 'fingers'.
210 MS *deus deus.*
211 MS *muette.*

et linivit oculos ceci nati et abiit et lavit et vidit et credidit Deo qui apperuit oculos ceci nati per suam purissimam misericordiam. Oculos istius .N. illuminare dignetur Domine sancte, Pater omnipotens, eterne Deus qui per sanctum Raphaelem, qui dicitur 'medicina Dei', sanasti oculos Thobie, ita et oculos istius .N. sanare digneris, in nomine Patris et cetera, Amen. Dic Pater Noster .iii. Pir sonus oculus filomene, cotidianis vestibus insutus aufert nimium saporem. Item: tere herbam que dicitur wakerwort[212] et jus mitte in oculos, crescit in blado, maxime in tritico.

[SLEEP]

[53] *Ad home que ne puet dormer: beve jus de mores e liez entour le chief le pastel chaud. Item: mettez souz son chef cestes letres escri[t]ez sur foils de lorer que il nel sache 'Exmael, Examael, Exmael, adiuro te per sanctum angelum Michaelem, insoporet homo iste .N.' Item: manjusce letusce e popi sovent. Item: beve fel de livre ars en pouder denz .i. techrs(?). Quant le voilez esveilier li mfifiz skskl en bb bpxchf.[213] Gardez que trop ne dprmf q'il purit mult tost morir. Item: mettez egrimoine desouz la[214] chewe de celui qui dort e il mfisf skskl frb devant que ce ert psts. Aut[re]: liez le trible souz sa giouye et cetera ut supra. Item: triblez maufes de cortel e .iiii. sprinkfis e de ce frptfz lfs dfns de le endormi; sachez de veire que ne se esveillera deke le aiez frps les denz de .i. psfe cix. Prové est. Cherme[215]* ut infirmus dormiat: 'Domine Deus, Pater omnipotens, qui per tuam clemenciam septem pueros + Malcum + Martinianum + Maximianum + Dionisium + Johannem + Serapion + Constantium + in monte Celyon dormire fecisti, concede propicius ut per eorum intercessionem hunc famulum .N. sompno quiescere facias atque eum ab omni malo liberes ut sibi sanitate redita tibi servire concede[at] contir ax ncl. Scribe in pergameno et pone super infirmitatem infirmi 'In nomine Patris oremus: sancte Blasii martiris tui atque pontificis quesumus domine nos omnino vivificet qui sacris virtutibus veneranda refulget per dominum nostrum Jhesum Cristum fi[lium] tuum mediatorem Dei et hominum qui [cum] te vivit et regnat in unitate eiusdem Spiritus Sancti, Deus per omnia secula seculorum, Amen. Sancte Leodegari, ora pro me ad dominum nostrum Jhesum Cristum, Amen.'

[54] Item *ad dormier* : succum jusquiani et succum mente tempera cum aceto et unge frontem et omnes pulsus, statim dormiet. 'In monte Celio requiescunt .vii. dormientes, Maximianus, Malcus, Martinianus, Dionisius, Johannes, Serapion, Constantius; Cristus vincit, Cristus regnat, Cristus imperat. In nomine domini nostri Jesu Cristi et in honore istorum sanctorum dormiat et requiescat iste famulus Dei .N., Amen.' Pone sub capite eius et dormiet. *Pur dormier pur le diabole: en chamle (?) en la cité la fuit seint Cristofore. Enz [q]ue le cok [n']eut chanté, issi[t] de la cité le malfé encontre, e sur luy anela(?), sur luy la seint croiez + mit, le malfé s'en fuit. In nomine Patris et cetera. Ditez .iii. Pater Noster. E[n] sur dorm[e]z de jur e nuit.* Ad eos qui nocte locuntur stulte: bibe in aqua benedicta reverenciam .iii. noctibus. Item: lilium cum vino vel cervisia

---

212 OED sub *wake-wort* gives only Palsgrave (1530) 'wakeworte: an herbe'.
213 Cipher is frequently used in charms.
214 MS *ces*.
215 Cf. *Pop. Med.* pp.80ff,84,89 and *NC* p.58 VIII.

bibe coctum. Ad eos qui per noctem loquntur id quod per diem audiunt: herbam reumaticam bibant per .iii. noctes in[216] [f.10r] aqua benedicta et amplius non faciet. Ad eum qui vexatur nocte fantasmate: rubeam petram que invenitur in habitudine serat in cerra virginea cum hiis nominibus in eadem cera scriptis : amey loun sodolomi. Item in nomine Patris et cetera. Adiuro vos, maligni et pessimi, per Deum vivum, per Deum verum, per Deum patrem omnipotentem et per Jhesum Cristum filium eius, unicum dominum nostrum et per descencionem et ascencionem eiusdem salvatoris ut recedatis ab hoc famulo Dei .N. Benedictio Dei et eius matris Marie et quatuor ewangelistarum Cristi et omnes benedictiones que in scripturis sacris sunt sint super te, benedictio patriarcharum per merita prophetarum et suffragia appostulorum et victuras (?) martir[um] et intercessiones omnium sanctorum sint super te. Item in nomine Patris et cetera on on, Agios Agios Agios, Deus Deus Deus, obsecro te, fili Dei vivi qui de virgine dignatus es nasci et per sanctam crucem tuam, ut protegas, munias ac defendas famulum tuum .N. ab omnibus insidiis et fantismatibus, pertur-bacionibus et illusionibus diaboli nocturnis, diurnis et ab omni temptacione[217] eius-dem inimici defendas et custodias. Conjuro vos demones per Patrem et Filium et Spiritum Sanctum et per summum nomen Dei + a + C + a + ut non nociatis hunc famulum Dei .N. nec illudas in die neque in nocte nec in aliqua hora diei nec noctis. In nomine domini nostri Jesu Cristi qui vivit et cetera. Item: *yiy d'chuh~ yis Jesus(ex-puncted?) nim ix bonen and writ on avereche yis ihc and say yeraftir .ix. Pater Nosters and ʒif him eche dai drenche yre and sai eche yis blesyns over ye man.* In nomine domini nostri Jhesu Cristi et salvatoris et in nomine sancte trinitatis et individue. In civitate Effeso in monte Celio ibi requiescunt .vii. dormientes, Maximianus, Malcus, Martinianus, Johannes, Dionisius, Serapion; sic requiescit dominus noster istos, Sic requiescat dominus noster[218] istum famulum suum .N. Amen.

[55] *Pur faies*: Conjuro vos, elves, per Patrem et Filium et Spiritum Sanctum et per sanctam Mariam virginem domini nostri Jhesu Cristi et per .xii. apostolos et per .xii. prophetas et per .xxiiii. seniores qui cotidie Deum laudant et per .iiii. ewangelistas Lucam, Marcum, Matheum, Johannem, et per .cxliiii. milia innocentes martires qui pro Cristi nomine passi sunt et per tremendum diem iudicii et per universas potestates Dei que in celo et in terra sunt et per virtutem sancte crucis in qua passus est dominus noster Jesus Cristus et per sanctum Johannem baptistam precursorem domini et per sanctum Sigesmundum[219] regem et per omnia corpora sanctorum qui dormierunt et surrexerunt cum Cristo ut non habeatur potestatem super istum famulum Dei .N.

---

216 MS *in in*.
217 MS *temperacione*.
218 MS *super*.
219 Gregory of Tours first wrote about Sigismund in Bk 3 of his *Historia* shortly before 576. On the association of the 6th-century Burgundian king, the first medieval saint to specialize in the cure of a particular medical condition, with the curing of fevers, see F.S. Paxton, "Power and the Power to Heal: the Cult of St. Sigismund of Burgundy", *Early Medieval Europe* 2 (1993), 95–110 and *id.*, "Liturgy and Healing in an early medieval Saint's Cult: the Mass *In honore sancti Sigismundi* for the cure of fevers", *Traditio* 49 (1994), 23–43. See the 'carmen ad febres' from MS Dijon 448 (s.xi in.) f.181r printed in E. Wickersheimer, *Les manuscrits latins de médecine du haut moyen âge dans les biblothèques de France* (Paris, 1966), pp.32–3.

Domine sancte, Pater omnipotens, sempiterne Deus, Jhesu fili Dei vivi et altissimi, Sancti Spiritus septiformis, sancta Trinitas, exaudi nos pro famulo tuo .N. in nomine Patris et Filii et Spiritus Sancti, Amen.

[BOOK III: THE EARS]

[56]   Passiones aurium quodam ab intrincicis causis et alie ab extrensecis. Quandoque ex humoribus, quandoque ex ventositate, quandoque a stomaco, quandoque a vicio cerebri. Si a vicio stomaci processerit, interpollata erit passio, si [a] vicio cerebri, continua erit. Vicium stomaci quandoque fit ex ventositate frigida et sicca, unde sequitur tinn[i]tus aurium et strepitus; quandoque ex ventositate frigida et humida, et tunc cum quadam temperancia ad modum rote molendini involumentis fit quidam sonitus in aure; quandoque ex ventositate ex frigida materia admixta ventositate ex calida materia procedente quadam melodia fit .i. cantus superior ex ventositate resoluta, a frigida materia fit cantus superior ut burdo. Si vero tinnitus aurium fit ex ventositate que resolvitur frigida, cum ex vicio stomaci, hec erit remedia. Primo minor est medicina melagoga ut theod[oricon] anacar[d]is, yera rufini, yeralagodion. Purgata materia hiis localis adiutoriis utetur: cepam cuiusdam perforabis sed non omnino et ipsam implebis oleo communi .i. olive. Bibito illo oleo iterum reimple et ita ter vel quater. Postea cepam exprime et illud quod exibit in aure tepidum pone et hoc frequenter facies. Si istud non profuerit, alleum coque in oleo et olium tepidum instilla. Vel aliter: accipe anguillas et frige in patella et accipe sagimen et misce cum tercia parte succi pori et instilla tepidum. Aut accipe parum euforbii et fac pulverem et misce calido oleo et pone in aure. Aut fac pulverem de pipere et oleo admixto [f.10v] pone in aure. Aut fac pulverem et cetera. Aut nitrum cum olio eodem modo pone in aure. Aut eleborum nigrum tritum cum melle et aceto et olio instilla. Aut, quod probavi, summe petrolium et instilla in aure. Aut lapidum persico[r]um medullam tere et succum attrahe et pone in aure tepidum, quod probatum est. Et idem valet contra surditatem auris.

[57]   Si ab extrinsecis causis, quemadmodum ex pulice vel pediculo ovino aut alio pediculo vel grano vel lapillo vel auriculari vel aliis habemus. Si pulex vel pediculus interfuerit, accipe vinum tepidum et instilla, deinde lanam carpinatam[220] appone. Si autem ovinus pediculus interfuerit, accipe panem calidum et auri appone. Si autem auricularis / erewike/, urinam propriam calidam impone [et] diligenter considera ad solem. Vel panem eodem modo vel epar ovis in aqua bene coctum auri eodem modo appone. Vel petrolium tepidum impone [et] diligenter considera ad solem . . .[221](et) [si] granum vel aliquid tale intra aurem fuerit, attrahe cum unco vel cornu vel calamo vel ventosa.

[58]   Ad aurium tinn[i]tum: betonica trita et in aure posita mire proficere creditur. Ad surdas aures: si vermis in aure natus fuerit, accipe barbam jovis, succus eius tepefactus ad solem in aure positus vermes necat et auditum reddit. Ad surditatem:[222]

---

220 MS caprinatam.
221 There is a blank in the MS.
222 This receipt reappears in Anglo-Norman in [59].

ova formicarum tere et per linthium cola et adde poligonie succum et in auribus pone. Vetustum emendatur et cetera. Si vulnus in aure fuerit aut si auditus graviter se haberet, urinam puerilem infunde tepidam, humorem desiccat et celeriter sanat.[223] Item: succus edere cum vino. Ad aurium difficultates: herbe millifolii succus cum aceto si bibitur, mire sanat. Item: bibat radicem millifolii jejunus. Hoc medicamentum surdis est auribus aptum: sempervive succo coclearia bina. Tandem sume olium quod prebet oliva, hinc ovi testa porrorum colige succum, lactantis pueri tantumdem simulo lactis. Hec tribus ad solis nitus suspende diebus et noctibus et totidem sub aperto desine celo. Ex hoc auriculem studeas infundere surdem, ut solis radium patiens assumat in aurem. Item: eder(e)a terestris, bruncus, betonia, species, mulsa, feniculus ante coquatur et inde lavetur. Enplasterizetur capud quod[224] sonus hiis renovetur. Item ad surditatem: *Querez [a]net savage la ou il crest, si le defouez e coup[é]s les coperuns desus, si les crucés e les enplez de seil, si remittez les coperuns desur e coverez de terre, la remaine .v. jours, puis le pendez sus e recev[e]z la degotture en un bacin. Cele medelez od jus de jubarbe. Totes surdesces poez ent garir. Item: jus de rue enfoundez ad*[225] *oreil.* Item: incide hideram in cruce et pone chutam in esthia (?), quod influit de hidera distempera cum modico vino, instilla in aurem. Item: jus .ix. foliorum magne nucis instilla in sanam aurem et si est surdus de ambabus, die tercio ponatur in unam et postea in aliam. Item: si nullo modo audiunt, fel porcinum cum lacte mulieris distempera et in aurem mitte per triduum et claude aurem cum lana succida.

[59]   Item ad surd[itatem] auris: *la greische de anguilles fresches quites em paste recevez en un veischel de veire e .ii. escales de oef de oile d'olive, quesez od gresse e le outime jour avant se seint d'un braz. Aprés i mette ad o(i)reil cele gresse, puis ad quinzime jour se seine de l'autre. Item: oefes de formies mettez en un vessel de veire e aseés en le fu desque seit decurable, puis le versez en les orelez. Item pur la dolur de orel:*[226] *jus tefe de mente versez en orel. Item:*[227] *jus de semence de siu enz versé amende la oizte. Item:*[228] *jus de yble versez denz, ke mult vaut ad ces que long ount esté surd. Ad mesmes ce: oefs de formies triblez, colez parmi un drap, ad ce mettez jus de poligonie e versez ad orel.* Item ad surd[itatem] : fel corvi destempera cum vino et inmitte in sanam aurem. Item: aures infunde jus fraxam (?) plena scala ovi et tantum de succo capitum porrorum et liberabitur. Item: instilla succum jovis barbe cum sagmine anguille. Item: urina pueri tepefacta in auribus infusa[229] humores exciccat.

[60]   Item ad auris dolorem: jus herbe jovis simplex inversa quod cum mihi(?) miseris, homo ipse fingat se masticare dum ipsum jus in aurem ingreditur. *Item:*[230] *jus de fenuil mettez. Item: si eles enflent, jus de betonke enversez, a merveile prophite. Si verm neische denz le orel, contre le soleil eschaufez jus de[f.11r] jubarbe e envers[ez]. Autre:*[231] *destemprez mentastre od vin e colez e tefe envers[ez]. Item: fac jus feniculi ke si il i ad plaie dedenz*[232] *o la oice vus greve, le jus de ere od vin tot freid vel urine tef d'enfant envers[ez]*

---

223 This receipt reappears in Anglo-Norman
     in [60].
224 MS *quod c. s.*
225 MS *od.*
226 LH 65.
227 LH 67.

228 LH 69.
229 MS *insusa.*
230 LH 68.
231 LH 66.
232 MS *ad de plaie denz.*

en les oreiles villoses, il seche(i)t e tout la dolour e sanet les plaies. Item: fel de buef od leit de femme enoinez, ce sanet les orelz rumpuz. Ad o(i)reil ou contre[233] *vermeine / jeo vous en dirrai medicine: / lait de chevre mettez od eiseil, / si garra tost de cel peril.*[234] *Item pur verme en orel: jus de jonke i mettez. Autre: ardez branchez de freine e la seue que en cort envers[ez]. Aprés, quant ben les poez ver, les ho[r]s trahez de un wndour. Item: versez leinz jus de mogwed e istrunt, trecerteine chose [est]. Ad irraine fer issir de orel: jus de foile de purretz enversez. Item vermes: jus de herbe que est appellé culrage enversez. Ad puce o poilz: fetes cu[m] une tente de drape linge, si le moilez en ta bouche de vostre salive e en mettez e cele part cochez vers val e la seine vers munt.*

[BOOK IV: THE NOSE]

[61] *Nes estoupé:* si quis nasum habeat abductum ut non possit sentire odorem nec flatum admittere, accipe zucariam et involve in percameno bombiceno[235] et impone super carbones et induc fumum eius per cannam ad nares. Ipsum fac cum mastico. *Ad estauncher deinz sank: mettez siu ad narilz.* Item jus apii bibe. *Item de mesmes: le saile ardez e fetes ent pouder e souflez en les narilez que il ne le sache, si est gariz.* Vel rasuram pergameni ustam naribus infla et musculos eius brachiorum circumvolve panno humifacto et enplastrum de aceto forti et argilla superpone et testiculi eius in aceto dependeant. Caprinum pilum ustum cum aceto mixtum mitte.[236] Ad sanguinem restringendum ubi volueris *cherme:* scribe in fronte ex ipso sanguine 'beronix', sed si est femina, 'beronixa'; aliter in fronte 'apernix' et in pectore 'beronix', sed si femina, 'beronixa', et si opus fuerit, in dextra aure dic ter cum Pater Noster '+ max nax pahp n c l s c l ʒ viii'. Item: 'Domine Deus propicius esto adiutor famulo .N. Sicut strincisti flumen Jordanus quando Cristus baptizatus fuit, sic restringas venas', cum .iii. Pater Noster, 'sepas rogas ranenas'. Probatum est. Item: scribe hoc signum in fronte .s. de ipso sanguine XX XX et dic eius nomen proprium, postea karmina. 'Miles quidam accepit lanceam et perforatus latus domini et continue exivit sanguis et aqua redemptionis et aqua baptismatis. In nomine Patris ne exeat sanguis, in nomine Filii restat sanguis, in nomine Spiritus Sancti non amplius exeat sanguis'. Pater Noster.

[62] *Ad poriture de naril:* semina rute et absinthii vel piretri[237] accipe et fac pulverem et in nares pone. Item:[238] *medelez ensemble jus de mente e de ere e mettez ad naril. Cel amendra e toudra la puor. Autre:*[239] *mettez jus de dragaunce.* Item:[240] *quesez roses en vin o en un poi de mel, si les colez, le jus mettez ad naril.* Item:[241] *soeflez leinz*[242] *pouder fete de escales arses des oefs dont les poucines sont escloses. Endement[e]rs que vous fetes ascune de cestes avantditz medicines fetes le bevre aloine destempré od mel. Item: jus preint de primerole mettez ad naril.* Item:[243] *rue e mente leinz mettez.*

---

233 MS *entre.*

234 PR 327–30.

235 MS *bambiceno.*

236 In the righthand margin is written *Aut radicem urtice tere et pone.*

237 MS *pitettri.*

238 See LH 41–2.

239 See LH 44 and NC 199ff.

240 See LH 43 and NC 195ff.

241 See LH 45.

242 MS *les leinz.*

243 See LH 41 and NC 187f.

[BOOK V: THE MOUTH]

[63] *Puor de la bouche*: folia fragis[244] manduca et pulegium et serpillum succum similiter et cum perexieris dormitum aceto bono lava, quod si nolit anelitus cum dormitum vadis, aceti boni ciatum unum per partes bibat. *Item ad aliene pulente: pernez jus de maruil.* Antidotum: [. . .] *de fevrefeue e bure medelez od mel e donez checun jour .iii. coilrez. Item:*[245] *destemperez peivre molu od blanc vin, si le tenez en vostre bouche et cetera. Item: lavez vostre bouche de jus de grant puliol e de*[246] *la menue. Item:*[247] *mangez le puliol sec.*[248] *Item: mangez cerfoil. Item:*[249] *bevez de puliol destemperez od vin .s. après manger. Ce fetes sovent e ce eschaufe e amende le entreil.* Item: si mulier haberit os fetidum causa stomachi vel intestinorum, [f.11v] fiat pulvis de meliori aloe quod inveniri potest et destemperetur cum jure absinthii, mane sole oriente accipiat ex hoc coclearia .iii. postea .iii. mellis. Hoc fiat sepe [eodem] modo quod supra.[250] Ad vicium oris, lingue et gutturis: quinquefolia pulverizabis et melle mixto os fricabis et fauces atque arterias purgat.

[64] Ad sudorem: quedam ultra modum habent fetidum sudorem. Istis facimus pannum intinctum in vino in quo bullieruntur mirti folia vel ipsa herba vel ipsi mastali .s. in illo panno ipsas se involvimus.[251] Ad sudorem recuperandum in cronicis egritudinibus: accipe sulphur et semen staphisagrie et eleborum album et pulverizatum subtiliter in oleo decoque et inde spinam fortiter unge. Sudores illi infirmi boni sunt qui per omne corpus manaverint, ad finem febre caruerint frigidi; qui circa faciem et cervicem [sunt] pessimi sunt et celerem mortem significant. Aliud refrigeratorium: crocum tere cum vitellis ovorum, cum olio roseo conmisce et stomacho induc, quod bonum est. Item ut sudes: bibe succum radicis feniculi et te cooperi bene ut sudes. Sub lingua quandoque crescit quedam caro superflua quasi esset alia lingua et quando crescit caro adherit superiori palato. Hoc modo curavi carnem adherentem superiori palato: primo attraxi dentem quia ad morbum aliter accedere nequivi, quo attracto apposui pulverem de tartaro, admixta calce viva, et sic frequenter feci quousque tota caro corosa fuit, post apposui desiccat[iv]um[252] ut thus et aloe pulverizatum.[253] Ita curavi carnem sub lingua quasi esset alia lingua: eundem pulverem apposui et in principio contulit, tandem accepi magnetem et tartarum et [. . .] virides ana et feci pulverem et apposui lanam carpinatam desuper.

---

244 LH 48 has 'foilles de fou', (Latin) 'folia fagi'.
245 LH 50 and NC 171ff.
246 MS *e de e de.*
247 For this ad the next receipt see *LH 47.*
248 MS *sicc'.* See *LH 47.*
249 See *LH 49.*
250 In the lefthand margin is written *Ad ulcera oris: cerum caprinum calidum diu in ore tene si kancer ibi est. Mel quam calidum [potest] postea in ore teneat.*
251 In the lefthand margin is written *Ad kancrum gingivarum: sal optime tritum superponatur, sed utilior est salgemma. Vel fricetur prius cum melle et lana succida et postea sal in ore teneatur et deinde cum vino abluatur.* This receipt is found lower down the page in the main text.
252 MS *desictatam.*
253 In the lefthand margin is written *Siliginem pone in testis duorum vel trium ovorum et combure, inde fac pulverem ad carnem superfluam sub lingua vel alibi corodendam.*

[65] Ad ulcera oris: plantaginis succum et eius folia in ore teneat. Ad gingivas corosas: accipe succum p[ar]itarie, salvie, pulegii et salis pulverizata et lavato ore cum aceto vel vino tepedo supersparge. Ad kancrum gingivarum: sal optime tritum superponatur. Utilior est salgemma. Vel fricetur prius cum melle et lana succida, postea sal in ore teneatur et cum vino abluetur.

[66] Est quoddam corpusculum quod in arabica lingua appellatur *nern* et in greca 'isophagus' per quod descendit cibus in stomacum. Illud corpusculum diversas patitur passiones, sed maxime .iii.: prima species passionum squin(i)ancie et secunda et tercia. Squin(i)ancia dicitur gule suffocatio. Prima species fit in sumitate trachee arteree[254] que laringa dicitur, cuius signa – tumor apparet in collo et extendet in cervice et hec valde periculosa non est nisi materia conversa fuerit ad interiora. Secunda dicitur peritunia .i. nodus in gula, cuius signa – tumor partim intra et partim extra apparet. Et hec est periculosior quam prima. Tercia fit in lacertis cordis et pulmonis et dicitur suffocatio quia suffocacionem inducit. Hec vix vel nunquam curari potest.[255] Cura generalis cuiuslibet speciei squinancie est fleobot[o]mia de utroque brachio. In illa specie que dicitur suffocatio nulla cura preter dietam. In aliis duabus speciebus ita operatus sum. In prima specie ligavi folium yrisilirice circa collum et materia non potuit descendere inmo recessit. Similiter in utraque specie dedi terram de nido yrundinum cum aqua calida et multum contulit. Item dedi de stercore canis albi cum aqua calida et multum contulit.

[67] Hec sunt phisicalia remedia et tamen curavi quendam yudeum per fleobot[o]miam de venis arteriarum colli. Consuevi apponere ephitimata maturata sicut de herba jovis cum visco malve et cum cilio et farina ordei. Et dieta comunis est frigida et humida et viscosa ut caro porcina, amigdalata.[256] Frellata et gargarismata dissolutiva necessaria sunt ut de mastico, [f.12r] piretro, pulegio, ysopo cocta etiam gargarizata. Ad guttam oris: cum vino calido os lavamus, fricamus[257] dentes et hoc in mane et in sero. Postea albumine rotundo circum ducamus per noctem et in brevi liberabitur. *Item ad mal de la bouche: lavez le de jus de plantainne.* Saliva si nimia a capite descendit: accipe zinzibra, juniperi ana .i., piperis .iii., confice cum melle, da coclearia .ii. vel .iii. cotidie donec constringat salivam. *Escaudure de bouche e del p[a]leis: launcelé boilez en vin rouge, cel vin aukes chaud tenez en la bouche sovent. Ad le hufet chei: oripiment eschaufez, si mettez sur un esclice, si le levez en osse* (?). Dic tribus vicibus hoc karmen et per singula exspue 'os gor bons basio'. Hec quoque sic ter vomes. Dicatur etiam de faucibus hominis vel jumenti os ana aliquid alium hesere potenter extrahit.[258] *Parole reciver: Respice ailurs la il parout de parlesie ke la tout .s. folon* (?). *Contre neresce: une vive aronde tot sanz plume ardez en poudre, cele od semence de cholet bevez en vin o en*

---

254 MS *arcecee*.
255 In the lefthand margin is written *Contra henfetum cherm: In nomine Patris et cetera*. 'Ex ore infancium' [Ps.8,3]. *In nomine Patris et cetera. Tunc insufflet in ore infirmi et postea dicat* 'Levavi oculos meos in [montes]' [Ps.120,1] *cum dominicali oratione .s. Pater Noster*.
256 In the lefthand margin is written *Recoverer la parol: jus de primerole mettez en la bouche. Item: o mettez aloen destempré od vin. Aut canis linguam cum cervisia vel succum marubii mitte in nares et statim loquetur qui subito obmutuit.*
257 MS *fridamus*.
258 Cf. above [48].

*cervise. Item: mange betunke.*Item bibe semen caulium in aqua. *Item: malad que trop beit donez li ad bevre centorie od ewe tefe, celi toudra seif e si li purgera le piz, si garra. Prové est.*

[BOOK VI: THE TEETH AND LIPS]

[68]   *Den dolour:*[259] *pernez planteine e le lavez / od siu [de] motoun, le estampez. / La face oinez de cele part. / Li verms istra, tropp li ert tart. Autre:*[260] *fetes autre medicine bele: / pernez de levre la c[e]rvele, / sicom li livre nus endite / ele d[e]it estre mult ben quit, / end[re]it de mal oignez adés / e si verms murrunt aprés. Autre: fetes poudre de es croscés [e] sechiés de nouyer e aube espeine e frotez les dens dehors e mettez le poudre sur, mesmes le jour serra*[261] *sein. Autre: mettez sur une tiule chaud semence de jusquiano e de orpree (?) e coveriz si ke la fumé munte par un tuel la ou les verms sunt. Pus bevez de l'euye e istrunt. Autre: sur autele tiule mettez une rouele de cire e dedeinz semence de chanilé e ut supra recevez (e) la fumé e charont les verms. Goute dé denz: maschés andre .s. bischopiswort et le pastel mettez ad la dent. Item : tenez jus de gletounier enz vostre bouche.* Dentes quandoque moventur ex frigore. Ad hoc bibe vinum in quo bullierunt gallanga et post ablucionem contra dentes pone pulverem olibani et si talis habet palatum excoriatum post appone allumen. Ipsum quere in Trota.[262] Item contra mocionem dentium: cinerem de corde cervi combusto in lineo panno appone ad dentes. *Oster denz: frotez les dentz de greines de ere od les foiles.*

[69]   Passiones dentium sunt plurime. Quandoque laborant dentes perforacione dentium, quandoque nigredine, quandoque laxacione dentium, quandoque corupcione gingivarum. Sed quia nigredo dencium turpissima est, curabis hoc modo: accipe radicem titimalli(s) et decoque in vino quousque ad medietatem et ex illo vino frequenter lava dentes. Vel aliter: accipe capud leporis et fac pulverem et inde frica dentes. Ad idem: accipe allumen, os sepie ana et fac pulverem et inde fiat dentifricum. Item: accipe .iii. dragmas galle et .iii. dragmas cucumeris agrestis et yeros .iii. dragmas et fac dentifricum. Et idem valet ad laxatos dentes. Dencium perforaciones fiunt de vermibus. Contra vermes attrahendos: accipe semen jusquiani et pone super carbones vivos et teneas desuper ore aperto et cadent vermes. Vel aliter: accipe dentem canis mortui et pone super dentem et orietur vermis. Vel fac crucem.[263] Sed hoc modo non curatur, cum ferro vel sine ferro hoc modo:[264] accipe lac titimalli et [f.12v] farina tritici et conmisce et superpone et per se cadet. Vel aliter: accipe radicem jusquiani et pone super carbones vivos et sic coctam et calidam pone super dentem et cadet per se. Caveat tamen ne ponat super dentes sanos, quia cadent quotquot contigerit. Ad idem: ungulam allei calidam super pone et cessabit dolor. Contra laxos dentes: accipe gallas et mirtillos et plantaginem et decoque in vino rubio et dentes lava frequenter.

[259] See PR 351–4.
[260] See PR 355–60.
[261] MS *sureinz.*
[262] The reference may be to the Salernitan 'Practica secundum Trotam', see Chapter Two, p.69.
[263] In the MS the rest of the line is occupied by a wavy line as if to mark the end of a section.
[264] The line has obviously been garbled through omission of material.

[70] *Ad dentz dolour: eschaufez milfoil triblé e mettez contre le dolour.* Ut dentes infantum sine dolore exeant: cerebrum leporis coque et frica gencivas. Ad vermes in dentibus et tineolas: semen jusquiani atque ceparum ponantur super tegulam calidam et fumus inde exiens ori aperto suscipiatur et quamdiu poterit sustineat. Et postea sepe abluat cum succo caprifolii et liberabitur. *Ad dent dolour:*[265] herbam millifolium cum butiro inpone, mire sanat. Item:[266] betonicam cum vino veteri ad terciam[267] decoctam atque cum aceto gargariza, dolorem dencium descutit. Item: herbe simphoniace radicem decoctam in vino austeri et teneat in dente que(m) dolet, mox sanabitur. Item: *tenez vostre bouche plein de jus de planteine. Ad goute dé denz: de ere terrestre e de orpyn ouelement pris e triblé, beve cel jus. Item pur dent dolour ad touzjours garier:*[268] *pernez la racine de la flaunbe .s. gladeine, si le triblez que hom puit hors attraire le jus, sil versez en le oreil vers la destre partie. (Ad) ceste medicine ne deit hom aprendre ad hom ne ad feme ne ad autre.*

[71] Item probatum ad conmotos dentes: fac pulverem de ossibus dactilorum et misce aliquantulum cinamomi et masticis et olibani et consolide majoris et super sparge. Vel cum succo expresso pampinorum circa dentes complastriza. *Une medicine i a de arondel. Quant il est primes esclos fendez la parmi la teste e le eschine e troverez .iii. parties ad le ventre; la blanche prophite ad dolour del chief, la rouje ad passions, la neire ad dentz. Par judi matin les pernez. Ad dolour dé dentz: cha(r)nillé e de la cire mettez sur une tiule chaude e coverez e recevez la fumé,* ut supra. Item:[269] *quisez la rasure de corn de cerf en vin e ewe, ce tenez en la bouche si chaud comme vous poez. Quant est refraidé, engettez e autre humez, issi fetes sovent. Vel mangez milfoil e bevez le jus sovent.*[270] *Vel bevez le racine de la chinillé e si la quesez en breszes,*[271] *si la reez de une coutel e cel rasure usez sur le dent; quant est refraid[é], i mettez autre.*[272] Item:[273] *quesez vetoine ad la tierce partie en eisel e en vin e tenez,* ut supra, *en la bouche. Item: boilez en estale cervoise semence de chanilé,* ut supra, *tenez en la bouche e de ce lavez les dentz.* Item:[274] *quesez en vin la raceine de verveine e de ce lavez sovent la bouche.*[275] Item: farina(m) frumenti, thus, succus urtice, de albumine ovi, totum misce simul et fac enplastrum mediocriter spissum et illine

---

265 See LH 54.
266 See LH 58.
267 MS *tercias*.
268 Cf. the Latin at the end of [70] below.
269 LH 51.
270 LH 56.
271 MS *bersize*.
272 LH 57 and NC 123ff.
273 LH 58.
274 LH 63.
275 In the lefthand margin is written a charm, as follows: *Beata virgo Apolonia, grave martirium pro deo sustinuit triaum(?). Primo traxerunt eam et fortiter ligaverunt et cum malleis ferreis dentes eius frigerunt. Et in illo tormento oravit Deum ut quicumque nomen suum pro dolore dentium i[n]vocaret, malum in dentibus non sentiret. Ora pro nobis sancta Apolonia ut digni et cetera. Domine, exaude orationem etc. Oremus: Domine Jesu Criste qui beatam virginem Apoloniam de manibus inimicorum liberasti et orationem eius exaudisti, te queso per intercessionem eius et beati Laurentii martiris simulque omnium sanctorum ut dolorem a dentibus famuli tui .N. expellas ut sanum et incolumem eundem efficias ut gratias tibi crescere valeat in omni tempore qui vivis et regnas et cetera.*

percameno et sic pone in timpore in qua parte est dolor. *Item:*[276] *peivre triblé e quit en vin tenez,* ut supra, *en bouche.* Item: manduca brasilium vel radicem millifolii et tresura aut *bevez le od vin e maschez le sovent, de rechef mangez le herbe alne, ce confirme les dentz.*

[72] *De dentz longement [. . .] ail quit en eisel vaut ad denz que doilent.* Item: *quesez la raceine de ere en vin e te[nez] en la bou[che]* et cetera, ut supra. Item: *leit d'eynesse chaude confirme les dentz e tout la dolor.* Item: *fetes ewe de fleurs de geneste cum l'em fet ewe rose e mettez en veire e quant mester est, lavez les dentz.* Item: *de menu pouder fet peletre, frotez les dentz. Vel mult masch[ez] le herbe.* Item:[277] *neir suffoine maschez vel maufe.* Item: *rue, planteine, launcellé, peivre, seell, ensemble ben triblez. Puis envolupez en une foile de cholet. Quisez le bien*[278] *en breses e si chaud cum suffre poez [mettez] sur la dolur.* Item ut unquam doleant: succum radicis flammule terendo extrahe et infunde in sinistram aurem. Cave ne alteri dicas.

[73] *Charme ad dentz:* sancta Maria supra petram sedebat, Spiritus Sanctus superveniebat et dicebat 'Quid tristaris Maria?' et dicebat 'Dolent dentes mei. Venit [vermis] migraneus et me mordit'. 'Adiuro te migranea [f.14r][279] gutta per Patrem et Filium et Spiritum Sanctum et per sanctum Gabrielem qui dicitur 'medicina Dei' ut non noceas famulo Dei .N. neque in dentibus neque in capite nec in ulla compagine membrorum, Amen. Pater Noster sicque carmina ter cum Pater Noster. Item *cherme:* Cristus super mare ambulavit, sancto Petro apostolo obviavit, et dixit ei Dominus 'Quid ambulas tristis, Petre? 'Domine, dolent mihi dentes. Venit vermis migraneus qui devoravit carnes meas et ossa mea'. Dixit ei Dominus 'In nomine Patris et Filii et Spiritus Sancti adiuro te, migranea gutta, Amen.' Item *cherme so(i)eflant: .iii. fiez seinez la jouye e dites* 'Sanctus Petrus sedebat supra petram marmoream tenens manus ad maxillas suas. Ait illi Dominus "Quid tristis es, Petre?". Dicit ei Petrus "Domine, dentes mei dolent, gutta et vermes tollent mihi dentes". Ait illi Dominus "Conjuro vos, vermes et gutta, per Deum vivum et verum et per omnia Dei ut modo non noceatis huic famulo Dei .N. Sanus sit hic famulus Dei .N. credens in Deum, Amen" '. *Cherem: par .iii. jurs et Pater Noster. Item escrivez en la jowe* + rex pax in ipso folio, Amen. Item: scribe hoc et suspende in collo suo: bou betu ual on. *Item: en noun del Pere e del Filz e del Seint Esprit Jesu sire Deus nous vous prioms que ceste institucion pusse prophiter ad vostre sergant.* +++ *tocassiam. Assuagez, sire Deus,*[280] *la dolour de ceste denz* +++ *e de tote la teste, Amen.* Item: in nomine Patris et cetera ++ Lucas + Marcus + Matheus + Johannes ++ u + boz + za + esse + u + mortuus est vermis. Deus eterne, nomine te invoco per invocacionem sancti nominis tui + Sother nominis theu et per signum sancte crucis tue, ut hanc infirmitatem et hanc guttam migraneam destruere et deficere atque recedere facias ab hoc famulo tuo .N. quia tu es benedictus in secula seculorum et preter te non est alius, qui vivis et regnas Deus et cetera.[281] Item: conjuro te dolorem dentium per .iii. magos Melchiar, Jespar, Baptizar, Sidrac, Midrac, Abdenago, joht,

---

[276] LH 61 and NC 131ff.

[277] PR 349–50.

[278] MS *c. bien le.*

[279] Folio 13, which deals with the stomach (see below [91]) is insititious, f.12v ending with the catchword *gutta* which begins f.14r.

[280] MS *denz.*

[281] In the righthand margin is written: *Ad dentes dealbandum: lana succida mell. . . illita dentes perfric. . . mire vero candorem cons. . .*

lohet, unhet ut habeas potestatem regnandi in maxillis ut in dentibus per Cristum dominum nostrum. Sanet te Deus Pater qui te creavit, sanet te Dei Filius qui pro te passus est, sanet te Spiritus Sanctus qui [pro] te effusus est, Amen. *Ad neire dens: fetes poudre del sarment de vin e de ce od charboun sovent frotez les dentz.*[282] Item: fiat pulvis nitri et salis usti et pumicis, cunicule mari[n]e(?), os [s]epie, coste, cum melle conmisce et dentes sepe frica fortiter. Item: de nuce maiori corticem bene mundatam ab illo exteriori quod viridet frica dentes. Si tamen prius abluti fuerint vino calido fricando sale si placet admixto. Item: fortiter et sepe frica dentes de veridis folii[s] corili.[283]

[74] *Levers*, ad rimas labiorum: sepe quando mingis de ipsa urina calida recipe et inde fricando bene lava. Item: ancerinus adeps aut gallinacius curat. Item: cissure labiorum sepe accidunt preter continuos amplexus amicorum et eorum suavia inter se labiis proiectis illa desiccata in mane propter calorem fissa inveniuntur. Has curamus sola inunctione de lilio facto unguento. Item: sunt alie fissure labiorum ex aere et vento et similibus causis. Hiis illinimus labia cum melle et postea picem grecam super aspergimus. Item: secundum magistrum Ferarium[284] accipe magnam nucem et sub cinere decoque et tere nucleum et ad fissuram appone vel crudum tere et fissure appone apposito tartaro et sanabitur.[285]

[75][286] Brachium cuius dolor: coque savinam optime tritam in bono vino. Postea liga ut enplastrum circa brachium invalidum vel aliud membrum fere mortuum et tunc primis suppositis calefac sepius per medium asserem minutim foratum ante dormitum. *Ke si le braz ou autre membre dorment: pernét le sumet de vermeil ortie et aprés le bainez [f.14v] en eble e de mesmes lour membres seit seint e est garriz. Ad hom que norit malvais sank: pernez femeterre, entrerusche de aube-espeine, poudre de crabe de mere, e destemperez od meske de leit de chevre e ly donez a bevere.*

[PHLEBOTOMY]

[76] Quid prodest fleobotemia? Mentem sencerat,[287] memoriam prebet, vesicam purgat, cerebrum contemperat, medullam calefacit, auditum aperit, lacrimas stringit, stomachum purgat, digestionem iuvat, leniorem vocem producit, sensum acuit, ventrem cohercet, sompnum munit, anxietatem tollit, tristiciam aufert, libidinem

282 LH 62.

283 MS *coridi*.

284 MS *.g. magistrum serarium*.

285 The following prescriptions seem insititious as well as so textually corrupt as to be virtually beyond remedy: *Barbe ad homme fer crestre o chewe: entre les orksches ad le bues creisent une derklue .s. un curesces sanz peil que luy creisent en ivern e en cest liu cheent e iceles ardez, si en fetes pouder, si le destemperez od veil oil [corr. oint?] e de ce oinez la ou vus vuilliez que peil veigne e cest oinement est tant vailant que, si vus envoiez ad une feme, le menton, ja [seit] ce que nature le vie, avra barbe. Omblil, si est mal escorché: farinam quam vermes a fustibus proiciunt tere cum olio et inunge. Si vermes fuerint in umbilico .s. circam postquam natus est, accipe sal indicum et tere subtiliter et destempera cum aqua. Postea illum per pannum lineum cola et da ei ad bibendum. Si sale indico cares, da ei sal commune. Item: in cisone umbilici in santoun (?) quod respice in Trota libro. Alias habet berbam ex una (ex) parte albam et ex altera coloris (est) alterius (hec) qui unum testiculum habet frigidum et alium calidum.*

286 This passage seems to be misplaced.

287 For 'sincerat'.

cohercet, sanguinem proprium nutrit, alienum eicit, longioris vite ministrat sanitatem.[288] Quando uti debes carsis et ventosis hiemis tempore quod incipit ab viii idus novembris et desinet viii idus februarii, tunc crescit fleuma ex quo nascitur frequenter omnibus fluor narium quod aliter dicitur catarrus, distillacio uve. Ideo mense novembris bonum est carsas et ventosas imponere quia in ipso tempore sunt omnes humores parate. Mense decembris venam cep[h]ali[c]am incide propter capitis vicia et oculorum infusionem; mense februarii venam de pollice incide quia tunc febricitat terra et omnia que in ea sunt.

[77] Isti sunt dies apti in quibus licet medico extrahere sanguinem ex vena: a xvii kl. maii usque pridie nonas junii et a xvi kl. novembris usque nono decembris que sunt c.(?) dies. Hiis diebus temperatus est aier et non multum caloris aut frigoris. Item isti non sunt apti: a xvi kl. februarii usque nono marcii et a xvi kl. augusti usque pridie nono septembris, continent dies c., quia in hiis diebus nimio calore et frigore sunt afflicti et est aer intemperatus. Ceteri vero nec laudantes nec vituperandi. Ut enim necessitas homini cogit, sic hiis diebus erit. Item diebus vitandis tres sunt in vobis auguste, decembre, aprile nomine, lunares et velud ydra dies prima dies primi postrema posteriorum. Isti sunt dies egipciaci in quibus nulla occasione licet homini vel pecori sanguinem minuere vel pocionem capere: prima dies est ultima dies lune in aprili, secunda prima dies lune intrante augusto, tercia ultima dies lune exeunte decembris.[289] Hii omni diligencia [ob]servandi sunt quia omnes vene tunc plene sunt. Qui in illis diebus venam inciderit, statim aut ante quatuor dies vel infra octavo aut xiiii morietur et si pocionem acceperit, ante xx dies mori[e]tur, quod si quis ex auca commederit, ante xl dies morietur. Item precipue observandum est ante exitum marcii illa dies lune. Hiis diebus omnes vene sanguine plene sunt: luna prima, secunda, quinta, xva xxa xxva xxxa. In hiis diebus a nono kl. junii non debes minui sanguinem. In inicio marcii .s. xvi die de brachio dextro minue. Et in principio aprilis ix die de sinistro brachio propter visum, in fine marcii in quarta vel quinta die de quocumque brachio volueris propter febres et si hec observes, unquam lumen amittes nec febres pacieris. Ver estas dextras, autumpnus, hy[e]mpsque sinistras. Cecos et mutos Ypocras iubet esse minutos.

[78][290] *Ore voile aprendre e aseiner / cum li hom se deit seiner./ Partout covent sen e mesure / ki vout ovrer solum nature. / Li fleumatic e le malencolien / ne se seinent mie la matin, / mes entre tierce hor del jour / e juns seient, ce dit le auttour. / Colericus ad midi se deit seingner,/ ce vus dit [. . .] / e qui est malencolien / ad noune o pus se seine ben, / kar solom les hores del jours / soleient regner les quatre humours. / Et pur les humours meime [. . .] / se deit li homme sovent seiner. / Hom ce deit seigner sagement / e garder se deit ensement, / de tout surfet se deit garder / e qanque est trop eschenier. / Et pus manger tele viande / cum sa nature demande. / Dont li covent aver bon pain, / le blanc levé est le plus sein, / les oefs moles quitz par tuoer(?) / Pur cors e chef reconforter / char de porc si est fine, / poucin, perdrez, fesant, gel(e)ine, / et seine est char de chapon / e char poudré de motoun;*

---

288   Cf. *Flos medicinae ed.cit.*, pt.8, c.x, ll.2655–65.
289   Bede has 'sed ex his tribus maxime observandi, octavo Idus April., illo die lunis, intrante augusto, illo die lunis, exeunte decembri, illo die lunis . . .' (*PL* 90,959).
290   What follows is an extract from a versified treatment of bleeding. For the only known Anglo-Norman poem on blood-letting see T. Hunt, "The Poetic Vein: Phlebotomy in Middle English and Anglo-Norman Verse", *English Studies* 77 (1996), 311–22.

/ *petit o nent manjut de fruit,* / *si ce n'est un poi par dedut,* / *su[e]if vin blanc [. . .] vin bevrat* / *o bone cervoise, si il ad(d);* / *ad manger lerra, si il est sage,* / *e auz e chaus lait [e] furmage* / *e le dormer e le veiler* / *e ce que affert ad doner* / *le travail e le corocer,* / *le trop penser e le veiler.* / *Que vous en dira[i] ge mes?* / *deuz jours ou .iii. plus se garde aprés.* / *En pes seit e en oscurtez,* / *k'il seit aukes recoverez.* / *E pur la veine reseiner,* / *q'il deit sur tote regarder* / *quant bracez enfle par seiné, seinez le de l'autre braçz, e si la pernez la issue, si fetes boiler en ewe e de cel ewe fomentez le [f.15r] (la) braçz malad e puis si querez la musse de keine e boilez en vin e en oile, si vous lavez e liez od la brace.*

[79] *Autre: e s'il doult,* faba cocta in vino vel in aqua tam diu ut resolvatur, adhicias sewm(?), quod, cum inducis in lintheo, pone desuper calidum, mirifice sanat. Aliter: mel, vinum, apium et farinam siliginis simul coque et appone calidum. *Autre: si la veine agurde, orties e sel defrotez en vos mains e sur liez a la veine. Estauncher sank de veine rumpue: ad veine rumpue restreindre* / *ne se deit hom nul feindre* / *et pur aver garison* / *planteine beve e karson.* Item: si de vena sanguis stringi non potest, plantaginem contunsam super liga vel ipsam herbam tunsam bibat. Item: in baculo quodam si masculus est scribe hoc vocabulum: 'beronix'; si femina, 'beronixa'. Et da effusori ut teneat et sic restringabitur.[291] *Cherem:* Sanctus Helias in heremo sedebat et dixit 'Domine, restringe'. Sic restringentur iste vene sanguine plene, Pater Noster .iii. Item: in nomine Patris et cetera. .N. max vax pax et Pater Noster, hec tribus vicibus et cessabit. Item: in nomine Patris et cetera. *Virgne femme, Virgne sint (?), Virgne enfant entre le bracz tient, virgne femme, virgne enfant, virgne veine .N. tein ton sanc.* In nomine Patris et cetera. Item:[292] *en flum Jordan .l. fontaines a e chescun home cinkant veines a. Le sanc .N. esta par la vertu ke Deus a.* In nomine Patris et cetera. Item: *en flum Jordan ou Deus cincens amsat(?), preum cel Deus ke il estanche la veine ke seinie. Seint Cosme e seint Damien [. . .] cum as tu a noun crestien?* Pater Noster .iii. Item sunt alia carmina, ut Longeus miles lancea perforavit latus domini et cetera.

[BOOK VII: THE HANDS AND FEET]

[80] *Mains que sont pocrus e ad peez vaut mult un bain fete en ceste manere: parnez saveine, lavender, mente, sauge, si quisez ben en ewe. En celle chaude ewe fumé des herbes tenge ses mains o ses peez que il seient sulenz e puis de l'oinement de esquinance les oinez. Qant ce ert fet, que serra le ewe refreidé, puis seit rechaufé od un fer chaud o od tiuls chaudes e de rechef oinez les e cum la char porra totes houres les oinez de poplion. Mesmes ceste mescine prophite ad lepros.* Ad passionem manuum vel oris torquentis: accipe tria folia de salgea et tria de garre vel moros eius vel brancias et tria genera pione et tres rotulas radicis gliris et da infirmo commedere cotidie et potus eius sit radix gliris et radix canis lingue. *Ad croulemen dé meins: ne les suiés pas multens quant les avrez lavé. Item: bevez toteveis une feiz parentre vostre potage. Item: ne mangez de nul teste e nomément de cervele. C[r]ulement avent de anguse e ire e de grant bevre. Crampe: ardez en un novel pot uint de tor, si li fetes manger, q'il ne sache. Roine dé mains: viltret vous prendrez en ewe, mout li*

---

291 See Hunt, "Anglo-Norman Medical Receipts", p.218 no.115 and *Speculum medicorum,* MS B.L. Royal 12 E xxii f.36r.
292 See *Pop. Med.,* p.362 n.149.

quisez, de cel ewe lavez les meins deke ben seient seinz. Et le ewe tele seit: ad vespre chaud, matin freid. Viltrit genus est herbe. Item: triblez encens e peivre e vif argent e veil oint e la racine de alne, de ce vous oinez ad le feu.

[81]   Item ad manus scabiosas: lapacium acutum et fu(l)mum terre ana et confice in modum unguenti cum auxungia porcina vel butiro facto in maio, quod melius est, et inunge. Item ad scabiem de salso flegmate que fit in manibus et cubitis vel facie vel quolibet loco et etiam ad dextras omnes: accipe succum lapaci[i] acuti et (et) acetum ana, unge ad solem fricando. Probatum est. Item ad scabiem manum et brachiorum aut aliorum menbrorum: *la racine de la rouge parele lavez, parez, menu la destrenchez, pus trebien le triblez. Aprés si versez atant de doutz let cum vous est avis que amontereit. Le jus de cele parele e de rochet*[293] *bien triblé issi remeine deke endemein, donke le colez, de ce oinez ad feu.* Probatum est. *Autre pur demanjure: ardez ensemble la racine de gletoun e foxesglove, si en [est] bon la pouder. Autre: emplastre de chauz e de savon. Autre ad blast que saut sur plein de rouges berbletes: frotez la bien de savon e seel. Autre pur demanjure e pur degrature: triblez la racine de rouge doke od bure de mai e od veil oint, mult ben le quesez, pus le colez, de ce vous oinez. Autre ad oster roine: bevez sovent femetere triblé od cerveise. Autre:* fiat unguentum de herba que dicitur fumus terre et oleo nucum. Ponatur pulvis fuliginis subtilis [f.15v] et conficiatur adiecto aceto et succo fumi terre in maiori quantitate quam de aliis et onguatur paciens. In balneo optimum est. Et nota quod herba fumus terre quanto fuerit viridior tanto melior, nam exsiccata nullius est efficacie. Huius succus ter in septimana datus purgat omnem inducentem scabiem. *Autre:* argentum vivum calidissimum et humidissimum est, ideoque pediculos necat. Mixtum cum litargio et aceto et oleo fit bonum unguentum ad curandam scabiem et postulas. *Autre: pernez la poume sauvatje,*[294] *si la quesez ben en estale cerveise e medelez ensemble, pus le pil[e]z*[295] *ensemble, pus le colez parmi un drap e cele quisez tant que seit espez cum oinement. Et de ce oinez.*

[82]   *Autre e ad goutte e ad parlesie:* Tolle salviam, savinam, rutam, agrimoniam, ypericon ana manipulum unum, tere cum butiro et oleo et ausungia et cera, coque omnia insimul et cola. Cum frigidum fuerit, usui reserva. *Autre* contra omnem scabiem: accipe sulphur et vivum argentum et masticum et oleum, confice et unge. Item: *les foiles de saxfrage quesez en ewe e de ce lavez. Item pur demanjure e degrature: pernez parele e mettez desur e triblez le ben od bure de mai e od mel e od oint de pork e colez parmi un drap e oinez. Et pur roin[e]:* eleborum tere cum adipe porci recenti[296] ad modum ung[u]enti, pista et inde corpus ad ignem unguatur. Et scabiem et postulas sanat in tercium diem. Probatum est. Item ad morpheas nigras et ad omnes carnis ulceraciones unguentum: sume cornu cervi et lignum savine, lignum coruli, lignum juniperi, frumentum, semen sinapis, omnia siccata, simul omnia in olla ponantur et calefac[297] in ignem.[298] Oleum inde fiat et ubi opus fuerit calefac et ute.

[83]   Ad formicaciones et cirones ubicumque fuerint in corpore et maxime in fronte vel facie: frumentum distempera cum vino et pulverem olibani appone et in modum enplastri ute. Item *cirons:* semen jusquiani super prunas ardentes pone, in fumo inde surgente manus fomenta et postea in aqua calida lava, deponet cironem. *Autre:*

---

293   MS *rechet.*
294   MS *sauviatire.*
295   MS *pilz lez e.*

296   MS *cum recenti cum a. p.*
297   MS *calore.*
298   MS *ignis.*

unguentum de sandenico et ausu[n]gia et modico argenti vivi inunge et sic dimitte duabus diebus, tercia cum calida lava manus et statim ad ignem extense videbis egredi. *Autre: semen jusquiani contunsum coque in aqua et ex ea manus ablue. Mettez sur .ii. foiles de aune,*[299] *del sanc des verues que plus serront meures e mettez la ou il purischent. Item: frotez les sovent del jus de amblette e quant les racines serront purriez, si encheirunt. Item: foils de ere terestre liez sur par .xii. jours. Item: si ce ne n'en taut, trenchez les, si mettez orpiment medlé od savon. Ce est esprové. Item: osilles e megke mettez ensemble e donez luy ad bevre del jus mesmes, si les oignez, si est garriz.* Item: testudines pone in vase, surmitte (sic) sal et exinde quod manet[300] unge et sepe frica et cadent. Si verucas vis alicui dare, accipe totidem lapillos cum folio edere, quasi aliquod bonum posueris, et ipsos sanguine verucarum intinctos prohice in tali loco ut ab aliquo inveniantur. Item: si habueris in uno loco plures verucas minutas, per noctem aspice stellas donec videas de qua ignem voluerit quasi lineam et eodem momento quo id videris tange eas verucas de quacumque re volueris. Hoc modo cadant omnes quod si manu tua nuda tetigeris, statim transferantur ad ipsam. Item: si tu ipse vel amicus tuus quamvis longe a te positus verucas habueris, ita eas deles: accede ad arborem juniperi tenens aliquam vergam in manu tua et dic Pater Noster. Cum dixeris 'sed libera nos a malo', percute de virga arborem fortiter ut fructus eius vel folia de arbore ista sic cadant. Omnes veruce hominis illius .N. de manibus vel pedibus aut alio membro suo omnes ipsa hora perdet. Item: hircus cum vino coctus et inpositus adligatus in quarto die verucas sanat. Idem facit solsequia cum sale vel agrimonia cum aceto aut urina asini cum fimo suo recenti vel de semine ebuli perfundantur. *Item: la racine de glejol liez .iii. jurs sur les verues. Item bevez la tere dé nis*[301] *de aroundes od ewe chaude.* Item ubicumque nascantur post prandium: accipe fel leporis recens et omnes verucas unge perfecte [f.16r] et desuper liga ipsas tenui percameno et (super) linthio fortiter per triduum. Si tunc sanus non fueris, iterum fac ut supra. Item: aprehende de terra limacem rubeum et inde tange ter verucas et repone ad terram ut supra aripuisti. Item: agrimonia cum aceto tunsa et inposita verucas tollit.

[84] *Ad ongles leprous: triblez staphisagre e mettez un poi de eisel e mettez le ongle dedeinz e leischez taunt que il secche e quant il s'en chet, le oinez de mel, si revendra. Item: fetes roules cum .ii. deners de racine de gletoner e metez sur le charboun e cum le purra chaud su(i)ffrier mettez sur le ongle, remuez, quant il serra freid, si le eschaufez dé jurs e dé nuitz, le fettes deke le ongle seit bien redoubé.* Item: *si ungle commeste sont kancré,* lava cum aceto, postea viridem grecum superpone, deinde pulverem verbene. Item: liga super radicem jusquiani donec sanus sis. *Contre freid pernez orties en soleil levé e quesez en oile, si en oinez la cors, ja n'avrez freid de tout le jour la ou serrez oint. Ad blauncher les meins e col:* recipe orola(?) dragmas .ii., nitri dragmas .iiii., tipsane unciam et de istis simul tritis et mixtis cum aqua lava. Item ad manus dealbandum et lenificandum: accipe affodilles et coque in aqua et bene movendo tartarum admisce et postea lava et ex inde frica. Item: coque lovesticum cum sua radice in aqua et lava.

---

299 MS *amne.*
300 MS *manat.*

301 MS *jus.* See *Pop. Med.,* p.277 no.78.

[BOOK VIII: THE MALE MEMBER]

[85] Vit:[302] *une medicine me remembre / que soleit valer ad mal del member: / la primerole me triblez / od orties e sur le mal mettez. / Item autre vous dirrai esprové / ke en Celerne est mult loee: / trente ofes ben les quesez / tant que seient dures asez./ Le aubon devez oster / les moueas ben tribler. / Pus les mettez en la paiele / ben escuré e bele, / ad petit fu les devés frire / e pus prendre com hee fait cire. / Cel oil que donc en ist / cel mal en une nuit gari[st]. / Mes que cel mal fuist enkancré, / par cest oile serreit garré. / Et si garrit en autre manere / goute enossé e goute aigue[re].*[303] De ista predicta curatus fuit quidam cuius testes et verga intumuerant et fuerunt ibi .xv. foramina. Semel vel bis in die minxit. Ad ulceratam virgam si fuerit recens, pulverem aloes tere cum succo mente et cum penna liniatur, semel in die unges et cum aqua calida lavetur. Item quidem sunt qui in virga virili paciuntur habentes inflationem virge et multa foramina et excolacionem sub prepucio paciuntur. Talibus bulli malvas in aqua et extorque eas ut nihil aque remaneat. Postea cum sanguine vel cum butiro aut oleo et (cros sub ligne?) appone super folia caulium et isto posito super pannum circumda virgam virilem. Tale fit ad inflacionem auferendam. Deinde prepucio inverso in aqua lava calida prepucii loca ulcerosa et pulverem de pice greca et carne vermium et rosis et radice tapsi barbasti [et] mirtilli superasperge et si cares mirtillis, illa quatuor sufficiunt. Et sic fiat singulis diebus bis vel ter.

[86] Quandoque ex alba corupcione inter pellem et virgam in priapo oritur quedam titillacio ut oportet vi titillacionis ipsum priapum fricare et exiet pruritus albus. Contra hec mingens extrahe pellem quantum potes ultra prepucium ita ut urinam retenias ut eat inter pellem et priapum sicque quam sepe fac fricando, bene lava. Crede mihi, *drap en oile en jus deliez e de ache e de aubon de oef. Item: fettez papeloz de ferine de segle e enplez un forel e dedeinz mettez le membre e ce si sovent cum mester est chescun jour. Item ad membre enflé: buletez bren de frument molu e medlez od leit de chevre o de vache e fetes pain, si le quisez ad cendrez e quant ert freid, fetes en pastel od novel bure e od mel e mettez sur le membre. Item: triblez betonk od vin, si mettez, pusantment san[era].* *Item ad mal de membre s'il est ranclé: premez le jus de ache e berle e jubarbe ensemble triblé, si assemblez od mel e siu de chastris e fereine de neile e eisel e si friez ensemble e metez*[304] *cum enplastre sur, si ert gariz. Mes si il est escorci e nurit malveis mal, triblez mel e ferine de segle e mettez entre quir e char, si ert gariz.* Item ad flegmonem prepucii: ausungiam porcinam recentem tolle et malvam ortensem vel radicem malve agrestis, simul coque et tere et decoque in patella donec bene dissolvatur et cola per pannum [f.16v] et cum frigidum fuerit, exinde penna super circulum prepucii linitur. Sepius fac hec usque ad plenam sanitatem. *Vit que seine,* ad fluxum sanguinis per virgam vel per alium locum: fac emplastrum de stercore porcino recenti et thure pulverizato. Ad fistulam: fac tentam (et) de auripigmento et sapone. Si vis ut ducat, adde pulverem elebori. *Vit eschaud[é]: un oinoun percez e enplez le de franc encens, si restopez le oinoun de ce ke einz i fut, si le quesez bien en breses, puis tant le estampez que seit come oinement, ce mettez sur si chaud cum il le purra siu(e)ffrer. Ce faitz matin e cere*[305] *tant ke il seit gariz. Item hom*

---

302 MS *vkt.*
303 MS *g. in aigue.*

304 MS *pietez.*
305 for 'seir'.

que git of femme e est malveis de son membre prengne de la souredoc e de seneçon e de veil vein, si en fetes enplastre e liez sur e ert garriz. Item yif scoldyng of ye man, nym saxfrage and morele and unbyl et cetera und botir in smere et cetera. Item postquam censeris te lesum, iterum vade ad ipsam et cetera et sic sanaberis. Item postquam comisceris cum aliqua si dubitas aliquam lepram, statim lava in sin brixe(?) cum aqua calida. Kancer fluit humore rubeo et festula plurima habet foramina. *Ad cancer del membre: pernez la neire crapoud e atant de racines de porrez et pres atant de ligne drap, si ardez tout en poudre en un novel pot e de cest poudre mettez sur le mal tant que moert seit, pus de sein de motoun freiz enoinez vos mains, si les eschaufés souz vos asceles e tenez le in sinbre(?) en voz meins e garrez.* Item stercus hirci sicca ad solem et fac inde pulverem et sal super ponatur. Si autem fuerit femina, stercus capre. Si autem infra corpus fuerit, cum vino idem pulvis bibatur vel pulvis cornu hirci. Etiam facta est cura. Item ad kancrum virilis virge vel alterius partis quod respice alias ut et cetera(?) in alio loco.

[BOOK IX: THE BLADDER]

[87] Vesice infirmitates: signa morbique pleni videntur cito et saturi. Sequitur inflacio ventris et creber strepitus. Videntur oscitari nec oscitant sed os deducunt. Fit urina livida et dari(?) odoris et vix erumpens. Tumescunt verenda et fiunt cauculosi.[306] Idropici dolore jecoris et renum vexantur atque dolore [. . .] vexantur .i. molestissime. Omnes cause vesice ex renum indignacione fiunt. Multe et varie [sunt] cause sicut tumor, duritia calculorum,[307]emoroida, trumbosis, vulneracio, pitiriacis, terciasim, atonita et sausudis, litiriasis, constrictio, stranguria, curia rivatissimo(?), diapne, sunt cause .xv. Vesicam purgat acorus, apozima, asarus, artiatos(?), evisci radix, attriplici semen. Ad omnia vulnera visice nucleos .xxx., admigdalinos .xx., dattulos .xv., dragaganti coclearia .iiii. tundes simul et da inde coclearia .ii. cum [vino] calido ubi coxeris mirtum viride et alia adiutoria que ad hoc pertinent.

[88] Ad vesicam petrosam millifolii .iii. manipulos et modicum savine et .iii. rodellas de radice tere et fac potum spissum et da bibere per .ix. dies mane et sero. Statim petram minget. Item: raffanum cum vino coctum bibe. Malvas et allea ad tercias decoque cum bono vino et da ei bibere. Ad petram que impedit urinam: *la terre de nés de aroundes bevez en ewe t[e]ve.*[308] Item: *gromil, rouge ortie e novele cerveise triblez ensemble e le bevez.* Item: *persil, ache, quinquefoil e saxfragie de chescun une poin[é] e de gromil e nouls de peres de cerises, de greines de ere tout estanpez ensemble, si quesez en bon vin, si en beve.* Item: *sanc de buke mettez en veire e en la nefime jour en la decurs*[309] *de la lune escorchez .i. levre e la pel tout sangle[n]te sechez ad fu que vous pusschez ent fer pouder e de la semence de anis une coileré, de persilz .ii. colerez, de safran .ii. colerez, de sanc de buke .ii. [coilerez], de la pel une coileré, triblez tout ensemble e destemprez od vin tenve e en beive le malad en .i. bain. Si volez prover que la medicine seit verraie, metez en cel bevre .i. pere quel que vous vuilliez, ad tierce jour si troverez depescé.* Item: hec frangunt lapidem: colofondera(?), squilla, lupinum, hircinus sanguis, saxfragia, millefolium. Item: accipe

---

306 For 'calculosi'.
307 MS *colculorum.*

308 See *Pop. Med.*, p.293 no.234.
309 MS *decrocis.*

saxfragia, *burnet, peres de cerises, spic, spica celtica*,[310] *spicanardi e greinz de ere, pervenke, persil, gromil, fenuil, boilez tot ben en stale cerveise [f.17r] e beve. Si medicine luy donez, ce seit insci; si garra.* Item: lumbricos terrestres tere, deinde cum cere [. . .?] nigro et glauco simul decoque et elixaturam bene colatam et infrigidatam da sepius potare; certissimum et probatissimum remedium est. Item: recipe radicem rafani silvestris manipulum unum et saxfrage uncias .iii., petrosilini uncias loc(?).ii., hipericum .iii., bulliant usque ad terciam. Adde parum mellis et bibe mane et sero; infra .ix. dies frangit. *Item: triblez ouel peis checu[n] par sei [de] semence de petrasilie, saxfragie, ache, e de alisander, pus les medlez e de ceste poudre pernez un coileré e destemprez od vin e eschaufez un petit, issi le beve .ix. jours matin e ser, si garra.* Item: vulpino sanguine [. . .] nervium inonge et lapis rumpitur statim. *Item: pernez mesgke e fetes quere en vin e en beve. Item: beve jus de ere e chescun jour manjusce baie ad jun tant q'il seit garriz. Prové est.* Item: *persel, egremoine, alisaundre, plantaine tot destemprez od leit de chevre e od cerveise e usez e garra.* Item: *pernez – cete, si la entendez, est la soveraine medicine – un vif buk de treis anz, mettez en un lieu deke seit defié e veudé de sa viande q'il ad mangé, pus la receivez la tierce urine q'il i piscera; cel tout chaud beve que ad la pier[e] e ce il feit deke quarante jours, la pere defiera e destrura tot ad nent,* sicut *testmoinent parfiz mires que ce ount esprové. Autre:* bibat sauxfragia[m] coctam in aqua vel in vino. Hoc fiat bis in die vel ter aut quater vel quin. Notandum quod si minxerit, datur vobis indicium quod vicio lapidis laborat, si sit in collo vesice: recipe malvam, cretan[um], caulicem agrestem, saxi-fragiam, pariteriam et seneciones, nastorcium aquaticum, et decoquantur in liquore cuius tercia pars sit vini, tercia pars olei, [tercia pars] aque marine ut facte salse cum hec decoctione fomentamus bene et maxime illas partes inducendo herbas. Hec cura liberavit quemdam habentem lapidem vesice qui post longam fecit sugendo extrahi, post fomentum circa peritonion fecit inungere caput virge cum unctione auree.

[89] *Estale.* Stranguria est dolor urine quam pacientes tam viri quam mulieres. Viris facimus nastorcium aquaticum super pectinem portare et in decoctione ponimus pacientem. Item hanc atque desuriam soluit incisio vene in talo. Item ad difficultatem urine interruscum de nigra spina cum aqua distempera et bibe. *Item: quesez ben en un bon vin la malve e ail ensemble deke la tierce partie, si bevez. Item: rue, persil, ache quesez en ewe o – ke meuz vaut – en vin deke a la meité, si bevez.* Item: leporis cerebrum cum vino bibe vel testiculos eius coctos commede vel vesicam verri combure et bibe cum vino. Item: accipe galbanum et inde fac enplastrum et pone in caput ubi frstrk[311] super foramen et statim minget, certissimum est. *Item: home ou feme que ne puet estaler: destempre alisandre e cerfoil saufage od vin blanc e beve matin e cere e garra. Prové est. Pur la chaudepisce: bevez gletoner par vinz jours e garra.* Antidotum ad eos qui urinam graviter cum dolore faciunt: recipe piper, petrosilium, semen sparagi, litus sperma,[312] lufestici at scrupulos .v. Hec omnia tunsa et tribellata cum melle dispumato confice et cum necesse fuerit jejunus cum lacte bibe. Certum adiuvat. Tamen si vis cognoscere virtutem huius potionis, mitte de isto pulvere super lapidem vivam in a[m]pula vitrea positum. Postea liquefiet et redigetur in pulverem. *Urine retiner: bevez la poudre de ungles.* Item: *cerv[e]lle de livre ben triblé e columbine od sa semence, la nepte od la semence de letuse en ewe.* Item: *bevez le entrerusch de neire espeine od la ewe en vin.* Item: *la cervele*

---

[310] MS *spicacencia.*
[311] Another use of cipher.

[312] I.e. 'lithospermon' or gromwell.

de levre quit e triblé od vin od la semence de anis o od letuse vel od pimpernel e puliol e [c]alamente od poi de mel e le quesez od vin, si le maungez. Item: vesicam capre vel ovis ustam bibe in pusca et sicciens se collocet. Item: bibe ciminum tostum. Sunt quidam qui mingunt de nocte velint nolint quoniam urinales meatus paciuntur paralisim. Has de calidis herbis fomentabis. *Contre estaler sank: plusours medicines valent ad ceus [f. 17v] que sanc estailent: la wedrof de cel bois poez cuiler a vostre chose, bevez ent chaut, ce est la fin, en bon cerveise .v. jours juin.* Item: *.v. chefs de auz od les racines quisez en l'ew e beve .iii. fez.*

[90]   Item et cum dolore renum sa[nguinem] mingit: amoniacum et olibanum ac mirra conmixta cum aceto et cum carta inducta apponatur tam diu renibus donec sponte carta decidat. Item: sanguinem meantibus fleobotomabis de matrice et vena brachii. Si fortis fuerit fmaū(?) imponenda est cucurbita super renes et detrahes eis sanguinem et spungeas cum pusca super pectinem et testes inpone super. Item: alliorum capita .vii. cum cimis vel foliis coque[313] in aqua in olla ruda ad tercias et singula per quatuor dies tepida bibe. Item qui sa[nguinem] mingit: centinodiam cum vino [je]junus bibat usque sanus sit. *Item: pernez liz /.s. liliel, gromil, saxfragie, planteine, lancelé, herbe beneite, herbe sancti Johannis, mogwort e quisez en ewe e mettez i mel, cet bevez matin freid e cere chaud.* Ut pruritus tollatur verendorum: salviam cum vino coctam [super] loca verenda scuta(?), omnes prurigines utriusque sexus emendat. Cpk.[314] fomentum ad testiculorum inflacionem: recipe malvam, maleviscum, cassilaginem, jusquianum, absinthium, archimesiam, caules veteres, hec omnia bulliant in forti vino, fomentabis bis vel ter in die et easdem herbas pista et misce cum melle bullito et istud panno lineo indutum superpone. *Item: herbe r[ecevez] ke est appellé regina, destemperez od leit e usez.* Item: ad testium tumorem et dolorem quecumque modo contingat: in novo cacabo coque fabas tritas cum urina pueri et admisce mel prout congruum fuerit, in panno inductum appone tumori. Castrare hominem sine ferro: 'Camphora per nares castrat odore mares'.[315] Est autem gumma cuiusdam arboris in montanis Indee frigidum et siccum in tertio gradu cuius odor asuescens libidinem extinguit. Item castrare homines: *triblez la racine de pastinace campestre e mettez deinz le forel, si serra chastrez.* Item ne testiculi crescant pueri nec mamille puelle erollissa[nt](?), tere herbam et inplaustrum fac et impone. Vel semen papaveris coque in aqua pluviali in lintheo appone tribus diebus.

[BOOK X: THE STOMACH]

f.13r–v

[91]   Constantinus Affricanus montis cassiniensis monacus scribens Alphano archipresuli ecclesie saler[n]itane dicit quod stomacus est cella in medio corporis posita et instrumentum est ad digerendos cibos habens duo ora, unum superius ad recipiendum, aliud inferius per quod fex cibi ad intestina descendit. Est autem stomacus sub pectore et corde positus. Stat enim infra epar et splen. Epar est inmittum(?) in dextro latere, splen in sinistro et a sinistra parte ei calorem tribuit.

313 MS *coquis*.   315 Walther, *Initia* 2336.
314 Another cipher?

Unde stomacus degerit cibum cum vapore que sumit ab epate, corde, splene et felliculo infirmato stomaco et a sua valitudine remoto et in digerendis cibis defecto et alimentis ab eo crudis et indegestis descendentibus et cum fleumate voluntatis puncturam facientis et ardorem lesio omnibus menbris datur. Videmus enim propter stomachi dolorem cephaliam, emigraneam, vertiginem, sonum in auriculis, oculorum tenebrositatem, cincopim cardiacam et alia multa ac diversa genera. Ipse enim est tocius corporis fundamentum quo in sanitate existente cetera menbra dicuntur sana. Cor etenim patitur stomaco paciente maxime si in superiori parte passus sit. Similiter et stomacus patitur propter cordis passionem causa vicinitatis et colligancie et propterea caloris parvitatem cibos degerere adiuvantis. Cibus a stomaco ad epar per venas transfertur, unde necessitas expetit ut cerebrum et epar propter stomachum paciantur. Similiter stomacus propter cerebrum et epar coegrotatur.

[92]   Cerebrum autem patitur propter os stomachi, nam in os stomachi de cerebro .ii. magni nervi descendunt. Passiones autem que nascuntur in cerebro propter colliganciam oris stomachi sunt[316] alienacio, stupor, oblivio, melencolia, cephalia, epilencia et vertigo .iiii. modis. Est autem propter dolorem nimium aut propter acutum sensum aut quia uterque nervus stomachi sensualiter est defectus et acutum habet sensum aut quia cerebrum naturaliter seu accidentaliter est defectum, unde velociter patitur. Cetere vero egritudines quas diximus pati cerebrum propter os stomachi non fiunt nisi propter fumos ad eum a stomaco ascendentes. Stomachus diversis passionibus laborat at sicut irracionali appetitu quod sicut fuit a Purfirio Galienus interogatus 'Quare pater comedes?' et ipse respondit 'Comedo ut vivam' et dixit Purfurius 'Magna differrencia est inter me et te quia vivo ut comedam'.[317] Item quesivit que essent summa remedia. R[espondit] Gallienus 'Abstinentia et non quelibet sed particularis' et non detur stomaco quando non appetit nec negetur cum appetit. Naturaliter est autem stomacus paterfamilias qui omnibus menbris ministrat, tum appetendo tum degerendo. Si ergo laborat, compaciuntur omnia menbra fastidium quandoque in sano, quandoque in egro. Quandoque in pregnante nascitur in sano, quandoque fit ex colera collecta in orificiis matricis stomachi quod testatur amaritudo oris, sitis continua, egestio colerica, cuius cura est colera evacuare cum predictis medicaminibus[318] ubi de quatuor humoribus diximus. Deinde utendum est triasandali, siropo acetoso, rosata novella, zucarata rosacea. Vel aliter, quod probavi in nobili viro, accepi rosas recentes et in siropo roseo per noctem sub divo distemperavi primo, ad solem disiccavi et rosas dulcorizatas ad masticandum dedi et appetitum recepit. Item: accepi nasturcium aquaticum et dedi cum zucarato aceto [et] melle, et apetitum recepit. Quandoque fit fastidium ex fleumate viscoso adherente multum stomachi, unde fit abhominacio et voluntas vomendi sine motu, sitis nulla est. Cura: purgetur fleuma ut superius hin sunt. Primo utendum est istis el[ec]tuariis diacitoniten, diatri(d)on pi[pereon], sale sacerdotali quod non tantum valet ad hoc, sed multum valet ad bonum anelitum sal sacerdotale. Ad raucidinem illum pulverem masticare debemus vel uti in cibiis vel in potibus carne assata, piscibus assatis quando homini non licet carnes comedere, vino

---

316   MS *est*.
317   This quip, which is not actually in Galen, is cited in the *Rhetorica ad Herennium* IV,39 (as an example of 'commutatio') and in many Latin sources is attributed to Socrates.
318   MS *medicamina*.

rubeo bono et forti clareto frequenter et moreto. Si autem fuerit fastidium cum egritudine sicut cum febre vel sicut cum fluxu[319] ventris, removenda est causa et removebitur effectus .i. fastidium.

[93] Irracionabilis appetitus quandoque fit in masculo, quandoque in muliere pregnante. Qui est in masculo dicitur bolismus .i. caninus appetitus quia incessanter appetunt. Ypocras curam indicat in **Afforismis** ut dicit 'Facilius est repleri cibo quam potu'[320] sed ibi potum appellat sorbilem dietam et ungtuosam utpote insellatam, unde hoc modo curavi. Cotidie feci eum uti offis de pane calido in melle cocto. Postea feci ciminum bene pingue et feci eum quoque uti cum carne, quandoque sine carne. Feci etiam uti cepis coctis in melle cum carne pingui vel sine carne et uti vino bono. Et ita fastidium induci ei in fine et ita curavi. Apetitus irracionabilis in pregnante fit ex retencione menstruorum. In inicio consepcionis si fleuma superhabundaverit, cretam appetunt et alba et consimilia; si autem colera rubea acerima, appetunt porros et consimilia; si sanguis, dulcia apetunt ut mel, poma et similia; si colera nigra, carboni-gros carnes [. . .] assatas(?) contra exhibenda sunt. Si cretam appetunt, fabas excorti-catas date ei, sed quia cito cessabit talis appetitus et dubitandum est ne fiat aborsus, dando talia nos debemus cassare. Item stomacus aliis passionibus laborat ut lienteria, dissenteria, diaria.

[94] Lienteria diversis modis fit ex debilitate virtutis retent[iv]e et ex stipticis interius receptis et ex viscoso [f.13v] fleumate adherente multum stomaci. Si autem ex debilitate virtutis, hec erunt signa: cibaria intus recepta aliquantulum moram faciunt, in z^a(?) mutantur, non in qualitate appetitus debilis, et tamen magis appetunt quam possunt degerere, sitis pauca vel nulla. Cura est cum dieta talis: primo loco confortat[iv]is atque calefactivis utendum est, quemadmodum diacitoniten, diantos, que usualia sunt et pulvere quo curavi multos qui pulverem recipit: cinomonum, gariofilatum, spicenardum, cubebis, (e)xilobalsamum, cassilaginem, maces, de hiis omnibus pulverem feci et feci uti in cibariis. Item quendam pulverem feci mutuo .s. et eo multos curavi. Illum pulverem cum vino rubeo feci uti. Si autem fuerit ex stipticis interius .s. receptis, vitanda sunt stiptica, et digestibilia et lenia sunt utenda. Signum est quod usum est stipticis. Si autem ex viscoso fleumate, signa sunt abhominacio et cibaria in tali quantitate et in tanta quantitate in qua recipiuntur evitantur et etiam viscosa. In lienteria fluxus sine mutacione ciborum in qualitate et quantitate. Prima cura est evacuacio viscosi fleumatis sicud per benedictam vel per aliam speciem blance vel aliter per polipodium et agaricum et coque cum gallina pingui et jus mane jejunus sumet. Tandem specialiter curare per vomitum catapucie vel magis[tri] Bartolomei vel magis[tri] Andree. Si hoc modo curari non potest, quod multociens probavi, accipe ovum crudum et eici albumen et pone cum vitello ovi pulverem satis et combure totum et fac pulverem et hec pulvere utetur in cibariis et vino rubeo. Item alio pulvere consuevi uti: accepi lupi aquatici maxillas et comburi et combusto toto et in pulvere redacto dedi cum vino rubeo vel aqua pluviali et non tamen in lienteria sed et in

319 MS *flexu*.

320 *Aphor.* Lib.2,xi (Articella 1523 f.24va). Martin de Saint-Gille, *ed. cit.*, p.59 'Les corps sont raemplis plus tost de boire que de viande'.

dissenteria contulit et hec de lienteria sufficiunt. Ad pectoris et stomachi dolorem: semen nasturcii . . .³²¹

[f.29r][95] Dissinteria est fluxus ventris cum extorciacione intestinorum et sanguinolentis egestionibus. Quandoque est ex salso fleumate, quandoque ex colera citrina, quandoque ex colera nigra [f.29v], quandoque ex vicio epatis, unde epatica dissinteria dicitur. Si autem ex salso fleumate cum autem inferioribus intestinis ut ab umbilico inferius vel a mediis vel a superioribus. Si autem inferioribus intestinis, hec erunt signa: dolor sub umbilico, punctio, torcio, egestio muscilaginosa et citrina ut aqua resoluta a carne salsa. Eius cura et dieta est: prius mollif[ic]atum fiat sicut de malva, furforibus, oleo vel pinguedine, deinde glisteriza. Constrictio huiusmodi: accipe parum calcis vive et cretam, unde pellipari utuntur et sumat mirtillos et decoquantur omnia cum sepo arietino optime in aqua, deinde colentur et inde fiat glistere non semel sed frequenter. Similiter subfumigationes debet fieri: accipe cuminum in aceto nocte infusum et thus in minori quantitate et sepum arietinum in maiori quantitate, pix, resina in eadem quantitate et super lateres candentes(?) ponantur in fundo olle vel patelle et preparetur ita ut fumus non possit intrare nisi per an(n)um. Medicina per os recepta ad hanc speciem parum valet. Dieta sit constricta ut caro arietina assata, faba cum corticibus, caseus assatus, vinum rubeum et stipticum plus valet. Tunc postea panis azimus, pedes porcini assati cum aceto, galline assate, pisces commedat assatos. Eadem cura circa intestina media nisi(?) quia per utramque regionem medicina sumitur plus probatur. Ad mediam illam et ad superiorem: recipe boli armenici, sanguinis draconis, balaustie, affacie, lapidis amatistis vel sanguinarii ana .z. .ii. Fiat pulvis ex omnibus et lacte caprino cocto vel cum vino rubeo et stiptico vel sapa vel succo plantaginis. Idem pulvis et eadem dieta valet contra dissenteriam que fit circa interiora intestinorum. In eidem intestinis fit dissinteria ex colera rubea, egestio citrina est expresse .i. flava, dolor acutior quam in alia, torcio et egestione maiori. Egestio quandoque spumosa. Cura et dieta: talis est cura: purgetur primo, si fortis est, cum trifera saracenica simplici vel cum clistere predicto (predicto). Et si inferioribus intestinis fuerit, item: vinum non adeo forte debet exhiberi in hac materia quam in aliis immo temperantur cum aqua celesti. Eadem dieta et remedia valent ad mediam et ad superiorem. Si aliquantulum ex colera adusta nigra est egestio, unde dissinteria inchoans e felle nigro mortale est et eam incurabilem relinquimus. Si autem epatica fuerit, hec erunt signa: post prandium inflantur et evacuato corpore venter vehementer appetit. Unde dum cibus in ventre tenetur dolet et evacuato se melius habet et statim appetuntur. Istam relinquimus incurabilem quia in ydropisim transit. Ex hiis que dicta sunt eleganceora collige ad curam dissenterie.

[BOOK XI: THE INTESTINES]

[96] De ruptura intestinorum.³²² Est quedam pellicula que dicitur sifac et sustinet intestina ne cadant in osseum et illa pellicula quandoque rarescit, quandoque rumpitur multis ex causis ut ex clamore, ex saltu, ex nimio onere, ex sublevacione inmensi

---

³²¹ The rest of f.13v is blank.   ³²² MS *intestinis*.

ponderis ex nimia replicatione intestinorum. Cum debilis fuerit illa pellicula ex rarefactione, tumor non debet descendere usque ad testiculos, sed ad superiorem partem membri virilis, cuius cura – et maxime si puer fuerit vel juvenis, caveat primo ab omnibus stipticis utere – ergo hec: recipe frequenter (recipe) pillocellam, consolidam maiorem, plantaginem, de hiis omnibus trahatur succus equaliter et utetur succo illo cum vino stiptico ubi due partes sint succi et tercia vini. Fiat ei ligatura talis .s. saculum de lineo panno, stuppis et lana impletum ut bene durum sit, sit quasi auricularis parvum et circa quatuor angulos pone ligaturas ut possit ligari ad bracale ne descendant ad inferiora intestina. Et sic cura[m] consolidat. Ita multi liberati sunt. Si autem intestina sunt in testiculis, incurabilis est egritudo, nec incidatur. De hac incisione ut inexper[t]us relinquo.

[97] *Prover si homme est rumpu: ard[ez] seu devant luy e son ventre croulera. Ad rumpture: fetes .xxix. pelotis de peil de levre en mel, si les engloutez un aprés autre tout lendemein .xxviii., issi un meins chescun jour. Issi le fetes que nul ne remeine. Item: fettes enplastre de soufre e de veil oint, si mettez en la plaie sur .i. tendre quir. Aprés ce qu'il ert bainé, si fetes un bevre de confirie e de consoude e osmunde, si ert gariz.*

[BOOK XII: THE KIDNEYS]

[98] De renibus et eorum passionibus. Renes et lumbi multis passionibus paciuntur, quandoque ex apostemate, quandoque ex opilacione venarum, quandoque ex viscosis humoribus vel calculo, ex opilacione grossi sanguinis. Si autem ex apostemate eadem cura ad[h]ibenda est que dicta est circa alia apostemata. Si ex grosso sanguine, ita medicina est precipua [f.18r] .s. fleobotomia de sofenis venis iuxta talos. Si ex arenulis vel ex calculo eadem cura utendum est diureticis et dieta subtili. Quedam diuretica usualia sunt ad hanc passionem .s. justinum, electuarium ducis,[323] licontripon, filiontripon, diaspermaton. Quidam pulvis probatus ad idem quid magister Bart[olomeus] ponit in Practica sua.[324] Quidam sanguine yr[c]ino triennale curantur. Quedam[325] autem alia remedia probavi. Consuevi accipere saxifragiam, filipendulam, ornnctam(?), semen petrosilini et apii atque anisi, coriandri, feniculi, masedonici, spicenardi, squinantum, ligustrum, anis et de hiis omnibus equaliter feci pulverem et feci eo uti mane et sero cum vino ubi radices diuretice cocte fuerunt ut petroselini graminis et multos curavi. Cum sola lingua avis multos curavi. Accepi eam viridem et terui in morterio optime et destemperavi cum vino albo et subtili. Deinde colavi et feci pacientem mane et sero uti. Ex hac tamen liberavi quendam militem Flandrie. Et eadem est cura [contra] arenulas in vesica et contra calculum nisi consolidatum fuerit. Calculus consolidatus non curatur nisi cum incisione ut testatur Gallienus in Organon, ubi ait 'Gracia perfecte curacionis est incisio'. Si autem ex opillacione viscosi humoris diureticam curatur et per vinum bonum et subtile, unde Ypocras in

---

323 MS *es'tuarium diutis.*
324 See Renzi, *Coll. Sal.* 4, pp.316,319 and 2, p.315.
325 MS *quidam.*

Afforisimis super hec ait.[326] Item si ex viscose humore fluxere debemus idem intelligere (rem).

[99]   *Ad dolour des reinz: bevez la racine de gletoun triblé od cerveise matin freid, seir chaud. Item: mel, peiz, bure boil[e]z e oinez le mal ad le feu. Item: semence de ache destemprez od vin, bevez sovent jun. Item: bevez centurie triblé od ewe freide, si garra.* Prové est. Item: semen plantaginis cum vino potatum renibus et vesice [prodest]. *Item ad reinz: triblez pigle, ailly vermail e metez sur les reinz e garra.* Ad neufreticos quibus lapides in renibus nascantur: occide yrcum annorum quatuor, recipe sanguinem, non primo nec postea, sed medium, et cum se coagulaverit, incide minutim in patella terre quam prius bulliat ad focum, ut tere saporem amittat. Deinde co[o]peri patella[m] linthio duplici et pone sub divo ut a sole et luna siccetur. Et cum siccus fuerit, tere et repone[327] in pixide et da cotidie. *Item pur frendre la pere si ce est deinz le home: pernez .ix. greinz de ere e persil e alisaundre e cerfoil saufage, ce bevre .ix. jours destempré od vin, pus si pese en un basin, si verez ad le founz ou ele ert menusement depescé.* Prové est.

[BOOK XIII: THE ANUS]

[100]   *Fundement:* D[e] exitu ani dicendum est quia morbus est communis tam viris quam mulieribus et facit sanguinem fluere. In restringendum sanguinem et in recipiendo fomenta cum vini decoctione in quo bulliat absinthium, postea inline eum totum cum incausto ad restringendum. Tercio pulverem factum de salice et eius radicibus et arista alicuius piscis salsi super asperge et repone in anum cum linthio. Sic fac .iii. vel .iiii. vicibus[328] in die et sanaberis. *Item: triblez les mouelles de oefs quiz durs en eisel o vinegre. Plus vaut od oile de lorer. Pus moilez un clut en cel pulte et fetes li malad ser sur tant que il seit sein.* Item: fac turtellos de pulvere radicis dracuntee et farina tritici et commedat. *Item: mettez desouz lin filee de linge .s. cru en chaud bain, si entra enz par la force del lin e par chalur de l'ewe, pus se seine. Item ad homme que ist le fondement: celidoine e oint de ver triblez ensemble, si mettez en .i. tenfe quir blanc, si le bot[e]z enz od tout le lequor.* Item sunt alii quibus non exit, tamen inde paciuntur maximum dolorem. Hiis aloen pulveriza et destempera cum vino calido et cum adhuc sit tepidum, lanam vel bombacem unge et in anum pone. Id mitigat dolorem inflacionem auferendo. *Item ad dolour del fundement: mettez l[e]inz lins moilé en mel. Item ad homme que le fondement le manjue: sancisues ardez en poudre e moilez leine en mel e aprés en la poudre e mettez enz. Si le*[329] *couste aler avant, distemprez mel e arnement ensemble e moilez deinz, pus le botez en le found.* [Prové] est e garra.

[101]   Contra curenciam et cum sanguis per fundum exit: conmisce acetum forte cum succo plantaginis equaliter et bene bulliantur. [f.18v] Deinde mitte ov[u]m .i. in mixturam illam et coque, ut fiat durum, et commedat infirmus et de mixtura illa bibat

---

[326] The reference appears to be to *Aphorism*, VI,18 'Vesicam incisam, aut cerebrum, aut cor, aut diaphragma, aut epar, aut ventrem, aut renes, aut intestinorum aliquod gracilium, mortale'. Cf. Martin de Saint-Gille, *Comm. ed.* G. Lafeuille (1964), p.167.

[327] MS *repc̄one*.

[328] MS *diebus his*.

[329] For *li* (*couster* is impersonal).

et sanabitur. Emoroide dicuntur ab emac, quod est sanguis, et rois, fluxus. *Pur le fondement et contre la meneisoun e pur les emeroides estufe: poretz e maufes mincez, pus boilez, si mettez desouz une sele percee que seit environ covert e sece le malad sur a receyvere . . .*³³⁰ *e se estufe ben, si sentent les veines, si est garri.* Item ad [. . .] sandex renat's(?) atramentum, herba fetida, vermem(?) molitum in illud equaliter teratur et sic calidum apponatur. Item: ovum galline, ordeum et sal equale pondus, omnia comburantur in rudi olla et pulvis inde fiat et ex eo emoroide aspergantur. Probatum est. Item: prius sanguisuge ponantur in unaquaque [. . .], tere sufficienter, detracto sanguine [pone] super enplastrum de pulvere galle et de pipere equaliter factum et de albugine ovi confectum et omni die laventur vino et iterum renovetur enplastrum usque dum bene sanentur.

[BOOK XIV: THE KNEES AND LEGS]

[102] *Genul ad mal de poleyn: liez ad genul fleur de forement boili en leit, si est gari.* Item si est inflatum: folia coruli vel eius corticem cum depentibus catulis coque in aqua usque ad terciam partem, inde cotidie te balnea jaumbes. Ad jambas pruriginosas sive ad omnem pruriginem: auripigmentum, sulphur, masticum, piper, ex omnibus equaliter fac pulverem, confice cum butiro ut sit strictus et unge et liga. Probatum est. *Item ad jaumbez e piez: veil formage trible[z] od mel e mettez.* Item ad inflacionem vel postulas tibiarum vel pedum: contere cum melle summitates salicis³³¹ et superpone ut enplastrum. Hii duo in triduo sanat. *Enfleure du pié: triblez ache e la mie de blanc pain e veil oint e mettez cel enplastre e sanera. Postume de pé: jus de ache, taneseie, sauge, planteine, ditaine, mel cru, ferine de segle, totes fetes si espés cum vus poez, si mettez sur le mal, si est garriz.*
[103] Ad malum mortuum unguentum: accipe edere terestris libram unam et de plumbo usto libras .ii., de sulphure vivo libras .v., argenti vivi libras .v. et de fructu silvestri plenum pungnum tantumdem de lentisco et de ligno cedrino unum coclear plenum et tantumdem de ligno aloes. Hec omnia simul in olla nova comburantur et cribretur pulvis eorum et postea cum aceto permixtus ad multam spissitudinem simul destemperate coligantur et tere in morterio cum olio diu et fortiter usque ad satis simul terantur et sic usui reserventur. Item: de succo cerfolii et sanguine recenti porcino et argento vivo, thure, mastico, repercutat humores inferioribus inunctis(?) et per salvam educit.
[104] Ad skabiem: album corallum et folia albe spine insimul tere. Postea accipe auxungiam veterem porci et argentum vivum que simul pistata cum pulvere supradicto unge. Item ad pruriginem: recipe litargiri unciam .i., ceruse unciam .i., sulfuris unciam .i. et s[emis], olei cimini quod sufficit, cum aceto exsolve. Ad scabiem vel impetiginem: herbam marubium cum aqua decoque et eius jure corpus lava et sic quod scabiem discuties et impetiginem. Item: desuper merubium cum melle coctum sumat, mire sanabit.
[105] Ad nervorum dolores et ad parilisum et nervos contractos et precisos: stipes brasice et caulis cum radicibus combure eiusque cineres cum aceto confice et dolori

---

³³⁰ MS illegible at this point.   ³³¹ MS *felicis.*

appone. Item ad nervos lesos et contractos: juniperum, edere terestris, ebulum, viscum de pomerio acernuo, avena, omnia in caldario coque cum aqua. Sella ubi sedere debet grande habet foramen et in hac decoctione stufet se infirmus et diligenter dolium sit coopertum et sanguine de mola molendini calefiat multum in igne et mittatur in illo balneo ut vaporetur infirmus. Item ad nervorum dolorem: petrosilinum tunsum et vice cataplasmatis impositum nervorum dolorem sanat. Item: herbe malve salvatice radices pistate cum auxungia veteri et imposite mirifice sana[n]t. Ad pedem si quis lassus cederit in langorem ad nervos et spasmum: herba(m) merubium cum oleo rosaceo permixta perunges eum, sine mora sanabitur. Ad coxarum dolorem: artemesiam tundes cum ausungia et aceto et impone et in [tercia?] die sanus erit. Ad nervorum dolorem: artemesiam tonsam cum oleo bene subactam impone et erit sanus. [f.19r] Ad nervorum dolorem et cetera [. . .] Ad tibias vel pedes inflatos: coque radicem ebuli in aqua, interuscum cum auxungia ver[r](icc)ina et panno induc tibiis vel pedibus impone et sanabitur sine mora. Item ad vulnera tibiarum vel tumore[m] vel duriciam vel vermes: mirre unciam .i., cere libram unam, sinapi, uncti porcini libram .i. circa fac moderamen, cum opus fuerit impone. De indignacione nervorum si fuerit ex percussione vel apostemate: prima die fac fomentum quod conficitur ex herbarum frondibus, visciole(?), volubilis, lappaceoli, brance ursine, jusquiani, cimarum rubri, sanbuci, cime ebuli, folia viole, radices ulmi, semina fenugreci, lini, omnia insimul coquantur et mane et sero fomentabis. Postea ungo unguatur quod recipit frondes evisci libram unam cenum, fenugreci, ana .i., pinguedinem anseris et gallinacii libram .i. vel minus, quibus tunsis addatur vinum et coquantur insimul usque ad consumpcionem vini. Postea addatur masticis unciam .i., cere albe unciam .i. que liquefacta depone cotidie, fomenta et unge cum supradicto bis in die usque ad curacionem. Memento tamen ut si vulnus fuerit in dimisso(?) fomento supradicto, ungento fusco curetur. Curato vulnere si nervi contracti fuerint, supradictis utere et eodem unguento stuppam superpone et liga cum fascia. Ad omnem skabiem ex frigidis humoribus, sic curabis: pulverem cecute et agarici unciam dimidiam dura . . . (?) ad solvendum [. . .] citrinarum unciam .i. pone in succo fumi[terre] cocto et dispumato et nocte ibi maneat, mane autem pulverem tollas et succum ad potandum tribue. Fiat hec ter vel quater. Ad scabiem pedum: arnoglossam cum aceto tritam pedibus appone vel unge cum abrotano trito cum ungulo.

[106] Ad podagram et ciragram: laureolam et cervi linguam, folia sinapis et cucorbite agrestis ac cucumeri agrestis, raphani atque sambuci, sulphur vivum et alumen. Ista terantur et cum olio olive coquantur et colantur. Cum opus fuerit utere sic: fac stupas cum fustibus sambuci et cum exsiccatus fuerit, unge. Postea incidantur vene que iuxta iuncturas manuum et pedum sunt et postea cum lato ferro coquantur et sic cartartico solutorio multociens purgetur et bis in die unguatur. Ad podagram: betonica decocta usque ad terciam, aqua potui data ipsaque trita et apposita mire dolorem linire experti sumus. Item ad podagram et ad omnem nervorum dolorem vel etiam tumorem: plantaginis folia contusa vel pistata cum modico salis et apposita optime facere certum est [et] exprobatum. Item: fimum caprinum in aceto acro mitte et coque et ubi consumptum fuerit acetum coquendo tolle a foco. Postquam acetum consumptum fuerit et stercus siccaverit, in morterio tere ut pulvis fiat. Adde mel et conmisce ut cataplasma fieri possit et pone ubi tumor vel dolor fuerit ut die tercio solvatur. Ad dolorem genuum vel tibiarum vel crurum vel ubicumque dolor fuerit:

herba simphoniaca facta quasi malagma tunsa cum stercore robillo(?) et modico aceto et imposita tumorem tollit. Ad podagram: betonica cocta ad terciam et aqua in potu data et ipsa trita et imposita mire dolorem linire experti affirmant. Ad calidam podagram: mustele sanguinem cum succo plantaginis inter ipsa nuntia linibis (?). Coriandri folia ana jusquiani teres eum diligenter et supermittes micam panis mundi et infundes frigidam aquam et simul teres iterum et conmisces adipis porcini recentis sufficientem modum. Aut pro adipere oleum arseum modicum mittes. *Item ad dolour dé pez podagrés: triblez ache vert od eisel e mettez.Item podagre:* caseus capre positus super pedes recens sanat. Item: muscus qui in aqua nascitur tritus et impositus prodest. Farina frumenti cocta cum aceto et imponetur. Item: *pijons de corbs vifs pernez hors del ni, si qu'il ne veient nul meisoun e les ardez en un novel pot. Cel poudre beve le poagré*³³² *e si est [garri] homme [qui] ad la goute aiue.*³³³ Item ad dolorem et tumorem podagri et calorem: [f.19v] succus morelle, curiandri et jusquiani ex quo conmixtus et unctus mirifice prodest. *Item: preignez une herbe que est appellé* **sourethestil et watercresces** *par ou[e]les porc[i]ouns e porke e boilez tout ensemble ovesque eus. Item pur faire ewe pur fevres: preignez sauge e avences, violet, tormentule e* **sowersthestilis**, *preignez d'ascune ou[e]les porc[i]ouns e stampez e preignez le jus de les herbes e mettés en une fiale issi que nul eawe poet vener hors. E preignez de cel jus en mati[n] trois 'sponful'.*³³⁴

[107] Ad pedes inflatos ex itinere: coque absinthium in aqua et intus quam calide potes tene pedes. Item: absinthium coque in aceto et inde circumliga. Ad scabiem coxarum sive aliarum partium: recipe enulam, acetum, olium, argentum vivum, secundum voluntatem imponentis conficitur sic. Munda et [s]cinde minutim radicem enule et coque in aceto postquam satis fiat decocta, tere cum ausungia in morterio, primo impone argentum vivum cum oleo et aceto in quo decocta fuerit enula. Destempera et hoc valet pruritu excoriatis. Cave ne intra os propter vivum argentum si superiora inde fovis. Ad impetiginem: frica locum cum radicibus lapacii acuti et pulverem colofonie vel coso(?) ferrum super aspergimus. *Ke vous ne seiez laz de aler: triblez rue en oile e de ce frotez voz piez. Item pur travail alegier: ambrosie destemprez od ewe au seir e bevez e si vous en aiez tout le jore laburé tout vous serra allegié(r). Ad verms du pé engetter: semence de jusquiani e de piretz mettez sur une tiule chaude, si ke la fumé munte ad verms.* Post aqua sumpta exient. Ad talorum dolorem vel tumorem: jusquianum cum radice sua tere et super pedes pone, mirifice prodest. Mulier non podagrizat si non deficiunt ei menstrua. Puer non podagrizat ante afroduliam . Podagra et marcaca in veere et autumpno moventur ut in pluribus et cetera. In itinere porta tecum artemesiam et non senties laborem. Item: canta Pater Noster super artemesiam et verven(d)am et fer tecum in via ut non fatigeris et cetera. Si pedibus quassata sunt ossa herba gladeoli segetalis superior pars trita sit a equis ponderibus et cum oleo rosaceo appone. Ad pedum³³⁵ dolorem: artemisia cum ausungia et imposita pedi dolorem tollit vel eius radicem cum melle de[bet?] manducare. Si ab itinere pedes intumuerunt, plantago contunsa cum aceto et imposita tumorem tollit. Ad talem dolorem: fimus caprinus cum aceto acro coctus in olla appone.

---

³³² *podre.*
³³³ See *LH* 135 and *Pop. Med.,* p.69 no.28.
³³⁴ The scribe seems to have written out the last four words again.
³³⁵ MS *pedem.*

PROGNOSTICS

Signa mortifera versus[336]

[108] Precinuit Gallienus in corpore humano quot signa sunt mortifera. Versus:
'Prima tibi facies occurrat, prima notetur,/ In se signa gerit, quibus egri cresis habetur;
/ Lumina si lateant, aut sint infusa rubore, / Signum mortis habent, vario distincta
colore. / Livida si fuerint, aut effugienda lumine, / Hec tibi designant venture mortis
acumen. / Auris pulpa rigens, frons arida, timpora plana, / Naris acuta, labo[r] in motu,
sompnia vana, / Algor in extremis, calor, sitis interiorum. / Hiis visis (h)abeas curasque
geris aliorum.'[337]

[Prognostica][338]

[109][339] Item bonum est invenire egrum iacentem in dextro aut sinistro latere et
in modum sani et manus et pedes atque cervicem non ut in spasmo distenta sed minime
rigida et totum corpus in sua dispositione flexibile que habitudo sanis[340] est et
familiaris et amica et iacere in modum sani melius est. Sed si iacuerit aperto ore, erecta
cervice et pedibus tortis aut rigidis, malum est. Item non est laudabile signum egrum[341]
iacere corpore supinato, brachiis ac pedibus (f)rigidis; malum est. Aut si iacuerit super
ventrem preter solitum, alienacionem et ventris dolorem significat. Si in augmento
egritudinis repente steterit hora in acuta egritudine et in pleuripleumonia, que est
pulmonis apostema, pessimum est signum. Si repente a capite lecti usque ad pedes se
iactaverit pessimum signum et valde angustiosum. Si in egro corpore sit antrax, quod
est venenosum apostema, sive precesserit [sive] egritudini[342] supervenerit, opus est
attendere, vel etiam si sit ibi carbunculus, qui est genus apostematis, considerandum
est si ex sudore siccatus sit et colorem lividum aut viridem sive citrinum habuerit;
malum signum est. Sudores frigidi qui circa cervicem et circa faciem emanant [f.20r]
pessimi sunt et celerem ac proximam mortem venturam significant.[343] Sed illi sudores

---

336 Written in the lefthand margin.
337 These well known lines, which are marked in the margin with the rubric 'signa mortifera versus'
appear in the *Flos medicinae Salerni* in *Coll. Sal.* 5, pp.60–1 (ll.2090–99). For an extensive survey
see R.H.Robbins, "Signs of Death in Middle English", *Mediaeval Studies* 32 (1970), 282–98.
338 What follows is a patchwork, often rather a jumble, of quotations from Hippocrates' *Prognostica*
(*Capsula eburnea*) which I have consulted in the 1523 print of the *Articella* and in MS Oxford,
Bodl. Libr., Latin misc. e 2 ff.27r–31v. Most of the material used is found in the Greek text of
the *Prognostikon* prepared by W.H.S. Jones (Loeb ed. *Hippocrates* 2), sections III, VI, II, XIV,
XIII. For an English translation see also G.E.R. Lloyd (ed.), *Hippocratic Writings* (Har-
mondsworth, 1978), pp.170–85. Note the material in *Flos medicinae ed.cit.*, pt.6, c.iv *et seq.*
339 Sections 109 and 110 consist mostly of excerpts from Bk 1 of the *Prognostica* in the following
order: ch. 16,20–1,17,22,23,25,29,10,15,13,14,10,14,27,24.
340 MS *sanus.*
341 MS *egro.*
342 MS *egritudinem sive s.*
343 Cf. Prog.148va 'Deterior autem sudor est qui est frigidus, postea qui est in capite et cervice' and

optimi sunt qui per omne corpus emana[n]tur et ad finem febre caruerunt. Sudor bonus et laudabilis e[s]t in omni acuta egritudine. Suaves fiunt [viz. sudores] si[344] in die cretico .i. die indicativo[345]emanant et egrum liberant et suaviorem et fortiorem reddunt.[346] Qui vero nihil horum feceri(n)t, sudor[347] mortalis est. Item si fuerint timpora plana, malum signum est. Si frons arida aut rubea et cutis intensa et dura, malum signum est. Si supercilia declinantur, malum signum est. Et si palpabre livide aut inverse, malum signum est. Et si oculi concavi et tremuli et instabiles atque lippitudinem sustinuerint aut eciam lumen effugiunt, [malum signum est]. Aut sinister oculus hominis et dextra mulieris minuitur[348] et minor altero aparuerit, [malum signum est]. Aut si eger nolens lacrimas effuderit aut aliter lacrimaverit aut foras tanquam in suffocacione pre[-e]minetur, malum signum est. Si alba oculorum in sanguinem conmutata fuerit [. . .] hec omnia periculosa et mortalia iudicabis. Si in sompnis sola alba oculorum videatur palpebrisque subclausis, malum signum est. Si iuvenis est et vigilat, si senex et sompno lentus, hec omnia signa oculorum mala sunt.

[110] Si aures [f]rigide aut contracte et parvicoli(?) contracti et aurium pulpe inverse, malum significat. Si nasi summus albificat malum signum. Si nares acute atque districte [. . .] neque solucio per se aut per catar[t]icum precesserit[349] neque ex consuetudine, si hoc non evenerit, malum signum est et mortis signum timebis.[350] Hiis signis solis sicque cum predictis omnibus mortem proximam iudicabis. Sanguis si emanaverit ex naribus infra .vii. dies, emanare bonum signum est.[351] Sed si anelitus frigidus ex naribus et ore exierit, mortem significat. Si cibum aut potum per nares exierit et vocatur [et] non respondit, pessimum signum est. Si labia livida vel alba aut pendencia fuerint, malum signum [est]. Si li[n]gua deficit et curtat, malum signum significat. Dentibus cum insania frenduere in febribus et hoc (non) preter solitum neque a puero hoc habuerit, mania est, que est quedam capitis passio, et mors vicina sequetur.[352] In omni egritudine sternucio cum reumate pulmonis vel coste malum signum [est]. Aposte[m]a in gutture cum acuta febre malum signum et si aliquid aliud malum signum ex iam dictis visum fuerit, mortale est. Item omne apostema magis in hieme quam in aliis temporibus evenit et amplius et si sanatur, non reciprocatur.

Et sunt hec indicia mortis et vite extracta de libro pronosticorum Ypocratis.

(f.148rb) 'Frigidus autem malus, peior si in cervice et in capite solo, qui quidem in acuta febre significat mortem'.

344 MS *ubi*.

345 MS *i. sive indicativo*.

346 The text in the *Prognostica* reads '. . . acuta egritudine qui in cretica die fit et egrum liberat. Est autem bonus qui fit in toto corpore et eger ex eo suavior et fortior efficitur'.

347 MS *sudoris*.

348 'oculus sinister minuitur' is contained in the celebrated verses on the signs of death found in MS Bodl. Libr. e mus. 219 f.81r.

349 MS *precesserunt*.

350 MS *timed*'. The lines garble *Prog.* f.145vb concerning the eyes: 'Oportet etiam videre quid de oculis in somno videatur: si enim solo alba videantur subclusis palpebris nec solutio aut per se aut per catarticum precesserit, neque ex consuetudine hoc evenerit, mortis signa videbis'.

351 *Prog.* f.149va has: 'Solet huic acute egritudini infra .vii. dies sanguinis fluxus ex naribus utiliter supervenire'.

352 *Prog.* f.147ra has: 'Frendere dentibus in febribus preter solitum neque a puero mortem vel maniam significat, quod si frendeat cum insania, mors sequitur vicina'.

[111][353] Item si fell nigrum ab ore cum omnibus egritudinibus emiserit, mortalis [est] et mortem significat.[354] Vel sanguinis quidem qualiscumque malum signum est. Vomitus si ut succus porri, viridis aut plumbeus sive niger, malus est et nuncius mortis. Sputum globosum [in]utile est, spumosum malum, et nigrum mortale. Spiritus[355] si frequens fuerit, dolorem et successionem significat in hiis que sunt super diafrangma et si magnus et cum[356] intermissione alienacionem significat. Spiritus vero bonus ex suo proprio ordine[357] cognoscitur[358] et habet evidentem salutis ostencionem in acuta egritudine que cum febre est cuius terminus in .xl. diebus [est]. Si mentum cadit, malum est.[359] Et sudor frigidus malus, peior si in cervice [et] in capite solo; qui quidem in acuta egritudine pessimus et mor[ti]s signum [est]. Si siccatus, color[360] viridis vel citrinus aut lividus, inde significat [. . .] quod si sic fueri[n]t,[361] in principio egritudinis oportet inquiri an vigilie precesserunt aut ventris multe soluciones aut jejuni[i] labores prius affuerint et si aliquid horum cognoveris precessisse, minus periculosum vere-bares,[362] quod si die et nocte precedentibus quicquam horum sustinueri[n]t, non multum periculosum sperabis. Si vero nihil horum cognoveris, mortis signum sperabis. Et [si] huiusmodi egritudo triduana fuerit, que precesserunt labores non minus per-cuntaberis et omnia que sunt inquirenda circa corpus in oculos perquiri [debes]. Si brachii rigidi, malum est. Si manus ut in spasmo non extensa,[363] bonum est. [Manuum mobilitatis signa sic pernotabis]: in febre acuta et in pleriplemonia et in frenesi non vera et in dolore capitis si manus ad capud tulerit tanquam aliquis positurus collectu-rusque[364] [h]ac illac aut quesierit seu detractaverit aut de vestibus aliquid advulserit aut festucas de pari[e]te deserpserit, mortalitatis signa[365] sic pernotabis. Pessimum [est]. Si in digitis et unguibus livor [f.20v] veridis admistus, mortem non dubitabis adven-ientem indicat. Si digitos sepe respexit aut aierem respexit, malum est. Si per pulsum sic probil . . . (?), si vena non batitat et pollex frigidus est, mortem significat. Vena agiliter baciens et pulsus iuxta impares mortis signa [sunt]. Vena cum virtute baciens et pulso cum virtu[t]e eius foras et pollex calidus bonum signum [est]. Vena debiliter baciens et pulso mixta una super aliam mortem significat. Vena urens et baciens batitura vero lenis et pollex calidus bonum significat.

[353] In this section the excerpts from the Hippocratic *Prognostica* occur in the order II,39, 46, 47, I,37, I,38, I,29, I,25, I,11, I,26.

[354] Cf. *Aphorism.* Lib.IV, c.xii / c.xiii (*Articella* 1523) f.66va: 'Egritudinibus quibuscumque incipien-tibus, si fel nigrum aut sursum aut deorsum exierit mortale. Quibuscumque ex egritudinibus acutis aut multi temporis aut abortibus aut aliter extenuatis, si fel nigrum exierit aut qualis sanguis niger, sequenti die morietur'.

[355] MS *species.*

[356] MS *sū.*

[357] MS *ordore.*

[358] MS *congruo.*

[359] Contained in the celebrated verses on the signs of death in MS Bodl. Libr. e mus. 219 f.81r.

[360] MS *calor.* The reference (see *Prog.* I,25) is to 'anthrax' or 'carbunculus': 'Si in egro corpore fuerit antrax aut carbunculus sive precesserit sive egritudini supervenerit, opus est attendere. Quod si exsiccatus fuerit et colorem viridem vel citrinum vel lividum pertulerit, mortem dicit proximam'.

[361] The reference is to a series of symptoms which the scribe has inadvertently omitted.

[362] *Prog.* f.143vb 'vereberis'.

[363] MS *existente.*

[364] MS *locaturque.*

[365] MS *singula.*

[112] Considerandum est in egris, ut ait Ypocras, color vultus, oculi, vox, taci-
turnitas, positio iacentis, et scema et corpus, habitudo [. . .] consideracionem corporis,
qualitatem regionis, aeris temperanciam, etates morborum, consuetudinem egrotan-
tium, corporis et animi vigorem, curam et originem animi an corporis vicio quo sit
nata egritudo: aut extrincecis venerit .s. potu vel cibo an coreptela aeris, si an ex
inmutate(?) cibi et potus, sanguinis est habundancia, si de etate fuerit, fellis nigri, si
senex est, fleuma illa nociva. Nihilominus et de temporibus intelligimus: si vero verno
tempore sanguis, si estate fel rufu[m], si autumpnus fel nigrum, si yemps fleuma. Si an
expascenda carne porcina pastus sit qui egrotat, fel rufum ex eo habundare scito. Si
vero ex bubula que dissimilia sunt nigri fellis causam scito. Si pulsus autem currerit,
mortem indicat. Si ventrem occuruat poentrem non fecerit infrigidasse in eo sanguis
ostenditur mortem. Si venter defugit et minuerit(?), mortem significat. Dentila
frigescunt et subtrahunt si est moriturus. Stercus viscosum, nigrum, viride vel fetidum,
et discenteria, si a nigro felle incoaverit,[366] et [nigri] egestiones, si a discenteria habito,
ut intestinorum carnes egerantur, mortale.[367] Egestiones nigre et quasi sanguis sponte
venien[te]s in omni febre et sine febre pessimum est et quanto colores plures sunt
tanto maius malum.[368] Quibus incipientibus si fel nigrum [aut sursum aut] deorsum
exierit[369] in omnibus egritudinibus mortale.[370] Ventositas cum sonitu laudabilis est.[371]
Sanguis [sursum] quidem qualiscumque fuerit [malum], deorsum bonum est – et si
sursum est, malum.[372] Si menuenda subtrahunt, mortalis [est]. Si urina aquosa, fetens,
nigra vel lutosa, mortalis et in utroque sexu nigra et pessima et mortifera.[373] Si pedes
non exstenti ut in spasmo, bonum est,[374] sed si pedes torti, rigidi, tepedi et nudi sive
frigescunt, malum. Et si pedes inordinate iactaveri[n]t, malum est. Repente hora stare,
malum est. Si aliquod malum signum ex iam supradictis visum fuerit, mortis periculum
iudicabis.

[113] *Experiment de mort ou vie: triblez ouel peis de chanilé e de mente damache, de*
cel aprés oinez le front de l'un oireile deke l'autre e le pastel liez sur le chef. Si tost aprés dort,
vivera, si non, morra. Et cestes mesmes profit[e] a ces qi ne puissent dormier. Item prufe de
mort ou vie:[375] *Oinez le plante destre du pié de lard tout del chef en autre. Puis le gettez al*
chen; si le manjut e ne vomit, si garra; si il vomit, morra. Item: metés la racine de orcie
ounce[376] *[en] une viole de veire e le malad si pise sur e coverez le souz la coverteure deke le*
seir. La nuit seit mis hors en une privé liu e si la urine al matin seit blanche, si morra; si verd,
vivera. Item: fetes une [. . .] de rue e liz e rose e reez le chef al malad e surmettez le pastel,

---

366 See *Aphorism*. II,22 (f.153rb).
367 See *Aphorism*. Lib. IV, c.24 (f.67ra) 'Dissinteria si a felle nigro inceperit, mortale . . .';
   [c.26](f.68ra) 'Nigre egestiones, si a dissinteria habito, ut intestinorum carnes egerantur, mortale'.
368 *Aphorism*. Lib.IV, c.xxi (f.66r) '. . . et quantumcumque fuerint colores plures, magis malum. Cum
   pharmaco vero melius et quanto plures fuerint colores, non malum'.
369 MS *exierunt*.
370 *Aphorism*. Lib.IV, c.22 (f.68va).
371 *Prognostica* II,24.
372 *Aphorism*. Lib.IV, c.25 (f.67va).
373 *Prognostica* II,32 (f.154vb).
374 *Prognostica* I,16 (f.145vb).
375 See *Pop. Med.*, p.293, no.233.
376 Correct *oculescunce* or read *ortie [e[[r]ounce*?

que si il esternue adprés les .vii. hures del jour, garra; si [non], morra. Item: quant il seine,
un poi del sanc mettez en un hanap plein de ewe: s'il descent enter al fonz del hanap, donke
ne mourra pas deinz le an e s'il departe e apert desus sicum goute d'oile, donke est perillouse.
Item ditez devant le lit(e) le malad quant il dort: 'Ancho eizi pancozerse' e s'il se leve quant
en veile, il vivera, si non, morra. Item: beve serpentinam triblé, que s'il le vomit, morra.
Item: mettez la urine al malad en un veisel e une femme que leite un enfant mad(e)le si
degoute leit de sa mamele sur. Si le leit flote desur la urine, morra hast[e]ment, mes si se
medele od l'estale, garra, que si est femme que madle seit norice de femme[377] *le face cum*
avant est dit. Item: herbe benete que ad le foile de raiz, savour de coste, issi charmez: 'Ge
vous conjur, par le tresgrant noun Deus toutpuissant que si icest hom doit vivere, mostrez le
moi' e ditez od ce .iii. Pater Nosters. Issi [f.21r] fetes .iii. jours. Pus[378] *si le foués sur de une*
trible feree e lavez en ewe nete. S'il deit viver, rouges serront les racines, si noun, toutes
seront pales.

[114]   Item:[379] *si le malades ad dolour [u] enfleure en la face sanc tus e s'il tient sa main*
senestre ad son piz e s'il frotet assudualment son nes, ad le vint e treszime jour morra. Uncore
si le malades frenetich – et ce est estordeisum[380] *del chef e derverie*[381] *– ad ambodeus gulinz*
rouges od sorre-enflure e neint ne ad le ventre soluble, le nefim[e] jour mora. Iceste enfirmité
commencet ad aveir[382] *freides suors e les oreiles freides e les dentz freides. Si les veines qui*
sont en col sunt estenduz e en travail e seiez[383] *cume surdes e eiez*[384] *brenetes /alias burbices?/,*
ce est malant petiz, sur les veines e une brenete seit entre les autres blanche e le infirme[385]
desiret chalour e bain chaud, el cinquantisme jour mourra. Iceste enfirmité vent ad ly qi totes
hours desiret chaut bain. Uncore cil qi ad mal oi l'uvet, si une brenete apert desouz la lengue
e il eit frischons en icel mal e une neire[386] *enfleur se apert petite el polce del piez, el seme jour*
murra. Uncore en fevre ague s'il ad une brenete oi ventril e el sinistre piz en la plante neient
haute mes vive e enfle de neir colour e nul talent n'eit(e) de nule rien ne [. . .] en la urine,
le secund jour mourra.[387] *Uncore si il ad mal en le poumoun o si sanc ly decurt de polce o si*
une bubette sang[u]ien en ist o s'il esternuet sovent o a tart, el seme jour murra. Uncore si
le feie dolet ad ascun e si el col en la grosse junte[388] *deus bubetes aperent de blaunche colour*

---

377 The incoherence of the text is due to material which has dropped out.

378 MS *pur*.

379 Here begins a translation of part of Ps.-Hippocrates, *Capsula eburnea*, MS Oxford,Bodl. Libr. e
mus. 219 ff.81v–83r (Explicit liber Ypocratis qui inventus fuit in sepulcro eius sub capite illius
in pixide eburnea') starting at f.82v line 3. I have also consulted the text in MS Oxford, Balliol
College 231 (s.xiii) ff.214va–215va. See also K. Sudhoff, "Die pseudohippokratische Krankheitsprognostik nach dem Auftreten von Haut Anschlägen, 'Secreta Hippocratis' oder 'Capsula
eburnea' benannt", *Archiv für Geschichte der Medizin* 9 (1916), 79–116.

380 MS *etrodeisum*.

381 MS *s'uerie*.

382 MS *ueuez*.

383 For *seit* referring to the patient.

384 See note 332 above.

385 MS *la infirmité*.

386 *neire* is a misreading of *magna* as *nigra*, the Latin having 'tumor magnus vel parvus'.

387 MS Balliol Coll. 231 f.214vb has 'Item in febre acuta et si in stomacho doluerit et si in sinistro
pede pustellam habuerit in planta non altam, sed equalem teterimo colore tumentem, et nullum
desiderium habuerit, .xx. die morietur'.

388 MS *justes*. MS. e mus. 219 has 'in gutturis iuncture'. Cf. Balliol Coll. 231 f.214vb 'In collo, hoc
est in gutture due pabule [= papule] vel .iiii. in juncte nate fuerint albi coloris'.

e si grant manjue surde el polce del destre piez o si en alet a tart o il piset sanc, el seme jour murra. Uncore qui unt mal al feie[389] unt cest signe – si treis bubettes neischent sur le umblil a destre e a senistre, le une blaunche, le autre aukes blew, la tierce aukes vermeile, el jour mesmes murat. Uncore si dolour neist en tot le corps[390] e si el surcil neist encement cum un noiz d'autretiel colour e ert le surcel pesant, al quart jour murrat. Uncore: si le esplein[391] li deut e si blaunces bubettes neiscent en la senistre main e si sanc decurt de par le nes escumous,[392] le dosime jour murat. Uncore scil qi ad longke curson o si ad autre enfirmetez se adjoste semblant[393] e si bubetes se aperen[t] en la senestre quische si grant cum gemme blanche e s'il estalez p[l]us ke il ne soleit, el ventime jour murat. Uncore si dolour neist en la veissie e si il pise ad grant grevance, si[394] ad senestre part desus le essele le [char] li enfle[395] ensement cum un poume e s'il veit en son dormant[396] cum pumes cheir e tener en sa main, le quinz[i]me jour murat. Uncore si le fundement li ist fors o dult[397] o si les rein(e)s si dulent o si il ad dolour el membre[398] o si devent bluef d'esparnement,[399] el quint jour mourat. Unco(quo)re s'il estaletz ad peine e sa urine est trouble e si bubetes aperent en la senestre oirele en manere de lentille e s'il froit sovent ses oiles,[400] el seme jour moura. Unquore cil qi rent sanc par le fundement e ad le fi seinant, si neires pubetes aperent en la senistre plante de pié, el vintime jour murat. Uncore sil qi vomisent sanc, si une bebete si grant cum un grein d'orge li neist el goi(s)terin e li rent mult salive, el vintime jour murat. Unquore s'il ad pubettes en sa plaie[401] o festre o kancre, o ascune manere de postune eit [o] de clou, o si multes petites bubettes en guise de lentille[s] blanches neischent o en ascun dé nerz e sur la serviz del chef e sur la umblil o sur le quer o sur la veine que cort par la espeine e si que les bubetes seient dolere[u]s e s'il covet ascun douce chose, el xii jour morat.

[115] *Item: en ceste guise esprovez la vie de ceus qi unt el cors le pleu[r]eisin, ce est mal al pomun: ce q'il escopent mettez sur les charbons, si le [f.21v] esrakeure puit, veirement morra[402] de cel mal. Item de mesme le mal: en un vesschel de tere mettez ewe, pus si le fetes enz escopez, si le escopurez noest, tot morra e si ele [v]a a fon dreit, si vivera. En quele enfirmité que li home seit, s'il suet de la peitrine en amunt, par iii jours li fetes enplastre, e s'il (ne) ceset de suer, si[403] poez desesperer.[404] Mes s'il suet tretot, donc ne li fetes null*

---

389 Latin 'colerici'.
390 Latin 'in corde'.
391 MS *le espeine*.
392 MS e mus. 219 has 'sanguis spissus', Balliol Coll. 231 'sanguis spumosus'.
393 MS Balliol Coll. 231 has 'vel passio alia similis addita fuerit'.
394 MS *sul*.
395 MS *lient*. Latin 'sub titillo caro tumuerit / stupuerit'.
396 MS *demant*.
397 Latin 'et non doluerit'.
398 Latin 'venter'.
399 MS *desparnenement*. Latin 'et si livor subtus factus fuerit in ipso morbo et si ova desideraverit fortiter'.
400 Latin 'fricat oculum'.
401 MS Balliol Coll. 231 has 'Vulnera si pustulas habuerint', whilst MS e mus. 219 has 'Si in vulva mulieris . . .'.
402 MS *mort*.
403 MS *siuz*.
404 Latin 'si non sudaverit, despera de eo'.

enplastre, ke ki unkes sei espamet, seit homme seit femme, si fevre li survent, si[405] *garist del pasmer e s'il ad fevre e il pamet, si est gariz de la fevere.*[406]

[116][407] *Si vous veiez le malade sovent turner sei ad le pareie, de cellui est dotaunce e s'il ad le(s) nes agudz o atenuetz e si les oils sont enfossez e les temples soient abeischés e les levres escorcez e les oreiles freides e reversees contre mont, ce est signum de morte. Item de eodem: Cum vous verrez le malade dormier, s'il ad oilz vertz*[408] *e la bouche overte, demandez s'il ad cursum o si ce fust sa custume endementers q'il fust sein, e s'il est issi, donke n'est une tel doutaunce, mes si il n'ad eu custume e si le senestre oil li remet e pluret, el tierce jour murat. Si le malades resaluez le meiz*[409] *e s'il mette ses meins ad son cap e s'il trahit a ses piés, de cel maladie eschapera bien. Et s'il se turnet qu'il remlt (sic) ad veer la nue, denz les .xxx. hours (deus) aprés morat. Si le malades turnet son chef ad piez de son lit e il perdet le dormier e sovent entent vers le eus de la meison, signum de morte. Si le malades fait desouz sei sa bosoine e s'il ad la ventre freid e s'il ne covet nulle liqu[i]de*[410] *e s'il ad freid suor, el nefim[e] jour morat. Si li ydropik pert sa seif e s'il ad talent de feves, el sinquantisme jour murat. Uncore: si en fevre ague seit la colour del malad vert neir o pal o plumbi[n] e tote la face horrible e les palpebrez blefs e les levres blefs, les oils nent establez et tremblans e seient enons(?), signefie peril de mort. S'il fremit ad deinz od freneseie cum devez la mort tost ensuit qi s'il est esechi? e eit(e) verte colour o cendren o blef, demusture la mort ad vener. S'il get sa mein e detreit a reume sza e la ce qui est entur li, mura. Si se aleine ist freid, mort sera. Suor ad chef e ad la cervice, mort sera. Mes s'il sue de doucz suor ad tot le cors, ce est bon signe. En icete maladie de fevre augue soileit deinz set jours sanc seiner del nes, ce est bon signe. Si les ongles dedeinz seient entremedlez de blef e de vert, signefie mort. Fente de malad si seit ventus, neir o vert o pulent*[411] *signefie mort. Item: s'il vomit vert cum jus de poree o neir o plumben, signefie mort. Item: pernez le jour quant le mal li prit e contez les letres de cel jour e lé letres del noun del malad e de l'age de la lune quant il comenc(er)a a(l)maladier; totes cestes letres roingés ensemble, departiés les issi disant par cescun lere 'Christus, Deus, homo'. Si la fin de les letres vent in 'Christo', il vivera, si in 'Deo', il est en aventure, si en 'home', il mora.*

[PERILOUS DAYS][412]

[117] *Item: qi chet en maladie le premer jour de quel meis q'il seit de l'an le tierce jour suiant fet a douter, que s'il pase, il eschapera desque le trentime jour; ki le secound jour, (ad) le .xiiii. jour est douté – s'il passe, longes eschapera ia ce qi languissant [seit]; et ki le .iii.*

---

[405] MS *sil.*

[406] Latin has 'Si vir qualescumque febres habuerit et spasmum non habuerit, m. subito'. MS Balliol Coll. 231 has 'Item si febres qualiscumque vir si spasmum habuit, mortem significat. Qui febrem habet et spasmum et post febris ei supervenerit, spasmum solvit et sanus efficitur. Item si plagam (?) habuit et spasmus non fuerit, mortem non significat'. Cf. *Aphorism.* Bk 2, c.26 'Febrem in spasmo melius est fieri quam spasmum in febre'.

[407] The source now changes to the 'Prognostica' attributed to Galen in the *Articella* of 1523.

[408] Latin 'concavos'.

[409] Latin has 'medicum'.

[410] Latin 'cibum'.

[411] MS *pubent.*

[412] The following is a translation of the text found in MS Oxford, Bodl. Lib. e mus. 219 f.83v under the heading 'Pronostica .G. dierum timendorum in incepcione omnium egritudinorum'. For

jour, en hast sera delivre sanz moleste. Et qui le .iiii., desque .xviii. jour serra malades, mes il eschapera; ki li quint jour, ja ce qui fort seit maladie, il eschapera; e qui le sime jour, ja ce q'il semble q'il amendie, nepurcant le .v. jour de l'autre meis murra; ki le setime, sanz moleste serra delivre; et qi la uitisme, moura s'il ne seit sein dek[e] al quinzime jour; ki la noefime, ja ce ki ad grant molest, il eschapera; ki le xme jour, sanz fail murra; ki la xie jour, en hast serra delivre; ki la xiie, s'il ne seit delivre dienz .xxix. jours, mura; ki le .xiii., malad serra desque .xxix. jour, qi si il les pasce, eschapera; ke le .xiiii. jour, s'il denz .xix. jours ne moert, eschapera; ki le .xvi. jour, ja ce qu'il [f.22r] par .xxviii. eit moleste, il eschapera; ki la .xvii., il eschapera desque xxviii jours; ki la .xviii. jour, sodeinement sanera; qi le .xix. jour, autresi eschapera; ki le .xx., eschapera cel meis, mes autre mura; ki le .xxi., si peril de moert ne encorge, denz les .x. jours de l'autre meis sera a delivre; ki le .xxii., ja ce que .x. jours fort [suffre], il eschapera; ki le .xxiii., ja ce ad moleste, demure, ad le meis serra delivre; ki le .xxiiii., ja ce qi ad le .xiiii. jour amende, en la suiant meis murra; ki le .xxv., ja ce ke auke suffre, il eschapera; ki le .xxvi., ne mora pas; ki le .xxvii., ja ce q'il suffre deske le .x. jour, en [le] suant meis sanera; ki le .xxviii. jour, de mort serra manacé; qi le .xxix., a l'autre meis auke sanera; qi le .xxx., doute est si eschapera o noun ausi del .[x]xxi. jour.

ITEM DE LUNA[413]

[118] Luna prima: in lecto qui inciderit diu languescet et gravem egritudinem sustinebit tamen vivet. Luna secunda: infirmus cito convalescet. Luna tertia: eger non evadet. Luna quarta: infirmus cito morietur. Luna quinta: infirmus cito periclitabit aut surget. Luna sixta: infirmus morietur. Luna septima: infirmus si medicatus fuerit surget. Luna octava: infirmus languebit sed evadet. Luna nona: infirmus diu egrotabit, sed evadet. Luna decima: infirmus non diu laborabit nec peraclitabit. Luna undecima: infirmus periclitabit. Luna duodecima: infirmus diu languebit, sed surget. Luna XIII: infirmus longo cubabit tempore. Luna XIV: infirmus laborabit sed surget. Luna XV: infirmus periclitabit. Luna XVI: infirmus diu languebit et vix evadet. Luna XVII: infirmus vix evadet. Luna XVIII: infirmus longo tempore iacebit sed evadet. Luna XIX: infirmus per medicinam sanabitur. Luna XX: infirmus cito sanus surget. Luna XXI: infirmus diu languebit. Luna XXII: infirmus angustiam pacietur. Luna XXIII: angustiam pacietur. Luna XXIV: infirmus diu languebit et morietur. Luna XXV:

Anglo-Norman fragments on the subject see P. Meyer in *Jahrbuch für romanische und englische Literatur* 7 (1886), 47–51 and *Bulletin de la Société des anciens textes français* 4 (1883), 93–5; O. Södergård, "Notes sur les jours périlleux", *Neuphilologische Mitteilungen* 55 (1954), 267–71. For English examples see M. Förster, "Die altenglische Verzeichnisse von Glücks – und Unglückstagen", in K. Malone and M.B. Ruud (eds.), *Studies in English Philology, A Miscellany in Honor of Frederick Klaeber* (Minneapolis, 1929), 258–77. See also G. Keil, "Die verworfenen Tage", *Sudhoffs Archiv* 41 (1957), 27–58 and Ch. Weissner, "Mittelalterliche Wochentags-Krankheitsprognosen. Eine Gattung laienastrologisch-iatromathematischer Fachprosa", in G. Keil (ed.), *'gelêrter der arzenîe, ouch apotêker'. Festschrift für Willem F. Daems*, Würzburger medizinhistorische Forschungen 24 (Pattensen / Hannover, 1982), pp.667–74. Compare the texts, all pre-1100, in Wickersheimer, *Les manuscrits latins de médecine*, pp.31,33,40,51–2,53,56(verse), 57–8,64–5, 139–40 (verse),151 (verse), 155–6 (prose and verse), 158 and cf. Beccaria, Index sub *Giorni egiziaci*.

413 For similar texts see Wickersheimer, *Manuscrits latins de médecine*, pp. 53–4,57,74,110.

infirmus sustinebit maximam injuriam et languebit usque ad mortem. Luna XXVI: infirmus langu[ebit] et convalescet. Luna XXVII: infirmus non diu langu[ebit], sed tristabitur et surget. Luna XXVIII: infirmus vel aliquis languebit et sur[get] sed sine multum(?) iacebit et morietur. Luna XXIX: infirmus morietur. Luna XXX: infirmus unquam sanus erit. *Item: frotez le front al malad de pain d'orge que si le chen nel vout manger après il moura.*

[PERILOUS DAYS]

[119] *Les meistres jadiz purvirent de males jors qi son[t] en le an ki [en] enfermeté charra ne resordra. Janver: les primer jour, .ii., .iii., .v., le .x., le .xv., le .xix. Feverer: le .xvi., le .xviii. Marcz: le .xiii., le .xv., le .xvii. Averil: .vi., .xi. Maii: .viii., .ix., .xv., .xvi. June: le .vii. Julie: .xv., .xx. Aust: .xix., .xx. September: .xv., .xvii. Ottober: le .vi. November: .xv., .xx. December: le .vi., .vii. e .xv. Le nombre de jours .xxxii.*

URINES[414]

[120] Urina est colamentum sanguinis et aliorum humorum de actionibus nature natum. Oportet considerare quot colores, quot egritudines, quot regiones sunt in urina. Tres sunt regiones, tamen et novemdecem colores. Qualis sueri ventus, talem solicitat humorem et qualis suere morbus talem movet urinam. Sanguis dominatur in vehere et sarcoden facit urinam. Colera dominatur in estate et rubeam facit urinam. Malencolia, que est colera nigra, dominatur in autumpno et nigram facit urinam. Fleuma dominatur in hieme et facit urinam pinguem et albam.

[121] Urina rubea, si dolor est in renibus, periculum significat. Urina in acutis febribus nigra, si modicus sudor venerit et toracem siccum habuerit, periculum significat. Urina in acutis febribus fellea et nigra, alba, spumosa, si sanguis de naribus fluxerit mortem significat. Urina in febribus acutis si in summo nataverit ut oleum,[f.22v] frenesim et mortem [significat]. Urina aquatica tenuis in febre periculum significat. Urina rubea et nebulosa vel cum spuma dolores cessare dicit. Urina sanguinea et nimis tenuis dolores venturos predicit. Urina intemperata ac parva cum fuerit mortem significat. Urina temperata aut supra protectionem longi temporis in morbo significat. Urina rufa et spissa cum plurima egesta solucionem ventris et medelam sanitatis promittit. Urina sangu[in]ea mortifera est. Urina nigra et turbulenta et veluti capillos aut rasuras aliquas habens mortem significat. Si animi egritud[o] est .i. ex tristitia aut ex cupiditate, urina eorum rufior invenitur quam in ceteris

---

414 See the works of Theophilus (Articella, 1523); Hippocrates; Isaac Judeus; Walter of Aguilon; Richard of Salerno; Alexander – the last four in MS Oxford, Bodleian Library, e mus. 219. See also Renzi, *Coll. Sal.* 3, pp.2–51 ('Regule urinarum magistri Mauri') and 4, pp.409–12 ('Regule urinarum secundum Johannem Platearium') and 506–12 ('De urinis secundum Mattheum de Archiepiscopo'); K. Wentzlau, 'Frühmittelalterliche und salernitanische Harntraktate', diss. Leipzig, 1923. An important study is G. Keil, *Die urognostische Praxis in vor- und frühsalernitanischer Zeit* (Freiburg, 1970).

effemeribus febribus. Item qui ex tristiciis et vigiliis atque cogitacionibus et iracundia; urina in hiis crocea est, venit extra consuetudinem ex colerico cum morsu ventris exiens.

[122][415] *Homme sera senz si sa urine seit blaunche le matin e devant manger rouge e aprés manger blanche. Urine grase e trouble cum pisace de adyner signifie dolour del [chef] primes a vener. Urine savereuse ad le .vii. jour terminé, si ad le seconde jour est rouge e ad le quart blanche, signifie garison. Urine [que] est grasse cum celle qui est de(s) multes humors signifie ad venir[416] la fevre quartaine. Urine sanclente[417] signifie [la vessie] estre blescé de ascune pureture dedenz. Urine cartive e blaunche e cum fut veluye signifie le mal dé reinz. Urine poudrouse signifie la vessie estre blescee. Urine for mise od perettes de sanc signifie grant mal denz le corps e nomément denz la veisseie. Urine qui chet par gotettes e si nouye pardesus sicum ampoiles signifie longe enfirmité. Urine que nouye desouz[418] une grasse rouele signifie auke longe enfirmité.[419]*

[PS.- HIPPOCRATES, DE URINIS][420]

[123] *Par.iii. maners puet home conuistre urines qi signefient enfirmité, ce est par une cerne que apert en la urine e par le fundriaile e par la sustance, ce est par le cors de l'urine.[421] Par le cerne est sig[nifié] la dolour del chef, quar s'il est en le soumet de l'urinal e s'il seit liz[422] e amples e hautz, donk signifie un vent que est en le chef. Icest vent tent totes houres vers [a]mount e trouble le cervele e de ce vent le grant dolour del chef. Mes si le(s) cerenes est tenues e plains, donc signifi[e] un petit vent que trouble le chef. Issi puiet hom conustre la enfirmité del chef par tiele cerne. Oncore puet saver en quel partie del chef est li dolours, quar li chef (est) ad .iiii. parties. Devant en la front converset le sanc. En la destre partie regne coilour rouge par la feie que est de cel part, en la senestre part converset la malancolie par la esplen qi est de cel part; detriés en la hatrel dominez li fleums. Pur ceo [que] li cernes [est] rouges sachez q'il signifie [que] la dolour del chef [est] devant; s'il est chaunes, sachez que li dolours est devers la destre; s'il est blefs o neirs, li dolours est ad senestre; s'il est blankes, li dolour est detriés.*

[124] *Ore ve(n)um de[l] cors de l'urine, c'est de la sustaunce. Si le urine est espisse e trouble[423] cum estal de kaval, ce signefie dolour del chef que vent de la fumee qui munte contremont del ventril. Par la fundril de l'urine q'est ad fonz repuit hom conustre la infirmité. Ce apele home la nuie pur ceo qi ad la fie(r) apert desus. Ceste nue s'il apert(e) desus ad le*

---

415   This pasage is found in the 'Lettre d'Hippocrate'; see *Pop. Med.*, p.109.
416   MS *advenit*.
417   MS *sanc lette*.
418   corr. *desure*.
419   The rest of the section on urines from the 'Lettre d'Hippocrate' follows after Hippocrates' treatise; see section [133] below.
420   I have used the text in MS Bodl. Lib. e mus. 219 ff.127r–29r.
421   MS e mus. 219 f.127r 'Triplici modo possumus cognoscere urinas infirmitates significantes: primo, per circulum qui apparet in summitate urine; per substantiam .i. per corpus urine; et per residentiam .i. per ypostasim vel sedimen.'
422   'latus'.
423   MS *trible*.

sumet de l'orinal signifie le dolour del c(e)hef estre de ventosité. Ore veum de l'urine que signefie la dolour del peitrine. Si le urine est trouble e oscure de la meité en amunt e de la meité en aval clere, donk signefie le dolour del piez qi vent de la fumé del ventril, li queus, cum il ne puet passer outre desque ad le chef, remonte al neke e va turneant e de ce si [. . .] si le dolours de la peitrine. Uncore si la meité de l'urine en amunt est rrouge e trouble ensement cum estal de roncin, dunke signefie pleu[r]eisin, ce est un clou devers destre de la poitrine e en ce posum agarder plusours choses, kar si le(s) clous est illuk, si faut le aleine e si ad touse e pert talent de maunger. Uncore en autre [f.23r] manere puet homme conustre dolour del piez en urine. Si hom veit durable escume desus, donk li deut la peitrine. E si vous veez vostre urine que seit jaune o ke el trahit ad jaune e que seit auke trouble, donc puet hom saver q'il ad pleu[r]eisin, ce est le mal del flanc en la senestre part del piez.[424] E par le rouge colour[425] pur ce ke (que) ele habonde plus en la senestre parte e le sanc ad destre, par tiel indice connut hom tiel mal par tiel urine e de cel pleu[r]eisin puit hom entendre que le flanc li dut e le chef e que les natureles espritz li faut, c'est le aline.

[125] Si le urine est rouge e espesse, donk signifie sinoce,[426] ce est un fevre que totdiz tent ouelment. E pur [ce] que il est rouge signefie chalour e pur ce q'il est trouble[427] signefie humours entremedelés.[428] Si vostre [urine rouge e espisse] est[429] blanch e clere, si que nul enfirmité ne seit devant terminé, donke signefie frenesye qui vendrat, ce est un esturdeisoun e (del) sufre del chef. Pur ce que tiel urine est blaunche signefie grand freidur. Si vostre urine est changé en blanche e en espisse, donk signefie litargie, ce est obliaunce, quar ce est une enfirmité que tout ad home sa memorie e tot se obliet e ce est pur ce qu'il est mult grevé e chargé de freid humor e espisse. Si vostre urine devent rouge e clere, ce signefie fevre terciene; pur ce q'il est rouge signefie chalour, pur ce q'il est clere signefie secheté. Si vous veiez vostre urine de la meité [amont blef et] contreval rouge, poez saver q'il resverat, car les humours sont troubles e sunt en une fumee que munte sus en la cervel e si le trouble, e de ce vent resverie, ce est cum la maladie susdit,[430] si folie non. Icele urine qi est aukes rouges e ardant par semblant e tenue signefie une fevre que ad a noun causon, ce est une fevre continuele que homme appelle 'gist' e de cel poez apersever qar il unt le bouche chaude, la lang[e] neire e grant sif e grand ardour e pur ce un grant chalur, qar ce vent de colour rouge, la neirtit de la lang[e] vent de grant sif. Si vostre urine est desouz espés e desus clere (e) cel urine signefie habundance e plenté de fleume que toutes houres descent vers val e signefie q'il ad enfirmité en parties de cors que sont vers val. Si vous veiez vostre urine rouge e clere cum piement, signefie grand chalour estre en le feie q'est en la destre part e par cel chalour est malveis e corumpuz. Si vostre urine est blew e aukes trahit ad blavor e seit clere o verte e clere, ce signefie dolour de l'esplen. Bleve [est] e [verte] pur la malencolie que ad son rescet en le esplen.

[126] Urine petit e pale auke trahit ad blanchor,[431] ce signefie grand freidour. Urine espisse e trouble e rouge signefie discenterie, c'est une enfirmité que li home cort hors totes

---

424 The Latin adds 'cum dolore cordis et anelitus gravitate'.
425 Latin has 'glaucus' (= 'jaune' in our text). The reference is to black bile ('colera nigra') being found in greater quantities in the left side, whilst the right side is home to 'sanguis et colera'.
426 MS sinepe with 'o' written over the second syllable and 'c' over the final letter.
427 Latin has 'spissa'.
428 MS funt m.
429 Latin 'deveniat'.
430 MS suedit.
431 Latin has 'livens'.

hours, une manere est de meneison, mes que ad assiduale [. . .][432] *La premere cursun ad a noun diarrié de cole rouge; la secunde discenterie que vent de sanc; la tierce lienterie, que est de cole neire que meine homme ad le mort. Urine que vent petite e est neire en fevre augue est mortel. Fevre augues [est] que vivement tent totes houres. Urine neire en fevre quart[eine] signefie deliverance de la fevre. Si la urine de homme seit neire*[433] *e il refuse q'il n'eit talent de maunger ne bevre, signefie la mort. Uncore: si home ad fevre e il trahit se aleine a(l) peine e li piez li su[e]t, [e] si le (vostre) urine est neire, signefie mort. Uncore: la urine neire est mortels en totes enfirmités fors en fevre quarteine e en femme que ad perdu les flours e en seus ki unt dolour en l'esplen e en celes que ont dolour en le penil. Urine q'est verte e grasse, ce est espisse, signefie arson de cole. S'il est od legere fevre, donk est il od defisement del cors. S'il(e) est od ague fevre, donc signefie esturdeison e resverie.*[434]

[127] *Les ypostases, ces sunt les nues de la urine. Si les esgarde homme en .iii. maners: o solum le liu en quel est, o sulum le colour, o sulum le temps en quel [deit] aparestre. Sulum le liu, car o ele apert el sumet de l'urinal o en le miliu o en le fonz; solum le colour, car il est blaunche o il est neire o ele est rouge; solum la forme o ele se [f.23v] entretent o ele est departie o ele est ru[n]die o de autre manere. Sulum le tens le esgardet hom car o ele (est) apert el commencement de l'infirmeté o en le jour q'il deit terminer o en autre tens. Si li ypostasie*[435] *seit blaunche e nepurquant seit amunt cume nue, signefie que la nature ad commencement de quire la matire de l'urine. Si la [y]postasie, ce est la nue, est en milieu, signefie que la nature ad quit la meité de urine. S'il est en le fonz, mustret que la nature ad quit tout la materie de l'urine maimement*[436] *si il est blaunche e seit plei[n]e e enterine [o] el commencement*[437] *de l'enfirmeté o en le jour terminable. Nepurquant si*[438] *ele n'est [en] un chescun houre ne en un manere, signefie [que] la nature commence ad quire la urine, mes nepurquant defant sei pur agyeitz de l'enfermeté, e maimement si sel nue [est] el sumet de l'urine, e si est rusette o del tout rouge o eit colour d'or, donc signefie agussement e asperté de l'infermeté. Si cel nue est ensement cum grosse ferine, donc signefie longe infirmeté. Si ele est neire, cel nue si signefie esturdeison e resverie. Nue neire en fevre que [est] entrelesch[é]*[439] *signefie fevre quarteine ad vener e nue ghaune, o que ad colour d'or signefie grand chalour e felnesse enfirmité. Nue rouge pur matire sanguine e quaillé, ce est humor de sanc espessé, signefie longe enfermeté e nepurquant n'e[st] mortel. Nue bleue signefie grand freidour e la colour de homme cum de mort.*[440] *La neire nue est tot la peure de totes e mesmement signefie mort car sempre signefie grant arson o grand freidour. Nepurcant deseverance ad entre eles, car cel que signefie chalour primes est en vert o tele cum soufre,*[441] *enprés devent neire. Cele que*

---

432 There is nothing to fill the gap in the Latin. MS e mus. 219 then has 'Nota: Tres sunt genera fluxuum . . .'

433 The Latin at this point has 'Si quis multum sudat et non appetit manducare neque bibere et urina sit nigra, mortem significat'.

434 In place of this and the preceding sentence the Latin has 'Si sit cum levi febre, significat frenesim venientem'.

435 MS *apostasie*.

436 MS *maunt*.

437 MS repeats 'el commencement'.

438 MS *si le est ele*.

439 Latin 'interpolata'.

440 Latin 'et virtutis mortificationem'.

441 After 'livida' there is a lacuna in MS e mus. 219 which is marked in red with the words 'Deficit hic'.

signefie freidour primes est bleue o tele cum plum, pus si est neire. Nue que est cum sanc o cum purreture signefie durable enfermeté. Nue que semble ad soufre signefie enfermeté de la veschie. Nue que est plentive e rouge si que le cors de l'urine seit cler ad jour del terminer signefie que la fevre amenuset e s'en vet. Nue qu'est cum bren est mal char, ce signefie que les veines sunt escorcez e sa vessie e ben puet homme veer de quel humor dé .iiii. ce vent, quar el est blanche [d]e flumme, rouse de col[e] rouge, e neire de cole neire, ce est de malencolie, o de sanc qu'est ars.

[128] *Si gravel i pert estre en le fonz de l'urine, signefie aver peres en la vessie o en les reinz. Si en le fonz de l'urinal i pert estre puriture, signefie que la kanel par oud le urine passe ad ecurceme[n]s e plais. Urine encoluré de sank que semble ewe, pur ce estuet coiler le urine vers le jour cum il est quit ben e veez ad le matin ad le rai de soleil, si doit homme noter illuk .iii. choses: la colour, le liquor, ce est le cler e la [y]postasie, ce est la nue, quar en le cors de hom sunt .iiii. qualitez, ce sont .iiii. vertuz ke conjuinent e lient la nature de l'home; les .ii. dé qualitez, ce sont les chalours e freidour, donent a le urine colour; les autre .ii., ce sunt sechetez e humiditez, engrossent le urine o tenvent e [. . .] ben saige que les .ii. li donnent colour, kar le chalour fet le urine ghaune o rouge o orine, ce est ti[e]l cum or, o citrine, ce est tiel cum cendre.*⁴⁴² *La freidour la fet blanche e neire o itel cum plumb o bleve. Des autre .ii. la sechetez fet la urine clere e delietz, e humiditez, c'est la moisture, la fet espisse e grosse. Ore si ce est chose que chalours e humidit[e]z dominent e sojurnent(?) en la nature de hom, la chalour fet la urine rouge o orine, la sechetez ferra la urine clere. Si freidour e humidit[e]z dominent, la freidour ferra la urine blanche e la humidit[e]z fra la urine espesse e grosse. Si freidour, secheté e la humidité dominent, la freidour fet blanche urine, la secheté clere, la humidit[e]z espisse e grosse.*

[129] *Par ces .iiii. humors sunt les urines de diverses colours, quar si le fleumes dominet, que est freide, e humidit[e]z la urine sera blanche e espisse, de la freidur blanche, de l'humidité espisse. Si ce est sanc ke est humide e chaude, le urine ert rouge e espisse, rouge pur la chalour, espisse par le humidité. Si ce est cole rouge, que est chaude e seche, le urine ert orine, ce est de color d'or e clere, de la chalour orine, de la secheté clere. Si ce est cole neire, que est freide e seche, le urine ert blanche e clere [f.24r], blanche de la freidour e clere de la secheté. Mes nepurquant ad la feie fet blanche colour e a la feie neire, kar cum il est freide e seche fet blanche colour, cum ele est chaud e seche, donk feit neire colour. Si les humors sunt uniement medlez, (e) les colours eren[t] uniez, mes si elles ne sunt mie uniez, les colours [n'erent uniez] – sicome voz poez veer en cest ensample. Si le sanc est medelez uniement od la cole rouge, donke est rouge e delié, mes si le sanc surmuntet la cole rouge, la colour est rouge e meins delié, e la cole rouge, si elle surmuntet [le sanc], donc ert la colour ghaune e delié la liquor. Si le fleums est medlé od la cole neire, donc si la mellance est unie, la colour ert sendrine, mes si li fleumes surmuntet, la color si ert plumbine, ce est tele cum plumb. Si la cole neire surmuntet e ele seit freid e seche, donc ert la colour bleve, mes si ele est chaude e seche, si ke il seit arse, la colour ert verte. Colour blanche si acordet od deli(t)ez [liquor],*⁴⁴³ *kar la blanc[h]or signefie grand freidour e ke la nature n'ad mie commencé uncore (ce) ad quire le humor e pur ce se acorde od tenve liquor, kar plus legerement puet la nature akes teindre la colour que espessier ce ke est deliez, quar enceis commenscet la nature col[or]er la liquor que troubler e espesser. E pur ceo en home sein si le urine est blanche e mult delié, (e) ce signefie*

---

⁴⁴² A surprising error, confusing 'citrinus' and 'cinericus'.
⁴⁴³ Latin has 'Color albus concordat cum liquiditate quia albedo significat magnam frigiditatem'.

grand freidour e la defisement de la naturel chalor qi deit quere les viandes. E ce de(l)falz o
el faie o el ventrel o es autres membres. Si ce defaut el feie, donc ert la colour de la face bleve,
e par se memement les lievres [e] les surcils sunt enflés e li feie est grevus. Si la naturel chalor
defaut en ventril, le ventre ert grevus e enflé e si routet /.i. ructat/ e la viande s'en ist crue.
Si ce est pur la naturel chalour que defaut par touz les membres, donc est enflé tout le corps
e memement la face e le piez, e les quises sont febles.

[130] *En enfirmeté longe sicum est gute caive e podagre e fevre quarteine (e), icel urine,*
si est blanche e soutil, signefie mal, kar ele moustre que la materie[444] *est crue e(n) la enfirmeté*
mult durat. Icel urine, si ele apert en fevre ague, s'il ad esturdeison e resverie, memement si
ce avent ad le quart jour, donc poez la mort attendre ad le seme jour. Uncore itel urine signefie
q'il ad peres e gravele es reinz memement si les reinz li maunjent e s'il ad dolour el pennil.
Uncore itel urine denunciet ydropisie ad vener meme[me]nt si li ghaunes li apert e signefie
que tot le cors li defit. Uncore si cest urine apert en megres hom, si(l) ele duret longement,
signefie la defection e defisement dé membres. Ice veit hom par la bla[v]or de la face e par les
oilz que sont crues e seches e ad enfastisement. Urine euouse e en sein[445] *e enferm pessime*
est, fors si ele vent en fevre ague, pus que il ad aparue rouge. E ce seit el jour terminable, si
que nue apert el sumet de l'urine, ce signefie que [le] malad turne ad santé. Nepurquant nent
hastivement ne purvent. Ad la fiez avent qu'il garrit tost si la nature [seit] forte o ke seit
apostume, ce est annete de pur[e]ture sicum est clau. Urine blanche [e][446] *espesse, si ele fut*
primes delié e pus apert grosse, ce seit al jour terminable, signefie que li[447] *enfirmetez*
terminerat par aposteme. Si tiel urine apert el jour determinable, donc terminera la enfirmeté
par apostume de[s]ur les oreilz, car ce est custume de fevre penuse qu'il termine par apostume
de[s]ur les oireiles o es ditz o es ortiz. Urine blanche e grosse od fevre sueffe signefie longe
enfirmeté [. . . e que] est medelé ad ague materie coleriene e ad grosse flematiene.

[131] *Urine qu'est tres rouge, pus dit estener(?) trouble, ce signefie que la nature*
domine(nt) en la [. . .] que cum e sulum la colour e sulum la liquor e s'il avent qu'il seit
sotel, ce est clere, donc est medlé od cole rouge e icel urine signefie dolour del chef e esturdeisun.
Urine rouge e grosse que v(e)ient e ne clarie(nt) od dolour des oreiles e od surdez e od dolour
del chef si les costes li tende[n]t e dulent, signefie q'il avra la ghaunice devant le seme jour.
Urine rouge e grosse s'il vent petit en ydropiseie, la mort n[u]nciet. Urine escumuse ensement
cum vessiettes qui surdent sur ewe cum[448] *pluvie qi chet de cel e s'il ne sent nul mal el cors,*
signefie enfirmeté ad vener. Urine s'il est clere e blanche e tenve e [noue] desur ensement
cum sein e (.i. pou de fericie?) ensement cum est .i. pou desus gelee signefie ad vener enfirmité
que muet de fleume. Urine blanche e sanz nue en toz homs signefie febletés e freid del cors.

[132] *En ver, c'est cum le temps [f.24v] renovelet vers averil, donkes deit estre trestote*
urine rouge e trouble pur le sanc que dominet (donke) q'est chaud e moistes, pur ce ert le
urine rouge de la chalour e trouble de la humidité. En (c)est[é] [deit l'urine estre] rouse e clere
pur la[449] *cole russe vel rouge que donc domi[n]et, rouse pur la chalour e (e)clere pur la*
secheté. En drain vers septembre deit estre vostre urine [. . . conflates with winter] [En iver
deit vostre urine estre] blanche e sec e espesse pur la fleume que donc domi[n]et q'est freid e
humides, blanche pur la freidour, espisse pur la humiditez. Urine as enfantz deit estre rouge
e espesse pur le sanc que dominet en eles e sunt qeinses en lur [. . .] [Lat. et infirmitate

---

444 MS *maladie.*
445 MS *seim.*
446 MS *b. ce est espesse.*

447 MS *il.*
448 MS *de.*
449 MS *purra.*

gravantur in vere]. Urine ad bachilers dite estre rouse e clere pur la cole rouse que domi[n]et enz eles {sic} e sunt qeinses anz esté. Urine de home que ad seisante anz deit estre clere e blanche pur la malencolie que dominet enz iles (?) e sent qeinses en heriiiis vers septembre, blanche pur ce qu'ele est freide e clere pur ce [qu]'ile est seche. Urine ad ceus qui passent cessaunte anz e ja vont declinant qui sont queinses enz yvern, lour urine deit estre blanche e espisse pur le fleume ke dominet enz eles, blanche pur ce que li fleums est freid e espisse pur ce qu'il est humide.

[133]   *Urine neire en femme que ad perdu ces fleur(e)s signefie bien, mes en totes autres enfirmetez, meme[me]nt s'i [e]lle est ague, signefie mal e [est] sovent mortel, mes en quant e en ceus qui (v)ont dolour en l'esplen e celes que unt dolour en la penil.*[450] *Urine ad femme (raié) pur e clere cum argent en la urinal [si] ele touse e vomit e pert de manger, signefie estre enceinte. Urine ad femme blanche e puant [e] pesant signefie dolour dé reinz e la marcie*[451] *pleine d'enfermité e freid. Urine de feme que est cum escume de sanc e est clere cum ewe signefie dolour del chef e aver perdu talent de maunger e beivre par enfleure de l'estomak. Urine ad femme que ad le colour de ferine espurgee*[452] *signefie la quartaine e que ele mora deinz le .iii. jour. Urine ad feme que est pesante e de la colour de plum signefie la marice estre purrie si ele est en la urinal puante. Urine ad f[emme] si ele est enflee e que eit touz e la menesoun, s'il seit de la flor*[453] *de lin signefie qu'il ne puet estre seine. Urine de fe[mme] que ad colour d'or e est clere e pesante demustre la femme aver talent de homme. Urine de femme o de home que ad fevre ague que ad neir [y]postasim, ce est une neire colour enz ad le urinal, signefie la mort. Urine de meschine seine que unque compaigne ne ot e[st] pure e clere sanz chescun teche.*

[MISCELLANEOUS]

[134]   *Ke maladie ne vous touche(s):* Si ambulaveritis inter egrotos ne tibi pestis contingat radicem eruce in ore teneas vel tecum habeas vel *portez sur vous la racine de alne, si n'avrez mal. Ad touz medicines que vous donez e charmez que vous ditez,* dites cest: "Sanctus Lucas per meritum quod habuit apud dominum tribuat ut conferat tibi hoc medicamentum'. Quo die ovum cum oleo frixum commederis, nihil mali pacieris. *Poudre fet de pellettre est bon ad cescun maladie que nest deinz hom.* Item: tolle de radice salvatoris .i. rege herbarum .s. alna .xiii kl. ante cathedram sancti Petri et cave ne vomat in domum tuam. Altera die seca herbam in melle tribus diebus et tribus noctibus et tercia die suspendetur ad siccandum sine fumo et fac inde pulverem et benedic nomen cruci(bu)s illam et manduca vel bibe pro omnibus doloribus et pro quacumque infirmitate detenueris et, crede mihi, proficere poteris super omnes medicos. Item: si vis per totum annum sanus esse et clarius videre et lumbricos et vermes a te proicere, absinthium, atanasium ortorum, betonicam, abrotanum, rutam, ysoppum, flambam /.i. flammulam/, apium, salviam, anetum per totum mensem maii bibe jejunus. Hec

---

450   The rest of this section is completed by that portion of the treatment of urines in the 'Lettre d'Hippocrate' which had not been completed in section [122] above.
451   I.e. 'matrix', 'womb'.
452   Cf. ed. Södergård, p.10, ll.16f 'se ele a ferm espurgement et a fievre quartaine'.
453   Corr. *color.*

potio non coquatur sed cruda bibatur. Item pulvis qui ad omnes infirmitates prodest: sicca bene eb[u]llam ad solem. Quando factus est pulvis, distempera in aceto et da infirmo ante prandium bibere, deinde colloca eum et bene cooperi ita ut sudet. Ita post prandium da ei similiter bibere, sed tunc non iacebit ut ante, sed ibit quo voluerit, sic tamen ut a frigore se custodiat. [f.25r] Hoc vero .iii. diebus datum infirmo bene faciet. Pocio cui nulla similis ventrem temperat, colera nigra et rubea et flegma deponet, cephalargicis[454] oculorum caligines et omnes humores deponit pleripleu-monicis, stomaticis, calculosis et omnes egritudines viris et mulieribus emendat, recipe hec: manipulos .ii. de radicibus feniculi, apii, petrosilii, pastinace maioris, mente nigre equaliter manipulos .ii., polipodii manipulum .i., munda et coque in vino aut cervisia et utere. Item pulvis amarus ad omnem infirmitatem cordis, epatis, spleni, utrumque molliens induratum cardiacis degestionem facit cephalargicis et paraliticis utile est: recipe hec: repontici, costi ana unciam .i., petrosilini, aneti seminis, aloes, genciane, centaurie, baccarum lauri, marubii, ana uncias .iiii., absinthii, lupini ana [. . .] .v., piperis, fenugreci ana uncias .iii. Fac pulverem subtillissimum et cum vino calido mane et eunti dormitum quantum .iii. degitis capere potest accipiat mirrum unciam ad vicium pulmonis et ad malam postulam et ad omnia mala que subito adveniunt corpori humano. Item quicumque dolor est infra hominem et ad omnem malum[455] pocio ista: genciana, aristologia .s. longa, mirra, (granem?) masticis, costo, fenogreco, baccas lauri ana [. . .] .iiii., tere et fac pulverem. Adde mel quod sufficiat, utere in modum fabe cum vino calido. Item el[ec]tuarium calamenti(?) faciens ad omnia vicia pectoris et corporis, ad in[di]gestionem stomachi, ad cordis dolorem, puncturam capitis et toracis descendentem; iecuri medetur, duriciam splenis tenuat, calculum solvit, et urinam movet, menstrua provocat. Hec etiam Galienus in precio habuit: recipe hec: lufestici uncias .ii., apii .ii., zinziber .i., nepte, siceleos, ysoppi, petrosilini, timi ana uncias .iii., piper et mel uncias .iii., manduca mane et sero. Item antidotum Appollonii Laudunensis ad dispmam[456] et ortom[i]am,[457] ad tussim et ad ventrem et ad omnes fere corporis dolores, ita ut anelitum infirmi cito pausare, videas, et datur in modum avellane cum aqua calida. Recipe hec: piperis albi coclearia .x. (?), cinnam[om]i coclearia .vi., jusqueani coclearia .iiii., tibappiri, spice, cardamomi, interiomum,[458] opii, mirre ana coclearia .iii., cere coclearia .vi., mel quod sufficit. Item el[ec]tuarium validissimum et probatissimum contra omnia malificia datur. Nuces maiores mundatas dragme .vi., rute folia dragm[e] .iiii., salis drag[me] .ii., scammonia .i. et tere diligenter, adde mel ut el[ec]tuarium conficias, ex inde accipies jejunus dragmam .i. et in illo die nullum maleficium erit tibi. *Item ad toz mals del cors*: fimus leporis cum melle coctus et tanquam faba cotidie acceptus omnia interiora vicia sanat et rupturas et tante virtutis est ut statim ficum sanat. *Item pur toutz mals: pernez demi livre de rubarbe e de aumbre le peis de .v. deners e de lingno aloes .v. d[eners] pe[is], de girofré demi once, atant de noiz muget, de galingal .i. once, autant de spica nardi e tant de cetrail e tant de kanele e tant de gingevere, atant de licoris e de cardomome, de cubebes, de esula, de carvi, de coriandre, de anise, de chescun .i. once. Medlés totes cestes especes ensemble e fetes poudre, fors le ambre triblez par sei od un poi de (d)eisel e donc le mettez ad la poudre des especes e*

---

454 MS *cephalargius*.
455 MS *illam*.
456 I.e. 'dyspnoea', a respiratory complaint.
457 I.e. 'orthopnea', asthma.
458 Corr. [*coloquintide*] *interioris*?

estuez en boistes e quant le voillez user, ce est une feiz en la quinzime, pernez ad commencement del diner pleine cuilere et cetera.

[135] Item ad dolorem et tumorem corporis: ciminum et folia caulium tere cum vino e asidueble (sic). Item syruppus valens contra omnes calidos humores sic fit: accipiantur .x. ofi pleni de succo fumiterre et buli usque ad medietatem. Post[e]a appone cifatum mellis dispumati et iterum bulliatur ad medietatem sicque usui reservetur. Item ad omnes humores depellendos de pectore et capite et a lateris dolorem et spineticos:⁴⁵⁹ recipe yreos scrupulum (?) .i., piperis grana .xvii., [cum aqua] calida, bibe jejunus. Ad passionem: fac panem acerime fermentatum de pura farina siliginis et cum forti aceto utere. *Ad esquinance: fente de ouye friez en frisch siu de motoun e mettez sur le mal si chaud cum le purra suffrer al seir e matin e beve herbe sein Johan e aloine quit en cerveise o en vin, si le seine de la veine cural. Item oinement ad se: grasse char de chat e o[i]nt de teisoun, greische de ver, resine, fenigré, sauge, la gomme de ere, cire [f.25v] virgine, tot ensemble detrenchez menument, si farsez une grasse ouye e quisez al feu, ce ke decura recevez e oignez. Item destrenchez od tote la bouele un grasse chat escorché e farsez une grasse ouye et cetera ut supra e si vaut ad goute e ad pocrous.* Item passioni puerorum que est quasi tussis et dicitur anglice 'chinke vel chekhost',⁴⁶⁰ ysoppum vel serpillum in vino coctum damus ad potandum. Singultus est anglice 'yiskynge'.⁴⁶¹ Adhunc constrictorium⁴⁶² cum succo mente distemperatum et haustum sine dubio stringit. Item facit nepta cum vino. Item: ambas manus in aqua calida teneat et pedes, postea aprehende spongeam, intinge in aceto et pone super stomacum.

[136] Ad omnia vicia stomaci el[ec]tuarium et per ventrem ponere humores, recipe hec: cinamomum, gingeber, gariofile, galingal, reuponticum, piper, zodar, spic seltica, scamonia, semina feniculi, lufestici, pulegii, apii, aneti, ana scrupulum (?) .i., in pulverem redige cum melle collecta, sume post cenam aut qua hora vis. Item ad febres stomachi et omnem vicium: rotulas lilii sine pausare in una phiala vini et hoc vinum bibe valde mane. *Item femme que ad dolour del stomak beve sovent ad matin e cer centaurie. Item [pur] purger le stomak: doxas allii⁴⁶³ distempera cum lacte et bibe. Ki vodra prendre bon poison sece al feu le seir e face .ix. piles de paulin od scamonie e mettez en .ii. oefs e transglout[e]z e bevez aprés un trahit de cerveise od un poi de chaud vin.* Si quis pocione non potest liberari superius neque inferius bibat rafanum cum sale tritum et vomet et liberabitur. Si vomitum provocare volueris, una die et nocte tempera in oximelle rafanum. Cum vomere volueris, ad modum .xx. denerarum commede et postea oximel plus parum tepidum distempera et bibe. Cibus vero fit jouta(?) de malva crassa cum solatria .i. morella admixta. *Item: bevez aeuye teve e moilez une penne [d']oile e suef si trahez par ce la vomite. Ad medicine doner que est appellé timbre:⁴⁶⁴ pernez ent un coleré o .ii. o .iii. sulum que le homme est e destemperez en chaud cerveise e se beve e si haster volet la medicine, beive un hanape de chaude cerveise e si tost cum est delivre, si manjusce. Ad vomer sulum vostre pouer: fetes poudre de .x. o .xv. o .xx. o .xxx. gra[i]nes*

---

⁴⁵⁹ Corr. *spleneticos?*
⁴⁶⁰ I.e. asthma and whooping cough, see MED sub *chinke* n. a) and b) *chinke-host*.
⁴⁶¹ See MED sub *siking(e 2* 'laboured and difficult breath, shortness of breath'.
⁴⁶² MS *costrorium*.
⁴⁶³ MS *illii*.
⁴⁶⁴ Winter or Summer Savoury (Satureia).

d'espurge e od un poi de poudre de timbre e mel e en un oef mangez jun. Si quis non potest bene commedere et cum fast[id]io cibos suos sumit quod per longam perhendinacionem sepe necessaria divitum evenit quia non egritant ut solent spaciatum vadunt et ipsi tali occacione sunt egrotantes ut post cibum illico vomant hoc faciant: centauria coquatur fortiter in vino vel cervisia forti et hoc bibat mane frigidum et nocte calidum per .viii. dies vel plus si voluerit et si hac pocione toto anno uteretur, pectus purgaretur et ipsum hominem sanum teneret. Ita hanc pocionem serva ut unquam sine vino vel cervisia sit. *Ad engrouté(r): pernez ferine od la semence de ache, si donez ad beivere la racine de gletoun ad la memite. Mestre medicine: li donez gerogodioforum*[465] *e garde ses dietes.* Ad ingrotatum: excuria[466] hedum virgium et coque bene cum istis ablutum in habundancia aque et ingrotatus nihil alium commedat vel bibat ant[e]quam. Totum commeda[tur] et aqua illa bibatur et convalescet. *Ki vomit e ne puet maunger:* argentum vivum et pionium(?) cum aqua benedicta aut vino alba disserta eius dentes et mitte in os et clausum sit os ut teneat et transeat et bibe valenciam et millefolium. Item: bibe val[e]rianum et millifolium. *Item: s'il vomit e ne puet retiner viande: quisez ensemble que seit ben espesse deus parties de jus de fennoil e la tierce de mel e beive cest ceir e matin e si vaut ad l'esplen e ad le pomon e ouste glette e vomite. Item: beive millefoil od eue tef e rue e la lu[v]ische autresi prophite.* Item: febrefugiam in ovo per triduum manducet. *Item vomite de sank qu'est appellé ficoal(?): coste, mentastre, e plantein beive od eisel. Item: fetez poudre de la crote de chefre e boillez farine d'orge en ewe e de la poudre mettez un coileré e manjusce sovent, si garra.* Item: millefolium aut consolidam minorem cum vino bibat. Item: qui nec cibum nec potum [f.26r] continere possunt sed voment, biba[n]t millefolium cum pipere tritum. *Item pur vomete: sumac triblé e quit en vin vermeil beive. Item: .i. oef quit dur (e) mettez en vermeil poudre de plum ars, si le manjusce. Ki enfle sovent aprés manger: (e) manjusce .iii. roueles de aundre .s. de la racine.* Ad vomete: mente, peivre, cerfoil quit en vin bevez. Item: betonicam coclearia .iii. et mel coctum conmisce et sic fac pilotas et utere ita jejunus cum aqua calida. Item: exprime jus portulace et plantaginis equali pondere et datur pacienti. Item: facta pocione cum melle, vino et pipere, quicquid comederis ea intinge. Item: polipodium cum eius [. . .] manducet .iii. [in] die. *Item, vomer fleume: mel e eisel boilez deke la tierce partie e mettez mince de la racine de rafanum e mangez jun plus que saulte e beivez tef ewe e mettez voz dites en vostre bouche e vomerez. Item: usez poudre de lauriol od mel, ewe tiefe o od vin e averez solucion.*

[137][467] *Ad dolur del piz e ad le espurgement e contre toutz mals veiez ci medicine verreie e esprové: triblez ensemble en un fort veischel une partie de purneles dé bois e cerveise novele. Cum ele est colee, medelez ovesque, si les enfondrez en un novel pot denz terre e les coverez ben. Pus gettez terre desus e seit illuk .ix. jours e .ix. nuitz e pus si pernez un hanap petit, si donez ad le malad le seir chaud, le matin freid. Ce fetes desque il seit garré e sachez que la medicine est verei. Item ad dolur del pez: fetes ad le fonz de un novel pot un lit de maril e sur cel lit un de bure. En tele manere replenez le pot, pus ben coverez, le mettez en une chaud[e]re plein de ewe desque ad le bouche, mes que le ewe ne i entre denz le pot. Illuc quisez desque le maruil seit ben quit, pus le purez forement parmi un drap, cel colure usez pur dolour e seche touse. Item ad dolour:* rutam, merubii, abrotanum cum melle tere et per triduum

---

465 Presumably for *geralogodion*.
466 For *excoria*.
467 For the first two vernacular remedies see *LH* 86 and 82.

utere .s. jejunus. *Item pur le pis: quisez en estale cerveise la escorce de neire espine, de houz, de pomer .s. savage, beivez chaud ad seir e matin freid. Item: enplez ad la meité un pote de cerveise furmentele, pus paremplez le pot de purneles e sufouez le souz terre .ix. nuitz. Pus le colez e ce beivez ad seir chaud e a matin freid. Item: mangez jun puliol e pur aleine pulente beive le jus. Pur destresse de aleiner: fettez poudre de orpiment e le ardez sur un tuile chaud e retenez la fumé si que voz la recevez parmi un chalmel. Autre: si fetes de vif sufre. Autre: sechez orevale ad le solail e fetez poudre e mangez in totes voz viandes. Item: beivez quit en estale cerveise deke seiez garré ysopp rouge, ache, moleine, blanc maruil e rue. Item: en autele quisez ysope, sauge, moleine, maruil blanche e licoris e bevez ad seir chaud, ad matin freid. Item pur dolour del chef e des oils: pernez la estred(?) de coudre, si le depessez en voz meins, de ce demi enplez un pote e parenplez le de blanc vin, ben le arzilez covert d'unes e le sufouez .ix. jours, pus de ce bevés matin e seir. Piz estoppé pur greische: beve rue quit en eiseil. Item ad ceus que sont trop gras: beivent semence de fenoil e en .ix. jours sanera.*[468] *Item ad engroischer: manjusce semence de karson e de femiterre par .xl. jours. [Pur] purger le piz:* ista sunt que incidendo humores mundificant et vocem clarificant: abrotanus, ysoppus, marubium, pulegium, feniculus, enula, apium, liquiricium. Omnia ista in vino cocta miro modo prosunt pectori. *Item [pur] purger le piez: triblez ouelment siu de motoun, seel /.i. sal/, ail. De ce oinez le piz ad le feu deke le odour del piz eisse par les nariles. Item: adecertes boilez en oint freis de pork poudre triblé de commin, pus le mettez en ewe quit od maruil e mel, e [bevez] tef le matin e ad cocher.* Item ad pur[gandum] et ad tussim removendum: tere fortiter marrubium album, tanum, reumac[em],[469] de radice frisgonis et elne et absinthii et gletinori, de granis juniperii, ysoppum, deinde coque in vino quantum carnem bovis, tunc proice jus herbarum, pastellum, munde, cola et in eadem olla quam coxisti pocionem [f.26v] servabis. Postea destempera butirum sufficienter in sartagine vel in patella, quod si butiro caris, accipe de sanguine porci recenti et infunde in patellam et cetera ut supra. Cum in mane ipsa uti volueris, move cum cocleario et utere frigidum et fere calidum. Item purgatorium et est optimum et mirabile: destempera cum aceto acerimo mirram et aloe et nares per .iii. infundes, capud et pectus ex flegma multum purgat. *Item ad le piz: boilez e escumez demi libre de melle e i mettez une libre de rafanum triblé en un morter e quesez ensemble e i mettez .i. once de zinziber, atant de ca[. . .], e atant de licoriz e atant de anis e autant de saxefrage. Tot cest mettez en pouder ad le avandit liquor e boilez le entendement e quant est refreidi, mettez en boistez e aprés vostre viande usez. Item ad dolour del piz e touse e encontre le quer oiez ci verreies medicines eprovez: quesez en estale cerveise maruil e en bure freches e triblez ben le marruil, si en bevez chescun jour jun, vel pernez .iii. baies, si quisez ben en vin e od (en) mel, si en bevez quant vous irrez coucher.*

[138] *Touse: lavez bien vos piez ad coucher e reez ben les plantes e frottez les bien contre le fu de leit de vache e bien vous coverez ad coucher. Ce fete[s] sovent. Item ad seche touse: bevez jun triblé od vin semence de ache e de fenoil. Item ad touse e ad le piz:* apio, ruta, puleio, salvia, nepta, marubio, cenecio, feniculo, satureia, plantagine, ysoppo, ex hiis omnibus manipulos singulos tere cum sexterio uno vini, super adde onciam .i. piperis et peretri dimidiam ; fac inde pocionem et mane jejunus et sero eunte dormitum cum melle et adipe porcino calidum utere usque sanus sis. Antidotum Filoxeni ad tussim diuturnissimam et ad pectoris vicia et ad empticos et ad vicium frag[oris](?): recipe

468 MS *eceniera*.   469 For 'rumicem', sorrel or dock?

hec: aristologie longe e rotunde oncias .ii., genciane oncias .xxi., prassi oncias .xii., simitinis(?) oncias .xxviii., mel da in modum avellane cum mulsa. Item *ad touse*: duas calices aceti et unum mellis dispumati lento ingne coque donec redigatur ad calicem .i. et refrigerato in vase vitreo pone et usui reserva, et proficit colericis et de viscato slante(?)[470] laborantibus terciane febre et causon appetiva atque dissolitiva virtute adiuvat. Item ad tussim periculosam: radicem feniculi tunsas in vino, da bibere per .ix. dies. *Item ad touse de poumoun malad: medlez ensemble la semence de ache e de anis e destemperez triblé od vin e quesez que seit ben espesses. Pus mettés en boistes e matin [e] seir usez ent .iii. coilers deke seiez garri. Item ad touse: pernez flour de furement e rouge tuile, jus de maruil, leit de chevre e fetes papelotes, si i mettez licoriz e bure de mai e le manjusce sovent chaud, e si est gariz. Item ad purger le piz:* ysoppum, centauriam, neptam, radicem elne et rafani, calamentum, apium, avanciam, et si volueris organa et organum excoque cum vino vel cervisia et per pannum exprime jus (per pannum) et pone .iii. partes huius juris et quartam mellis [de]spumati et coquatur lente in igne ut aliquantulum spiscetur et coclearium mane sume. Item ad tussim et posin et cardiam; cardian idem est quod hoc cor et inde venit cardiacus (testatur cardian est cor): accipe lelifer, herba que (est) crescit in flumine, et fert quasi ollas et ipsam coque bene in albo vino vel in cervisia optima facta de frumento, post contere et iterum coque in eodem liquore ut carnem bovis et cola jus per pannum et inde utere usque melius habeas. *Tussick* ad tisicos qui purulentum ciciunt: herbe betonice dragmas .iii. et in pulverem redactas cum melle coclear .i. per triduum jejunus edat et sanabitur. *Item ad tusick: vert lin si en fetes joutz e leinz hakés la greische de geline e mettez ent le jus ou quit seit enz la geline la quele ben quite coupez e i mettez, ke si vus ne n'avez lin, fetes memes ce de commin. Pernez oefs quitez en brese e triblez od veil oingt e fetes enplastre e mettez al ventril e aprés roistiez blanc pain e movez en jus de mente e le poudre de commin e de mastic e fetes un bevere de baluc,*[471] *maruil, isoppe e licoriz. Toutez choses que piz delivre sont bones ad tesick. Gardez [f.27r] ke freisches choses seient quites en rost de ci ki il seint laxatif. Aprés qu'il serra turné ad garrisoun ses viaundes quesez en ewe.*

[139] Raucedo sine impedimentum vocis fit multis causis, sed tamen hiis principaliter: siccitate, humiditate ex defectu spiritualium virtutum. Ex siccitate dupliciter: aut meatus aeris constringente et humiditate, similiter duobus modis, aut ex humiditate in vasis et maxime in sanguine aut in flegmate a superioribus adinstillante aut ex humiditate instrumentum vocis infundente. Hec autem humiditas aut in fleumatica vel sanguinea que cum a capite descendunt et instrumentum vocis infundit et planitatem aufert loquendi et aliquando vocem omnem extingunt. *Ad enroure: ache quisez en ewe, de ce vous estuffez e s'il est de freide nature, use diadragantum calidum, si de chaude, diadragantum frigidum. Aprés face un beivre de racine de gletoner, de moleine, ysoppe, sauge, fenuil, poudre de la boce de keine, maroil blanc e licoriz, quisez en estale serveise e beivez matin freid, chaud seir. Item: quisez savine en vin e usez.* Item ad fauces et ad pulmonem curandam: de marrubio, nepte, senecionis, betonice, plantaginis, de unoqoque manipulum unum, trisicalam[i] et piperis quantum sufficit et vini sunt (?) .i. bibe cotidie mane. Item ad raucidinem: gargariza succum por[r]i. Item: fabam aut pisum coctum cum olio calido bibe. Vox, ad vocem clarificandum: .s. bisantinum pigra

---

470 Corr. *flegmate?*   471 From 'ballota', Black or White Horehound?

utere. *Item: centorie, ysoppe, organe, ache, rue, maruil en un novel pot quisez en estale cerveise. Quant ben serront quitz, mettez licoriz, kanele, girofre, e reboilez bien. De vermeil maruil sur rouge tuile enbrasé se estufe e .ix. jours aprés si en beive. Item ad esclarer {MS esclarez} voiz: maruil e lard gentil triblez ben e quesez en ewe en un veischel de arein deke la meité e premez le jus e engettez le pastel, puis requisez cel jus ke seit espés cum mel e dunc i mettez la tierce partie de mel, pus requisez deke la tierce partie, ce usez jun. Item: commin, peivre, calment, kanele, peletere [e]galment .i. once, tot triblez e mettez miel tant que suffice. Cest usez matin jun une coileré e autre ad seir. Item: bevez jus de mente. Autre: mente damasche e blanc marruil triblez e quesez od bure de mai e colez e ce usez.* Item: savinam coctam cum vino et melle bibe. Item: apium, serpillum, marrubium album, cenecionem, neptam, equali mensura cum vino bibe. Item: allium coctum in socco aut per se tritum cum melle et caseum improtum(?) commede, probatum est. Item ad vocem probata medicina: accipe .iii. manipulos ex .iii. herbis .s. nepte, betonice, marrubii albi et tonde bene et comprime succum earum et misce cum olio et vino et cum pi[n]guedine veteris lardi conmisce .iii. calcibus et jejunus calicem per .ix. dies sume. Item: pulverem cimini cum jure mente et rute sive cum albumine ovi distempera et ori stomachi superpone. Item: succum porrorum pleno stauppo, mell coctum et acetum similiter coque simul ut spissum sit et cotidie bibe .i. coclear i. jejunus. *Rume: quisez tot dure un oef, pus si li escalez e tout si chaud cum unke le purra soufrer liez sur le vertiz del chef, si estanchera la reume.*

[140] *Quer [qui] ad la paumesoun .s. contre les pointz del cuer que fet home paumer: pernez la menue escorce del coiner, si maschez le bien, si souchez le jus. Item ad mal de coer que longement ad duré e ad mal del ventre: depescez un oef e ostez la gleire e ad l'encontre mettez al novel autant de seel e le movez bien e quisez dour en breses e le mangez. Ce face par .ix. jors, si vous gardez longement de beivre e mangez devant ce que vous beivez, si garriz par la grace de Dieu. Prové est. Ad coer arçoun: poudre [de] commin e creie usez en vostre viande [. . .] de toutz maus que neisent deinz hom.*

[141] *Splen, mal de esplen [. . .] vent[r]e freid ad quele pernez le maulard tout vif, si le destrenchez .i. veine sur la chef, quant la sanc qui ist avez resceu serra tote fleue, destemperez le od girofre e kanele en vin e donez lui a beivere. Autre: quisez mult bien en ewe les racines de fenoil, lovesche, alisaundre, persil, cicurie, ache e coopere /.i. livrewort/, pus le doucez od mel e sugre. [f.27v] Icest est bon bevre autresi pur la feie. Ad seir bevez chaud, ad matin jun, freid. Prové est.* Item: les escorces de fust de ferine quesez en vin e bevez chaud ad matin deske seint seiez. *Et si vous vuillez, pernez [. . .] d'un purcel, donez le ce .iii. jours ad beivre. Le quart jour le tuez e in troverez esplen [e] feie echaufé(?). Oinez voz de popilion e mangez suer e rosee*[472] *e seingnez de la veine de la feie.*

[142] *Pomoun,* ad pulmonis vicium: tere marrubium album et exprime jus in lacte caprino, ita ut tercia pars sit de succo et due de lacte et simul bulli et exinde accipe tepidum. Cum primum ceperis manducare si .N. fuerit tanta infirmitas ut non remanserit nisi parum de eo, totum recuperabis si hoc frequente feceris. *Asceles, ad dolours d'asceles: mangez jun foiles de ere o les triblez e bevez ad coucher. Coste,* ad dolorem lateris: betonica, agrimonia, millefolium, frisiarium, centinodium, revolam(?), lanceolata, acero, yppericum, pimpinella, de hiis omnibus equaliter tere et cum pipere et

---

[472] MS *suere rosee.* As I have printed the text it could mean 'pig and rose pottage'.

vino da calicem unum jejuno. Item: ista pocio ad plures dolores valde utilis est et maxime ad illam quam vulgus appellat punctas, hoc est quando diversi vel crebri ictus contraquatiunt latera vel aliqua membra habentis. Ad lateris dolorem: herbam malvam silvaticam decoque in aceto et postquam distringes folia, in morterio teres, in panno induces et appone per triduum et emendabit dolorem: recipe hec: piperis dragma .i., alia costis fenogreco .iiii. Probatum est. Epar est giser, ad epatis dolorem: centauria cum absinthio equali mensura ex aqua cocta, ipsa aqua jejuno potui data liberat. Item ad epatis dolorem (doli) et ad omnes dolores et duricias, indignaciones, inflaciones corporis: rutam viridem, ortensem vel agrestem, oncias .vi. cum ausungia oncia tere et fac cataplasma et induc vel aluta et pone ad latus ubi dolor est et statim san[abitur]. *Flanc, ad mal de flanc: beivez quinquefoil quit en cervisie e contre la cengle vaut ice quit od herbe seint Johan. Bon est e verrei. Item ad le flanc: triblez burnette e saxefragie e destemperez od vin beive matin freid e ad seir chaud. Ventre, pur le ventre turné: quisez vetonie en leit de chevre, si le mangez od seim de pork. Prové est.* Si fuerit fistula in ventre et cetera [vide] ubi agitur de festris: si quis pocionem sumpserit et non potest liberari superius vel inferius rafanum cum sale tritum in vino bibat et vomet et liberabit.

[143] Ventris passiones in intestinis sunt multe et varie ut illa ylliaca, colon, colica nec iste due passiones differunt nisi loco. Tamen ex eisdem causis in eadem sin[t]homata nisi quia illa intestina gracilia sunt et inde yliaca et colon illud grossum intestinum quod et culcitra dicitur et inde colica fit autem yliaca quandoque ex ventositate et tunc dolor vagatur, quandoque fit ex stipticis ut mespilis et piris crudi et caseo, quandoque ex apostemate. Si autem ex ventositate dolor vagans et ideo turpis est illa passio quod cogit pacientem vomere stercus per os. Eructatio, difficultas mingendi, constipacio ventris: cura talis sicut diaciminum, diaspermaton, diacarvi. Precipua cura est distere[473] de herbis istis et istud clistere distemperetur cum benedicta, vincietur. Emplastrum super calefactum: recipe ciminum, carvi, anisum admixto pauco aloe, coquantur semina in forti vino et deinde conterentur et addetur pulvis aloe et fiat enplastrum et superponatur tepidum. Apostolicon superpositum valet. Cum[474] diaterasco unguentum ungetur [vel] cum agrippa [vel] marciacon .s. unguentum diaforeticum et cetera. Eadem cura ex ventositate ad colicam. Si autem ex stipticis vomerit quia usus est illi et diu non assellaverit, prima cura est clistere mollificatum vel acre clistere hoc modo fiet: accipe catapucias .s. ipsam herbam et non semen et cum furfure coquantur, adiecto oleo vel sanguine inducto, sume per os pillulas aureas et pillulas 'sine[475] quibus esse nolo' vel benedictam vel catart[icon] imperiale. Alii faciunt ex sale gemme subpositoria, faciunt ad modum degiti et inponunt, alii ex melle et oleo vel sanguine decoquentur insimul ad spissitudinem formant et supponuntur. Si ex apostemate febris commitatur, dolor intollerabilis, vomitus continuus, difficultas mingendi et egritudo periculosa est ita quod in .viii. dies interfecit. Tamen quedam remedia possunt poni exterius sicut unctio de populeon vel oleo rosaceo et enplastrum de frigidis herbis: barba jovis, jusquianum. Quidam apponu[n]t clistere ignora[n]s causam morbi et magis ledunt [f.28r] quam conserv[a]nt quia nihil per . . . nihil per illam regionem, sed expectandum est domini(?) auxilium ventrem habentibus

---

473 The scribe consistently writes *distere* for *clistere*. I have silently emended from here on.
474 MS *c'cmum*.
475 MS *super*.

obstrusum tere ebulum, exprime succum per lineum pannum, duo coclearia plena et tercium cocliar lactis conmisce in sartagine, calefac et bibe continuo, largam solucionem habebunt. Ad ventris pruriginem: herbam pulegium tritum diu mittens in aquam ferventem donec bibi possit, optimum est. Ad ventrem stringendum: plantaginem in aceto coctam coclearium unum jejunus bibit et stringit. Si ventrem constipatum habuerit, utetur siro[po] violaceo, si flux[ib]ilem, siropo rosaceo et potest commedere herbas frigidas – lactucas, portulacas, pira, sirasia, nisi dolorem capitis habuerit, quia capiti sunt nociva. *Ad celui ad ki enfle le ventre aprés manger: mangez .iii. roueles de la racine de aundre, si en seez. A estresse del ve(l)ntre: beivez sovent rue triblé e destemperé od vin o cerveise. Trenches del ventre: quisez vetoine en leit de chevre od seim de pork, si mangez. Item: eschaufez aveine en la teie de oriler e cochez e mult chaud sovent ad le ventre.*

[144] *Verms denz le ventre:* abrotanum cum auxungia tere et superpunctus appone spīam(?) tunc et dolorem tollit. *Item: pernez milfoil e commin e eisil o egre vin ensemble, fortment les quisez, sur un doubler les mettez enplastré e garrira de peril qi chaut le met sur le omblil. Les verms que sont deinz le cors vifs o mortz isteront hors. Item [ad] verms que sont appellez 'lumbriks': une mesure de douz leit bevez .ii. jours, le tierce jour triblez foiles de pescher, si destemprés od douz leit, si en bevez e de ce en beveront les verms angussement e morront, si est gari.* Item: olei partem .i., aceti .ii. da bibere et parum de felle taurino si sumere possunt. Item ad lumbricos et tineas necandum: vetonice herbe pulverem in aqua calida datam potui, lumbricos et tineas eicit. Item ad tineam: *tenez le sumet de sauge en vostre mein e .iii. fiez le ben quiez disant* In nomine Patris et cetera, Argo Mergo Gor Guus at(?) super aspidem et cetera, Pater Noster .iii., *pus le mettez sur le chef xlaemu(?) rouez e ditez* 'mentem sanctam spontaneam honorem deo patrie liberacionem' *e face chanter une messe pur touz les feuls Jesu Crist e de ce[t] omme chescun jour desque seit sein. E si ce faut, adjustez autre ad ce.*

[145] Fich per totam manum: bibat milefolium cum aqua et sine dubio amplius non pacietur. Item contra ficum occidendum: accipe .iii. cocliaria mellis et .iii. salis et .ix. grana piperis et tere simul et utere per .iii. dies et liberabis. Probatum est. Item: tartarum sub cinere coctum et allium et piper simul mixta et involuta stuppa ano intromite. Item a ficum qui sanguineat et quando homo non potest ire ad exitum: accipe [. . .] .iiii. equali mensura, (id est) unum ovum quod die jovis positum [est] confringe, parum caput gracile ipsius ovi et excute in scutellam totum quod interest. Sume tunc testam predicti ovi et imple sale et mitte cum ovo sicque totidem farine siliginis atque de pulvere cornu cervino pistri diligenter et coque ad mensuram in foco calido mediocriter sic paulatim cotidie jejunus eo utere donec deficiat. Item ad ficum ardentem curentem sanguinolentem: fac gluten de houz(?) et ipsum cum albo ovi et farina siliginis. Fac curtellum et coque in foco et manduca contraria die pensum maioris nucis donec sanus sis. Item ad ficum qui sanguinat: fac pulverem de atrimento, creta pariter et da ei in cervisia nova de tercio in tercium diem sepcies et abstineat se a carne recenti. Item: sicca bene folia de amblette et fac pulverem et serva quid manducez (sic) paciens cum suppis in aqua temperatis cotidie et non statim aliud manducet, sed aliquantulum se abstineat.*Item ad hom qui ad fich corant: triblez .ii. parties de planteine e la tierce de cenecion, si le bevez destempré od novel cerv(i)eise .vii. jours en decurs e .vii. en descresant un tortel de segle e de arnement pestri e quit.* Item ad ficum sanguinentem et contra vermes in ventre: da ad potandum post prandium et ante

sanicle, avence, weibred et elfane et cetera cruda. *Charme pur le fiche: voit le malad ad muster e face [f.28v] chanter une messe de Seint Esprit e offrei. Pus .ix. jours beive lait de vache e ne beive autre chose, si garra sanz faile. Prové est.* Autre: 'In nomine Patris et cetera. Sint Job verms out: .ix. out, .viii. en out, .vii. en out, .vi. en out, .v. en out, .iiii. en out, .iii. en out, .ii. en out, .i. en out, nul en out. Si verraiment cum Dieuz garisout Job de verms e dé maus[476] qu'il out, si verreiment garrit iceste home de verms e de mal qu'il ad. Pater Noster'. Ce face Deus pur quanke il vout qui home la sue merci prit [e] requirge e pur touz ces feus Deus e par totes almes que furent confés que ad eus verrei merci lour face e Deus pur amour garise cest crixtien .N. de ces verms e de ces mals qu'il ad. Pater Noster. Qui [de] cest charme est charmee deit juner .ix. jours en pain e (e) ewe e nent vereil(?) que le charma en ces jours e si se garde totes de kanker un pez sur merde de pouz e de puz.*

[146] *Ydropisie: pernez rue, persil, ache e quisez ensemble en cerveise deke la meité e donez a beivre e garde qui autre chose ne beive; plus i eit de rue que des autre herbis.* Item ydropicis qui subito intrinsecus egritudine incurrunt: sambuci corticis mediani succi coclearia .iii., vini coclearia .iii., mellis coclearia .iii., olei coclearis .i. et conmisce et in balneo bibat. Probatum est et pocio mirabilis. Item qui portaverit lapidem gagaten liberabitur et cetera. Item vomitu canino: unge ventrem contra focum et bibat assidue semen feniculi cum vino veteri et pipere. Item: fimo vitulo venter illinietur. *Item ad femme que ad dropisie: beive stafisage quit en ewe.*

[147] *Menesoun de ceste curacion saver s'il murra o non: pernez semence de creison peisant de .i. dener, si manjue par .iii. jours, puis beive .i. viole de tef vin e autre de tef ewe e s'il ne estanche, il murra.* Si quis cum conatu velit egere et egerat cum sanguine quod et probatissimum est ad ficum, ut supra dictum est magis. Ad corendiam: de felle porci masculi plantas pedis hominis (per) ter fricabis, statim restringit. Item ad flux de ventre: accipe pulverem masticis et cum ovo sumatur, mirifice stringit. Ad omnem fluxum ventris: coque glandes in aqua et depone cupes et coque poma acerba et appone farinam ordei et sepum arietis. Hec omnia bene tere. Hoc enplastrum calidum super ventrem pone, sed utere nomine et enplastrum pone in pannum lineum. *Item flux de sanc res probata:* interuscu[m] de alba spina [et] corticem pulverem fac et exinde cum vino bibat. Si febricitanti dederis cum aqua, miraberis effectum. *Ki seine de fundement: sein[e]z de ambedeus les braz ad le .iii. jour le bainez, si estanchera. Prové est.* Item charme ad flux de sanc: 'In nomine Patris et cetera. Libera me de sanguinibus .N. Deus, Deus salutis mee et exaltabit lingua mea justiciam tuam. Hoc breve ligetur sub umbilico femine pacientis. *Menesoun ad le quelez pernez mies de pain wastel, si les dunez si menument cum vous purrez, pus les quisez mult bien en vin vermail, si le liez del moel de oef e requisez que seit espés cum gruel, si en mangez tot chaud. E pernez restebuef e quisez en ewe cum char de buef, destemprez ses pes leinz si chaut cum il le purra soufrir, si garra. Item: jus de pleinetaine, purnels dé bois, si ne avez purnels, donke pernez le escorce [de . . .], quisez en cel jus, pus le premez [en] .i. gros boletel e mettez i autant de bel mel boili e poudre de perche de cerf arse, tot boilez que seit espés e mettez en boistes, si donez a manger e garra. Item: fugere boilez en ewe, de ce frotez les plantes des piez de malad si chaud cum le purra suffrier. Item: fetes papelede de cler furment e dedinz mettez .i. piece de cire virg[i]ne que illuc tout defie e ce manjuce. Item: destemprez fente du cheval od jus de planteine e ewe de*

476 MS *mankes*.

marle, ce beive, qu'il nel sache. Si ce est femme, la fente de jument ut supra. Item: roistiés
feves que bin seient crevees sur charbons en .i. teches, pus les friez en mel, de ces prenge
chescun jour .vi. jun. Item: bainez lé pes en ewe quite od arestebuef que si ne estaunche,
l'endemein les mettez desque dimi jambe e si uncore ne estaunche, ad tierz jour [f.29r] les
bainez desque desus les genoills e estanchera. Item e ad vomite: sumac triblé quisez en vin
vermeil, si le beive. Item peres qi(ls) gisent en ewe corante enbrasez en fu que seient totes
rouges, pus les esteinez en leit de chevre d'une colour e cel li donez beivre. Item discenterie
que est medlé od sanc: triblez spodium le peiz de une mai[l]e o ad plus de une dener od eue
freid e donez ad bevre. Il restreint meneson e chescun flux. Item ad meneisoun certe chose:
destemprez bren en eue tot nuit e en eisel commin endemein, de ce qui chet del brin ad fonz
fettes papelotz od leit de vache de une colour e del commin sichi en un teches fetes poudre e
le poudre[z] desus e si mangez vigerousement, que certe chose est. Costivure[477] *ad la quele*
quant homme ne ose doner beivre, triblez ben porretz od tot le chef e tout la tere e de ce une
bone poinz laver sanz, si le mettez sur un drap bien eschaufé. Liez bon pose ad le ventre, si
destempre[z] e garra. Autre: v'eine? megk quit sz pilrai sovent vel chirnelad aut cicer egre.[478]
Item ad solucion: lardonz fettez ad la manere de .i. deit e les voutrés en arrement triblé, si
les mettez ad exil. Item ad tunbanum(?) : radicem huius herbe lava et inde crude rotulas
et in furno aut sole sicca et tere cum melle spumato aliquantulum ultra spissitudinem
illius. Et si placet, semen apii, petrosilini et levestici, feniculi, gingeber et piper
aliquantulum misce ut magis valeat et ad quantitatem magne nucis in tepida cervisia
vel in cibis pone. Sine periculo sume. Item: sale ternam lavatam cum radice distempera
tritam cum vino et melle et bibe. Item: carnem porcinam valde recentem et pinguem
coque in aqua cum malva quousque omnis pinguedo decurrat, deinde micam panis
clare conmunis(?) desuper et sic comede. Item: *quisez herbe maufe e mettez novelle*
cerveise od la geste dedenz, si mangez demei[n]tenant, si guarrez. Item: si quis non potest
egere, pone vetus unctum cum atramento atritum in eius fxudbm~t. Item *distemprer*
ventre: triblez od sein de porc la racines de chennillé e liez ad plantes dé piez e chaufez ben
les plantes ad le feu, si destempera. Et si vous vuilliez restrandre, sikés sur le pé meimes.
Item, sed solummodo in marcio, accipe equaliter jus de interrusco radicis sambuci et
jus ebuli et ad solem siccare fac dum coagulat et misce pulverem mastice aut fulgeriole
quantum tibi videtur et postea fac pillulas quinque aut .vii. Item si vis solucionis
pocionem accipere, .i. die antequam ipsam accipias hora tercia cibos quos solibiliores
poteris sume non ad satoritatem cum et ea die amplius ne commedas, bibere si volueris
non prohibemus. Sequenti vero die in aurora accipe cum aqua tritam sicut piperatam
spissam an(?) cum de pillulis cum lagana .i. nebulis p̄p̄a(?) vero die nec manduca nec
bibe usque dum solucio terminetur, sed postea manduca, bibe et dormi et a frigore
cave et tercia die post acceptam pocionem accipiat reconsiliacionem .s. adriani maioris
ante egie grece[479] aut tyriace. Quarta autem die balnieris, sexta vero sanguinem minue
et usque ad .x.am digestabilibus cibis utere et pocionem custodi nec in equm ascendes.
Item: *donez medicine pur malad hom deliverer ben e aler ad chamber sanz dolour e sanz*
trenchesons: pernez le pesant d'un dener de scamonie e autant de parietre e atant de gingebre

---

477 MS *costrue.*
478 The sentence seems to be irremediably corrupt.
479 I.e. 'ygia greca', AN 51.

e autant de girofré e autant de licoriz e medlez autant d'entonas(?), destemprez od mel e medlez od blanc vin e donez ad malad ad bevre et cetera. Restreindre ventre: beive cheferfoile espés primes e forces par .iii. jours fetes, e pus si beivez ce beivre e aprés bainez. Item venter sistendo: fimus columbinus cum melle ventre illinire. Item ad vert formage quit en vin vermeil mangez et estaunchera le ventre.

MEDICINE IN MEDIEVAL ENGLAND:
SELECT BIBLIOGRAPHY[1]

J. Alford, "Medicine in the Middle Ages: The Theory of a Profession", *Centennial Review* 23 (1979), 377–96

D.C. Bain, "A Note on an English Manuscript Receipt Book", *Bulletin of the History of Medicine* 8 (1940), 1246–8

G. Beaujean, "Fautes et obscurités dans les traductions médicales du moyen age", *Revue de synthèse* 89 (1968), 145–52

A. Bell, "A Thirteenth-Century MS Fragment at Peterborough", M.H.R.A. (*Bulletin of the Modern Humanities Research Association*) III,vii (June, 1929), 132–40

H.S. Bennett, "Science and Information in English Writings of the Fifteenth Century", *Modern Language Review* 39 (1944), 1–8

M. Benskin, "For Wound in the Head: A Late Mediaeval View of the Brain", *Neuphilologische Mitteilungen* 86 (1985), 199–215

W. Bonser, *The Medical Background of Anglo-Saxon England: A Study in History, Psychology, Folklore* (London, 1963)

W.L. Braekman, *Studies on Alchemy, Diet, Medicine and Prognostication in Middle English*, Scripta 22 (Brussels, 1988)

L. Braswell, "Utilitarian and Scientific Prose" in A.S.G. Edwards (ed.), *Middle English Prose: A Critical Guide to Major Authors and Genres* (New Brunswick, 1984), pp.337–87

M.L. Cameron, *Anglo-Saxon Medicine*, Cambridge Studies in Anglo-Saxon England 7 (Cambridge, 1993)

M. Carlin, "Medieval English Hospitals" in L. Granshaw and R. Porter (eds.), *The Hospital in History* (London, 1989), pp.21–39

H.P. Cholmeley, *John of Gaddesden and the 'Rosa Medicinae'* (Oxford, 1912)

R.M. Clay, *The Medieval Hospitals of England* 2nd ed. (London, 1966)

J.B. Colton (transl.), *John of Mirfield (d.1407), Surgery: A Translation of his Breviarium Bartholomei, Part IX* (New York, 1969)

M.P. Cosman, "Medieval Medical Malpractice and Chaucer's Physician", *New York State Journal of Medicine* 72 (1972), 2439–44

W.C. Crossgrove, "The Forms of Medieval Technical Literature: Some Suggestions for further Work", *Jahrbuch für Internationale Germanistik* 3 (1971), 13–21

W.R. Dawson, *A Leechbook or Collection of Medical Recipes of the Fifteenth Century* (London, 1934)

M. Deegan and D.G. Scragg (eds.), *Medicine in Early Medieval England. Four Papers*, University of Manchester, Centre for Anglo-Saxon Studies (Manchester, 1987; corr. reissue 1989)

L. Demaitre, "Scholasticism in Compendia of Practical Medicine, 1250–1450", *Manuscripta* 20 (1976), 81–95

W. Eamon (ed.), *Studies on Medieval Fachliteratur*, Scripta 6 (Brussels, 1982)

---

[1] For herbals and plants see bibliographies in T. Hunt, *Plant Names of Medieval England* (Cambridge, 1989) and W.F. Daems, *Nomina simplicium medicinarum ex synonymariis medii aevi collecta*, Studies in Ancient Medicine 6 (Leiden, 1993).

id., "Books of Secrets in Medieval and Early Modern Science", *Sudhoffs Archiv* 69 (1985), 26–49

A. Eccles, "The Reading Public, the Medical Profession, and the Use of English for Medical Books in the 16th and 17th Centuries", *Neuphilologische Mitteilungen* 75 (1974), 143–56

M. Faribault, "La Chirurgie par rimes: problèmes de compilation de recettes médicales en français", *Fifteenth-Century Studies* 5 (1982), 47–59

A. Fonahn, *Arabic and Latin Anatomical Terminology chiefly from the Middle Ages*, Videnskapsselskapets Skrifter. II. Hist.-Filos. Klasse. 1921. No. 7 (Kristiania, 1922)

P. Fordyn (ed.), *The 'Experimentes of Cophon, the Leche of Salerne': Middle English Medical Recipes (MS Add.34111, f.218r–230v)*, Scripta 10 (Brussel, 1983)

E.F. Frey, "Saints in Medical History", *Clio Medica* 14 (1979), 35–70

R.M. Garrett, "Middle English Rimed Medical Treatise", *Anglia* 34 (1911), 163–93

F.M. Getz, "Gilbertus Anglicus Anglicized", *Medical History* 26 (1982), 436–42

eadem, "John Mirfield and the *Breviarium Bartholomei*: The Medical writings of a Clerk at St. Bartholomew's Hospital in the Later Fourteenth Century", *Society for the Social History of Medicine, Bulletin* 37 (1985), 24–6

eadem, "Archives and Sources: Medical Practitioners in Medieval England", *Social History of Medicine* 3 (1990), 245–83

eadem, "Charity, Translation and the Language of Medical Learning in Medieval England", *Bulletin of the History of Medicine* 64 (1990), 1–17

eadem, "The *Method of Healing* in Middle English" in F. Kudlien and R.J. Durling (eds.), *Galen's Method of Healing: Proceedings of the 1982 Galen Symposium*, Studies in Ancient Medicine 1 (Leiden, 1991), pp.147–56

eadem, *Healing and Society in Medieval England: A Middle English Translation of the Pharmaceutical Writings of Gilbertus Anglicus*, Wisconsin Publications in the History of Science and Medicine 8 (Madison, 1991)

J.R. Gilleland, "Eight Anglo-Norman Cosmetic Recipes. MS Cambridge, Trinity College 1044", *Romania* 109 (1988), 50–67.

R.S. Gottfried, *Doctors and Medicine in Medieval England 1340–1530* (Princeton, 1986)

P. Grymonprez (ed.), *'Here Men May See the Vertues off Herbes': A Middle English Herbal (MS Bodley 483, fols.57r–67v)*, Scripta 3 (Brussels, 1981)

M.-R. Hallaert, *The 'Sekenesse of wymmen'. A Middle English treatise on Diseases in Women*, Scripta 8 (Brussels, 1982)

E.A. Hammond, "Incomes of Medieval English Doctors", *Journal of the History of Medicine and Allied Sciences* 15 (1960), 154–69

H.E. Handerson, *Gilbertus Anglicus: Medicine of the Thirteenth Century* (Cleveland, Ohio, 1918)

H. Hargreaves, "Some Problems in Indexing Middle English Recipes" in A.S.G. Edwards and D. Pearsall (eds.), *Middle English Prose. Essays on Bibliographical Problems* (New York, 1981), pp.91–113

M.P. Harley, "The Middle English Contents of a Fifteenth-Century Medical Handbook", *Mediaevalia* 8 (1982), 171–88

P.H.-S. Hartley and H.R. Aldridge, *Johannes de Mirfield of St Bartholomew's, Smithfield: His Life and Works* (Cambridge, 1936)

F. Heinrich, *Ein mittelenglisches Medizinbuch* (Halle a.S., 1896)

G. Henslow, *Medical Works of the Fourteenth Century together with a List of Plants recorded in Contemporary Writings, with their Identifications* (London, 1899)

C.B. Hieatt and R.F. Jones (eds.), *La Novele Cirurgerie*, ANTS 46 (London, 1990)

F. Holthausen, "Medicinische Gedichte aus einer Stockholmer Handschrift", *Anglia* 18 (1896), 293–331

id., "Zu den mittelenglischen medizinischen Gedichten", *Anglia* 44 (1920), 357–72

T. Hunt, "Recettes médicales en vers français d'après le manuscrit 0.8.27 de Trinity College, Cambridge", *Romania* 106 (1985), 57–83

id., "The Botanical Glossaries in MS London, B.L. Add.15236", *Pluteus* 4–5 (1986–7), 101–50

id.,"The Medical Recipes in MS Royal 5 E VI", *Notes and Queries* 231 (1986), 6–9

id., "The 'Novele Cirurgerie' in MS London, British Library, Harley 2558", *Zeitschrift für romanische Philologie* 103 (1987), 271–99

id., "Horses and Courses", *French Studies Bulletin* 22 (1987), 1–4

id., "Early Anglo-Norman Recipes in MS London, B.L. Royal 12 C XIX", *Zeitschrift für französische Sprache und Literatur* 97 (1987), 245–54

id., "Materia Medica in MS London, B.L. Add. 10289", *Medioevo Romanzo* 13 (1988), 25–37

id., "The Trilingual Glossary in MS London, B.L. Sloane 146 f.69v–72r", *English Studies* 70 (1989), 289–310

id., *Plant Names of Medieval England* (Cambridge, 1989)

id., *Popular Medicine in Thirteenth-Century England* (Cambridge, 1990)

id., "An Anglo-Norman Medical Treatise" in G. Runnalls and P.E. Bennett (eds.), *The Editor and the Text* (Edinburgh, 1991), pp.145–64

id., *The Medieval Surgery* (Woodbridge, 1992)

id., "Anglo-Norman Medical Receipts" in I. Short (ed.), *Anglo-Norman Anniversary Essays*, ANTS Occasional Publications Series 2 (London, 1993), pp.179–233

id., *Anglo-Norman Medicine* 1 (Cambridge, 1994)

I.B. Jones, "Popular Medical Knowledge in Fourteenth-Century English Literature", *Bulletin of the History of Medicine* 5 (1937), 405–51, 489–88

eadem, "Halford 16: A Mediaeval Welsh Medical Treatise", *Etudes celtiques* 7 (1955), 270–399

P. Murray Jones, "Harley MS 2558: A Fifteenth-Century Medical Commonplace Book" in Schleissner (q.v.), pp.35–54

id., "Medical Books before the Invention of Printing" in A. Besson (ed.) *Thornton's Medical Books, Libraries and Collectors: A Study of Bibliography and the Book Trade in relation to the Medical Sciences* (Adershot, 1990), pp.1–29

E.J. Kealey, *Medieval Medicus. A Social History of Anglo-Norman Medicine* (Baltimore / London, 1981)

id, "England's earliest Women Doctors", *Journal of the History of Medicine* 40 (1985), 473–7

G. Keil, "Magister Giselbertus de villa parisiensi. Beobachtungen zu den Kranewittbeeren und Gilberts pharmakologischem Renommé", *Sudhoffs Archiv* 78 (1994), 59–79.

G.R. Keiser, "Epilepsy: the falling evil" in L.M. Matheson (ed.), *Popular and Practical Science*, pp.219–44

id., "Reconstructing Robert Thornton's Herbal", *Medium Aevum* 65 (1966), 35–53

C. Kren, *Medieval Science and Technology: A Selected, Annotated Bibliography*,Garland Bibliographies of the History of Science and Technology 11 (New York / London, 1985)

M. Kurdziałek, "Gilbertus Anglicus und die psychologischen Erörterungen in seinem *Compendium Medicinae*", *Sudhoffs Archiv* 47 (1963), 106–26

S.J. Lang, "John Bradmore and His Book Philomena", *Social History of Medicine* 5 (1992), 121–30

M. Löweneck (ed.), *Peri Didaxeon. Eine Sammlung von Rezepten in englischer Sprache aus dem 11./12. Jahrhundert*, Erlanger Beiträge zur englischen Philologie 12 (Erlangen, 1896)

R.W. McConchie, " 'It Hurteth Memorie and Hindreth Learning': Attitudes to the Use of the Vernacular in Sixteenth-Century English Medical Writings", *Studia Anglica Posnaniensia* 21 (1988), 53–67

L.M. Matheson (ed.), *Popular and Practical Science of Medieval England* (East Lansing, 1994)

C.F. Mayer, "A Medieval English Leechbook and its 14th Century Poem on Bloodletting", *Bulletin of the History of Medicine* 7 (1939), 381–91

P. Meyer, "Les manuscrits français de Cambridge", *Romania* 32 (1903), 18–120

id., "Notice du ms. Bodley 761 de la Bibliothèque Bodléienne", *Romania* 37 (1908), 509–28

id., "Manuscrits médiévaux en français", *Romania* 44 (1915), 161–214

G. Müller, *Aus mittelenglischen Medizintexten. Die Prosarezepte des Stockholmer Miszellankodex X.90*, Kölner Anglistische Arbeiten 10 (Leipzig, 1929)

J.K. Mustain, "A Rural Medical Practitioner in Fifteenth-Century England", *Bulletin of the History of Medicine* 46 (1972), 469–76

J. Norri, *Names of Sicknesses in English, 1400–1550: An Exploration of the Lexical Field* Annales Academiae Scientiarum Fennicae, Dissertationes Humanorum Litterarum 63 (Helsinki, 1992)

B. Odenstedt, *The Book of Marchalsi: A 15th C. Treatise on Horse-Breeding and Veterinary Medicine edited from MS Harley 6398 . . .* (Stockholm, 1973)

M.S. Ogden (ed.), *The 'Liber de diversis medicinis'*, EETS OS 207 (London, 1938; reprint with revisions, 1969)

L.B. Pinto, "The Folk Practice of Gynecology and Obstetrics in the Middle Ages", *Bulletin of the History of Medicine* 47 (1973), 513–23

O. Riha, "Gilbertus Anglicus und sein *Compendium Medicinae*. Arbeitstechnik und Wissensorganisation", *Sudhoffs Archiv* 78 (1994), 59–79

C. Rawcliffe, "The Profits of Practice: The Wealth and Status of Medical Men in Later Medieval England", *Social History of Medicine* 1 (1988), 61–78

R.H. Robbins, "Medical Manuscripts in Middle English", *Speculum* 45 (1970), 393–415

id., "Signs of Death in Middle English", *Mediaeval Studies* 32 (1970), 282–98

S. Rubin, *Medieval English Medicine* (London, 1974)

M.R. Schleissner (ed.), *Manuscript Sources of Medieval Medicine: A Book of Essays*, Garland Medieval Casebooks (New York / London, 1995)

H. Schöffler, "Gedruckte mittelenglish-medizinische Texte", *Archiv für Geschichte der Medizin* 11 (1918), 107–9

id., *Beiträge zur mittelenglischen Medizinliteratur* (Halle a.S., 1919)

N.G. Siraisi, *Medieval and Renaissance Medicine. An Introduction to Knowledge and Practice* (Chicago / London, 1990)

O. Södergård, "Recettes pour les femmes", in K.B. Flemested et al. (eds.), *Mélanges d'études médiévales offerts à Helge Nordahl à l'occasion de son soixantième anniversaire* (Oslo, 1988), pp.187–96

A.C. Svinhufvud, *A Late Middle English Treatise on Horses edited from British Library MS Sloane 2584 ff.102–117b* (Stockholm, 1978)

E.W. Talbert, "The Notebook of a Fifteenth-Century Practising Physician", *Texas Studies in English* 21 (1942), 5–30

C.H. Talbot, "A Mediaeval Physician's Vade Mecum", *Journal of the History of Medicine and Allied Sciences* 16 (1961), 213–33

id., *Medicine in Medieval England* (London, 1967)

id. and E.A. Hammond, *The Medical Practitioners in Medieval England: A Biographical Register* (London, 1965)

L. Thorndike, "Notes on Medical Texts in Manuscripts at London and Oxford", *Janus* 48 (1959), 141–202

H.E. Ussery, *Chaucer's Physician. Medicine and Literature in Fourteenth-Century England* (New Orleans, 1971)

L.E. Voigts, "Editing Middle English Medical Texts: Needs and Issues" in T.H. Levere (ed.), *Editing Texts in the History of Science and Medicine* (New York / London, 1982), pp.39–68

eadem, "Medical Prose" in A.S.G. Edwards (ed.), *Middle English Prose: A Critical Guide to Major Authors and Genres* (New Brunswick, 1984), pp.315–35

eadem, "Scientific and Medical Books" in J. Griffiths and D. Pearsall (eds.), *Book Production and Publishing in Britain 1375–1475* (Cambridge, 1989), pp.345–402

eadem, "The 'Sloane Group': Related Scientific and Medical Manuscripts from the Fifteenth Century in the Sloane Collection", *The British Library Journal* 16 (1990), 26–57

eadem, " 'A drynke pat men callen dwale to make a man to slepe whyle men kerven him': A Surgical Anaesthetic from Late Medieval England" in S. Campbell *et al.* (eds.), *Health, Disease and Healing in Medieval Culture* (New York, 1992), pp.34–56

eadem, "Multitudes of Middle English Medical Manuscripts, or the Englishing of Science and Medicine" in Schleissner (q.v.), pp.183–95

B. Wallner, "A Note on some Middle English Medical Terms", *English Studies* 50 (1969), 499–503

INDEX OF MANUSCRIPTS CONSULTED

(Vols.1 and 2)[1]

BASEL

Universitätsbibliothek D.II.11   9;

BOLOGNA

Bibliotheca Universitaria 2836   8;

CAMBRIDGE

Corpus Christi College	511	154;
Gonville and Caius College	159	154;
	401	154;
St John's College D.4		18; 12
Trinity College	O.1.20	17ff,24ff;
	O.5.32	195ff
	O.8.27	12
	R.14.30	155;
University Library	Dd.iii.51	154;
	Dd.x.44	155ff;
	Ii.vi.39	154;

EDINBURGH

Old Advocates Library (NLS) 18.6.9 129ff

LONDON

British Library

Additional	34111	10f
Harley	2390	7n
Royal	12 B II	154;
	12 B III	144,154,263f;
	12 B XII	76n
	12 C XIX	13
	12 E XXII	7f,216n,235n
Sloane	14	158;
	146	12
	240	13ff,24ff;
	371	153;
	420	153,263f; 7
	1124	150ff,156f,162,256; 69
	1610	76n
	1615	24ff;
	1977	11ff,24ff;
	2454	153;

---

[1] Page references before the semi-colon are to volume 1.

GENERAL INDEX

(Vols.1 and 2)[1]

1 Page references before the semi-colon are to volume 1.